The Treatment of
Medical Problems
in the Elderly

CURRENT STATUS OF MODERN THERAPY: VOLUME 3

The Treatment of Medical Problems in the Elderly

Edited by

M. J. Denham

SPRINGER-SCIENCE+BUSINESS MEDIA, B.V.

British Library Cataloguing in Publication Data
The treatment of medical problems in the elderly. – (The current status of
modern therapy; vol. 3).
1. Geriatrics   2. Therapeutics
I. Denham, M J   II. Series
618.9′7′06   RC953.5
ISBN 978-94-011-6225-8   ISBN 978-94-011-6223-4 (eBook)
DOI 10.1007/978-94-011-6223-4

REDWOOD BURN LIMITED
Trowbridge and Esher

Contents

List of Contributors   vii

Consultant Editor's Note   ix

Preface   xi

1 Clinical pharmacology and the elderly patient   1
   K. O'MALLEY, M. LAHER, B. CUSACK AND J. G. KELLY

2 Antibiotic practice in elderly patients   35
   P. J. SANDERSON AND M. J. DENHAM

3 Treatment of cardiovascular disease in the elderly   77
   R. W. STOUT

4 The management of hypertension in the elderly   117
   B. MOORE-SMITH

5 Treatment of the elderly diabetic   159
   R. A. JACKSON

6 Management of Parkinson's disease in the elderly   215
   MARION HILDICK-SMITH

7 Drugs acting on the central nervous system   259
   M. IMPALLOMENI AND F. M. ANTONINI

8 Cerebral activating drugs   295
   D. E. HYAMS

9 Management of malignant disease in old age   333
   A. E. KARK AND D. F. GUÉRET WARDLE

   Index   419

List of Contributors

F. M. ANTONINI
University of Florence, Italy

B. CUSACK
Department of Clinical Pharmacology, Royal College of Surgeons in Ireland, Dublin, 2, Eire

M. J. DENHAM
Northwick Park Hospital and Clinical Research Centre, Watford Road, Harrow, HA1 3JUJ, Middlesex

D. F. GUÉRET WARDLE
London Oncology Centre, 109 Harley Street, London W.1

MARION HILDICK-SMITH
Nunnery Fields Hospital, Canterbury, Kent

D. E. HYAMS
Merck, Sharp & Dohme Research Laboratories, Rahway, New Jersey 07065, USA

M. IMPALLOMENI
Royal Postgraduate Medical School, Hammersmith Hospital, London and Italian Hospital, London

R. A. JACKSON
Highlands Hospital, Enfield, London N21

A. E. KARK
Northwick Park Hospital and Clinical Research Centre, Watford Road, Harrow HA1 3UJ, Middlesex

J. G. KELLY
Department of Clinical Pharmacology, Royal College of Surgeons in Ireland, Dublin 2, Eire

M. LAHER
Department of Clinical Pharmacology, Royal College of Surgeons in Ireland, Dublin 2, Eire

B. MOORE-SMITH
The Ipswich Hospital, Heath Road Wing, Ipswich IP4 5PD, Suffolk

K. O'MALLEY
St Laurence's Hospital and the Charitable Infirmary, Jervis Street, Dublin 1, Eire

P. J. SANDERSON
Northwick Park Hospital and Clinical Research Centre Watford Road, Harrow HA1 3UJ, Middlesex

R. W. STOUT
Department of Geriatric Medicine, Queens University of Belfast, Lisburn Road, Belfast BT9 7BL, Northern Ireland

Consultant Editor's Note

CURRENT STATUS OF MODERN THERAPY

The *Current Status of Modern Therapy* is a major series from MTP Press with the purpose of providing a definitive view of modern therapeutic practice in those areas of clinical medicine in which important changes are occurring. The series consists of monographs specially commissioned under the individual editorship of internationally recognized experts in their fields. Their selection of a panel of contributors from many countries ensures an international perspective on developments in therapy.

The series aims to review the growth areas of clinical pharmacology and therapeutics in a systematic way. It is a continuing series in which the same subject areas will be covered by revised editions as advances make this desirable.

As the diseases of youth and middle age are cured, so the proportion of elderly people in the population of industrially developed countries rises. This means that more general and medical resources must be devoted to geriatric care.

Hence *The Treatment of Medical Problems in the Elderly*, Volume 3 in the *Current Status of Modern Therapy* series, edited by Dr Denham, comes at an opportune time. In this book, with a galaxy of talent among the authors, he shows that we are moving out of the period of care of the elderly as just an art, to care of the elderly as a science and an art. Previously geriatric medicine was the Cinderella of the medical specialities. Now it is coming into its own as studies of the type described so well in this book show how we can add not only years to the life but more importantly life to the years.

J. MARKS
Girton College
Cambridge

Series Editor

Preface

It has been said that geriatric medicine is the last stronghold of those physicians whose interest is general medicine. Although some diseases are rarely seen, a wide range of illnesses do occur, and indeed the non-specific presentation of disease in the elderly, with the associated problems of diagnosis, is one of the attractions of the specialty. It is increasingly recognized that medical care of the elderly requires special expertise and the fact that the patient is old is not, of itself, a reason for diagnostic or therapeutic lassitude or nihilism. Elderly people deserve and should receive the best medical care available, given with discernment, enthusiasm and kindness.

The extensive nature of illness in the elderly means that the physician in geriatric medicine has to keep up to date with advances in knowledge, management and therapeutics in a wide range of subjects, not only in his own speciality, but also in other spheres which have implications for the treatment of the older person. The selected topics in this book aim to give informed comment in areas where there have been developments, controversy, or where the geriatrician may not be an expert, but where correct management and treatment is essential. It is hoped that the subject matter will appeal not only to physicians in geriatric medicine, but also to physicians and surgeons who are increasingly likely to have to treat elderly patients due to the rising proportion of older people in the population.

M. J. DENHAM

1

Clinical pharmacology and the elderly patient

K. O'Malley, M. Laher, B. Cusack and J. G. Kelly

INTRODUCTION

The elderly patient differs from his younger counterpart in many important ways, not least with respect to drug therapy. As an almost inevitable part of ageing, the elderly suffer from many degenerate disorders and in addition are susceptible to other diseases. The resultant signs and symptoms not infrequently elicit the 'prescription reflex' by which the doctor attempts alleviation of all or most problems. The large scale of prescribing puts the elderly at increased risk of developing adverse drug reactions. The elderly patient may exhibit altered pharmacokinetics (absorption, distribution, metabolism and excretion of drugs) and pharmacodynamics (the time-course and magnitude of drug effect). Matters are complicated further by the attitude of the elderly to medical intervention. In addition, infirmities such as confusion, poor sight, forgetfulness and failure to comprehend instructions militate against the patients adhering to a therapeutic regimen, both pharmacological and otherwise.

In the present chapter we shall discuss adverse drug reactions, compliance, pharmacokinetics and pharmacodynamics as they pertain to the elderly patient. The clinical importance of these and possible means for taking them into account will be examined.

ADVERSE DRUG REACTIONS

Adverse drug reactions are difficult to monitor and the reported incidence varies from 0·4%[1] to 35% of patients[2]. Papers which report very low incidences of adverse reactions have been based on retrospective studies which rely on reactions being reported to the investigators or on reports being entered in patients' notes. Studies which show higher incidences have been prospective studies where investigators have actively sought adverse reactions. Retrospective studies probably underestimate the incidence of adverse reactions as only serious or life-threatening reactions are included. Prospective studies on the other hand include many trivial reactions and because of observer bias non-iatrogenic disease or placebo effects may be mistaken for adverse drug reactions[3]. Many studies contain numbers too small to allow assessment of age as a factor in the causation of adverse drug reactions.

Reactions requiring hospital admission

In some well-known studies the incidence of adverse reactions leading to hospital admission has been prospectively examined. Hurwitz[4] examined 1268 patients admitted to hosptial and found that 2·1% were admitted because of adverse reactions to drugs taken for therapeutic reasons. Although there was some indication of a correlation between reactions and age, she did not give detailed figures and when allowance is made for the fact that admission to hospital for *all* reasons was correlated with increasing age the data relating age to incidence of adverse reactions becomes less convincing. Caranasos *et al.*[5] examined 6063 admissions to hospital over 3 years and found that 2·9% of admissions were due to drug-induced illness. Results from this study, adjusted to show the incidence of adverse reactions as a percentage of all admissions in the relevant age group, are shown in Table 1. A modest increase in this incidence may be seen from 61–80 years.

Table 1 Hospital admissions due to adverse drug reactions (modified from Caranasos *et al.*[5])

Age range (years)	All admissions (no.)	Adverse reactions (%)
11–20	394	2·8
21–30	782	2·4
31–40	746	2·7
41–50	1006	2·1
51–60	1225	2·7
61–70	1213	3·6
71–80	546	4·8
81–90	139	2·2
91–100	12	0

In a recent study[6] 1998 patients who were admitted to geriatric departments in the United Kingdom were assessed for adverse reactions. Of these, 12.4% were judged to have had adverse reactions. Hospital admission was due solely to adverse reactions in 7·7% of cases. Hypotensive agents and antiparkinsonian drugs were most likely to produce adverse effects.

Reactions occurring in hospital

Most investigators report a 10–12% incidence of adverse drug reactions in hospital in-patients. In most cases there seems to be an increased incidence with advancing age. Hurwitz[7] showed a significant correlation between increasing age and adverse drug reactions from a total of 1160. The incidence in those aged 60–69 was twice that observed in those aged 30–39. Patients aged 70–79 had four times the incidence of those aged 30–39 (Table 2).

Table 2　Adverse drug reactions observed in hospital (from Hurwitz[7])

Age range (years)	No. given drugs	% with adverse reactions
10–19	64	3·1
20–29	100	3·0
30–39	122	5·7
40–49	159	7·5
50–59	222	8·1
60–69	252	10.7
70–79	178	21·3
80–89	59	18·6
90–99	4	0

In a similar study Klein *et al.*[8] indicated that there was an increased incidence of adverse reactions with age and although no detailed statistical analysis was attempted the results suggest that the incidence of adverse reactions in those aged more than 60 years was about three times that in patients aged less than 60 years. Part of this difference was due to a large sex-linked component whereby women aged more than 60 years had a much higher incidence of relatively mild adverse reactions.

Siedl *et al.*[9] also showed an increased incidence of adverse reactions with age although the difference between young and old was not as marked as in some other studies. Again elderly women accounted for a large proportion of mild or moderate adverse reactions (mostly intestinal side-effects).

Problems in assessing the incidence of adverse reactions

Most studies published show some increased incidence of adverse drug reactions with increasing age, but in many cases good statistical analysis is lacking. It is sometimes difficult to assess genuine age-related differences in the incidence of reactions since hospital admissions for *many* causes contain a disproportionately large number of elderly people. When defined populations are monitored continuously little attention is paid to the fact that the population is constantly decreasing since patients are leaving at intervals and therefore, bias in the population readily creeps in. Where studies are prospective, investigators who examine patients may find it difficult to retain objectivity.

While there is little dispute that older patients tend to have a moderately higher incidence of adverse drug reactions more work needs to be done in the field of assessing the clinical significance of these reactions. In particular the relative incidence of serious or life-threatening adverse reactions in the young and old requires further investigations since even in fairly large studies, numbers of these are too small to allow adequate correlation with age. We suspect that the higher reported incidence of adverse reactions in the elderly may in part at least reflect greater drug consumption in this group.

COMPLIANCE

No matter how carefully drugs are prescribed, patients will not derive full benefit from their medication unless they adhere to an appropriately prescribed regimen. A substantial literature has accumulated concerning the magnitude of non-compliance and although it is extremely difficult to assess compliance accurately, results indicated that non-compliance is a major factor in determining a response to a therapeutic regimen requiring self-administration[10]. In a review of published studies Blackwell[11] suggested that 25%–50% of patients did not take their medication at all. Sackett[12] summarized the results of 14 studies on compliance with long-term drug regimens and stated that on average about one-half of these patients are compliant. Compliance with short-term medication was extremely variable and studies were not reproducible.

It would seem reasonable to assume that errors of intake of drugs are common in the elderly patient, as they may not fully understand instructions, they often have impaired hearing or sight, they may suffer confusional states, etc. Decreased manual dexterity may lead to difficulties in opening containers particularly the childproof type. However valid this kind of intuitive reasoning may be, objective measurements do not always support the view that the elderly are less compliant than the young. Haynes[13] reviewed studies in which associations between demographic characteristics of patients and compliance were examined. Of 37 studies reviewed only seven showed a positive association between decreased compliance and increasing age.

Failure of compliance can be difficult to detect as Caron and Roth[15] demonstrated when they found that a group of 27 physicians could not adequately assess compliance of individual patients. Questioning the patient and pill counts gives some information, but can be misleading. Measurement of blood or urine drug concentrations in suspect patients is the most direct way of assessing compliance but obviously has limited general application.

Various methods for improving compliance have been tried, among them counselling, written instructions, the use of calendars and single tablet dispensers. Most attempts to improve compliance using one or more of these techniques have reported some improvement[14] but their effects on outcome of treatment have not been adequately assessed. In general, published studies describing attempts to improve compliance do not deal specifically with the elderly. One study in the elderly[16] showed that over a 14-day period patients given tear-off calendars made fewer errors in medication than those with a tablet identification card. Both methods were better than standard verbal instruction. Despite our lack of hard evidence in this matter, commonsense suggests that the following approach may help in minimizing non-compliance:

(1) A simple regimen involving as few drugs and as few doses as possible should be prescribed. A simple explanation of the treatment should be given. A regimen containing three drugs is said to be a reasonable maximum for an old person to manage[17]. This statement is based on a subjective conclusion in one study, but it has an intuitive logic.

(2) Help in supervising a patient can be sought from a neighbour, relative or health visitor.

(3) The necessity for compliance should be emphasized and the instructions repeated at follow-up.

(4) The pharmacist should provide well-chosen easy-to-open containers, with clearly written or preferably typed instructions. The pharmacist can also emphasize the dosage instructions verbally.

PHARMACOKINETICS

Introduction

There are many changes in body composition, blood flow and physiological function (Table 3), commensurate with ageing, which may alter pharmacokinetics. In this section a number of pharmacokinetic terms are defined. This is followed by a consideration of each of the pharmacokinetic processes – absorption, distribution, metabolism and renal elimination – in relation to ageing.

Table 3 Physiological changes and ageing

Parameter	Change	Reference
Lean body mass	↓	40
Total body water	↓	41
Body fat	↑	42
Cardiac output	↓	43
Renal blood flow	↓	44
Hepatic blood flow	↓	45
Cerebral blood flow	↓	46
Renal function	↓	47
Plasma albumin concentration	↓	33

The plasma half-life of a drug $(t_{1/2})$ is the time taken for its concentration in the plasma to fall by one-half. It is usually calculated from the terminal portion of a graph of log plasma concentration versus time. The plasma half-life is a guide to the time taken to reach steady state concentration during chronic dosing and the time taken for elimination after cessation of such dosing. In each case the time is approximately four half-lives.

The degree of drug uptake by tissues relative to that in blood or plasma determines the volume of distribution (V_d). It is the apparent volume of body water into which the amount of drug in the body (A) is distributed to provide a given plasma concentration (C).

$$\text{Thus } V_d = \frac{A}{C}$$

Clearance is the volume of plasma which contains the amount of drug removed from the plasma per unit time and its units are those of volume per unit time. The relationship of clearance to half-life and volume of distribution can be expressed as follows:

$$Cl = \frac{V_d \times 0.693}{t_{1/2}}$$

It is apparent that a change in $t_{1/2}$ with a corresponding change in V_d need not necessarily result in a change in Cl (see section on diazepam, page 17).

During chronic dosing when a dose (D) is being administered at time intervals (T) and F is the fraction absorbed, the average steady state concentration (C_{av}) is determined by:

$$C_{av} \propto \frac{D \times F}{Cl \times T}$$

Thus Cl and F are the pharmacokinetic factors which determine average steady state concentration.

Absorption
After oral administration many factors affect drug absorption from the bowel. The disintegration time and dissolution rate of the preparation determine the rate at which the drug becomes available for absorption. These depend on drug formulation and physio-chemical characteristics but in addition may be affected by age-related changes in gastrointestinal physiology. Gastric pH rises with age[18] and this may change the degree of ionization and thereby the lipid solubility of some drugs. However, the rise in gastric pH may hasten gastric emptying[19], and in some cases this tends to enhance absorption. Splanchnic blood flow[20] and small bowel mucosal surface area[21] decrease with age. These changes would tend to delay or reduce absorption.

Changes in active absorptive mechanisms appear to occur with advancing age. The absorption of galactose[22] is delayed and 3-methyl glucose absorption[23] appears to be reduced in older persons. D-xylose is also actively absorbed, but in this case absorption seems not to be impaired in the elderly[24]. Studies in animals indicate that the absorption of calcium, iron, thiamine and dextrose is diminished with increasing age[25]. However, as most drugs are passively absorbed, data pertaining to actively transported substances whether from animal or clinical studies, are of little value in predicting the possible effect of old age on absorption of drugs.

Drug absorption must be considered under two headings – rate of absorption and extent of absorption. These two parameters are not necessarily related. The absorption rate partly determines the time to peak and the height of peak drug concentration in the plasma. Rapid absorption is important where early and high peak plasma concentrations of drug are required for clinical effect, for example with antibotics, analgesics and hypnotics. Extent of absorption is particuarly important in chronic dosing, since it is a major deter- minant of drug steady state plasma level and therefore of magnitude of drug effect. These two pharmacokinetic parameters, particularly extent of absorption have been little studied in the elderly.

Rate of absorption
The effect of increasing age on the rate of absorption of certain drugs is shown in Table 4. There are no age-related changes in the

Table 4 Changes in rate of absorption with advancing age

Drug	Change	Reference
Acetylsalicylic acid	→	48
Acetylsalicylic acid	→	49
Chlordiazepoxide	→ ?	50
Digoxin	↓	27
Indomethacin	→	51
Paracetamol	→	28
Phenazone	→	52
Practolol	→	53
Propicillin	→	31
Propoxyphene	→	52
Quinine	→	47
Sulphamethizole	→	28
Tetracycline	→	29

rate of absorption of most drugs studied to date. It is noteworthy that some antibiotics and a few commonly used analgesic drugs are in this group. The delay ($1 \cdot 05 \pm 0 \cdot 86$ h) in absorption of digoxin as measured by time to peak concentration (Figure 1) is probably of little clinical significance since the peak action of the drug occurs well after the absorptive phase[26].

Because of the wide scatter of values in the young a difference in the rate of absorption (absorption rate constant) of chlordiazepox- ide between young and elderly groups did not quite reach statistical significance[50]. However, the data does suggest that chlordiazepoxide may be more slowly absorbed in the elderly.

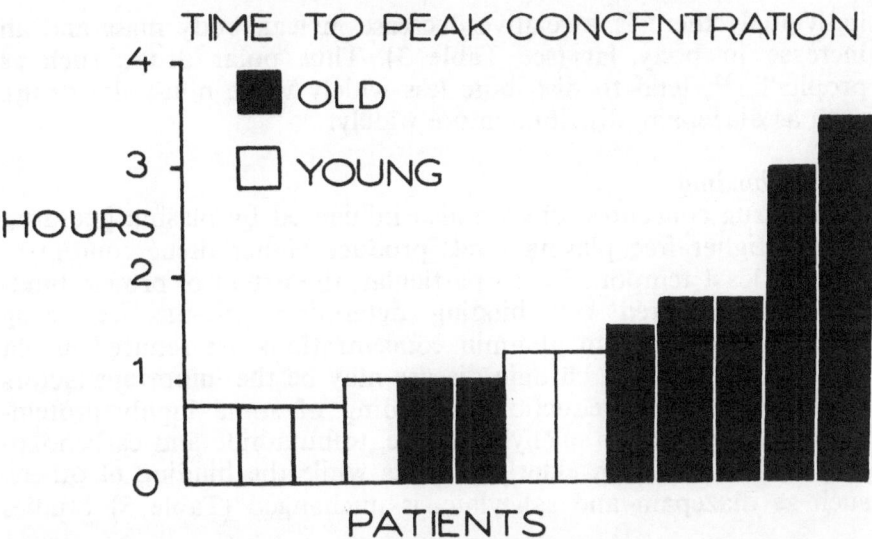

Figure 1 Time to peak plasma digoxin concentration after oral administration in old and young patients (from Cusack *et al.*,[27], with permission)

Extent of absorption
Studies on absorption of five drugs – digoxin[27], paracetamol and sulphamethoxazole[28], tetracycline[29] and theophylline[30] – failed to show significant alterations in the extent of absorption. The extent of digoxin absorption in the elderly patients (76%) was reported to be slightly lower than that in the young (84%) but the difference did not reach statistical significance. Such difference is unlikely to be of clinical importance either. In the case of other drugs the extent of absorption was found to be insignificantly reduced in the elderly group.

Although information is lacking on many drugs we may tentatively conclude that the rate of absorption of most drugs is unchanged and the extent of drug absorption is also probably not significantly altered.

Drug distribution
The pattern of drug distribution is obviously an important factor in determining the concentration of free drug available at its site of action. Distribution of a drug depends on its physiochemical properties and on certain patient characteristics. In broad terms, a non-polar drug distributes selectively into lipid tissues. The distribution of polar drugs tends to be confined to the lean body compartment and such drugs cross the blood–brain barrier poorly. In older

individuals there is a relative decrease in lean body mass and an increase in body fat (see Table 3). Thus polar drugs, such as propicillin[31], tend to distribute less widely while non-polar drugs, such as diazepam, distribute more widely.

Protein binding
Tissue drug concentrations are also influenced by plasma free drug levels. Higher free plasma levels produce higher tissue concentrations at least temporarily. In particular, the extent of protein binding and also red cell binding determines plasma free drug concentrations. Serum albumin concentrations are reduced in old age; immobility and chronic disease may be the important factors which cause such reduction[33]. Binding of some highly protein-bound drugs such as phenylbutazone, tolbutamide and carbenoxolone is diminished in elderly subjects while the binding of others, such as diazepam and salicylate, is unchanged (Table 5). Studies

Table 5 Changes in protein binding with advancing age

Drug	Change	Reference
Carbenoxolone	↓	54
Chlormethiazole	↓	36
Desmethyldiazepam	→	32
Diazepam	→	55
Lorazepam	→	56
Penicillin	→	57
Pethidine	↓	35
Phenobarbitone	→	57
Phenylbutazone	↓	34
Phenytoin	→	57
Phenytoin	↓	58
Quinidine	→	59
Salicylate	→	34
Tolbutamide	↓	60
Warfarin	↓	61
Warfarin	→	62

concerning the binding of warfarin and phenytoin have produced conflicting evidence. Technical differences in method may have accounted for these disparities. One study has also shown that competitive binding of drugs to plasma proteins causes greater drug displacement in the elderly with an increase in plasma free drug concentrations[34].

However, the effect of reduction in protein binding may only be transient and of little importance with chronic dosing as a new steady state is achieved quite rapidly in which total plasma drug concentration falls but the concentration of free drug returns to initial values. Decreased red cell binding of pethidine[35] and chlormethiazole[36] in older subjects, with resultant higher plasma levels, may augment drug action when single or widely spaced doses are used.

Volume of distribution
Age-related changes in apparant volume of distribution of some drugs are shown in Table 6. It is interesting to note that the apparent volume of distribution of certain lipid-soluble drugs, such as diazepam and lignocaine, is increased. The volume of distribution is the main pharmacokinetic determinant of the loading dose of a drug, the dose being proportional to the volume. Thus the absolute

Table 6   Changes in apparent volume of distribution of drugs with advancing age

Drug	Change	Reference
Chlordiazepoxide	↓	63
Chlordiazepoxide	↑	50
Chlormethiazole	↓	64
Desmethyldiazepam	→	55
Diazepam	↑	32
Digoxin	→	27
Ethanol	↓	65
Lignocaine	↑	66
Lorazepam	→	56
Oxazepam	→	67
Paracetamol	→	28
Phenazone (Antipyrine)	↓	68
Phenazone (Antipyrine)	↓	69
Phenylbutazone	→	68
Propicillin	↓	31
Quinidine	→	59
Theophylline	→	30
Tolbutamide	↑	60

loading dose of digoxin required by an elderly patient is less than that required by an younger patient[27]. However, since the weight-corrected volume of distribution of digoxin is unaffected by age, the required loading dose/kg in adults is independent of age.

Regional distribution

While the apparent volume of distribution is a useful kinetic concept relating plasma level to amount of drug in the body, it tells nothing of distribution to various organs or within various organs. Such changes in regional distribution in themselves may alter drug effect. For instance, one might expect that the effective single dose of diazepam would be greater in an old patient since the apparent volume of distribution of diazepam increases with age[32]. However, one study has shown that the dose required to produce sedation for cardioversion is smaller in older subjects[37]. In other studies increased sensitivity of geriatric subjects to central nervous system-acting drugs, such as nitrazepam[38] and morphine[39], has been observed. One possibility is that distribution of these drugs to the brain may be enhanced due to increased blood – brain barrier permeability. Such aspects of possible changes in regional distribution with advancing age have not been studied to date.

Metabolism

There are multiple pathways and sites for drug metabolism in the body. While some drugs are metabolized in the plasma, skin and various organs the main site of drug metabolism is the liver. As the liver size and liver blood flow decreases with age, alterations in metabolism might be expected.

Most metabolized drugs are inactivated by metabolism and are changed to more polar compounds which can be more readily excreted in the bile or urine. The rate of metabolism is a major determinant of the duration and intensity of effect. The metabolism of relatively few drugs have been studied in the elderly and where data is available the kinetics of metabolized drugs is assessed by measuring plasma clearance, half-life and occasionally steady state data. While these data are available for a number of drugs the precise implications for drug effect in the elderly frequently is not clear.

Most drugs are metabolized by the microsomal enzymes and perhaps the most widely studied drug in relation to age is phenazone (antipyrine). This is a model drug used in studies of drug metabolism as it is completely metabolized, is not significantly protein bound and is well absorbed after oral administration. The plasma half-life of this drug is prolonged (Figure 2) and clearance is reduced in the elderly[68–71]. Two points emerged from these studies. Firstly, there is wide interindividual variability in elimination of antipyrine so that a relatively small prolongation in half-life of say 20–40% in the elderly, while statistically significant, is associated with con-

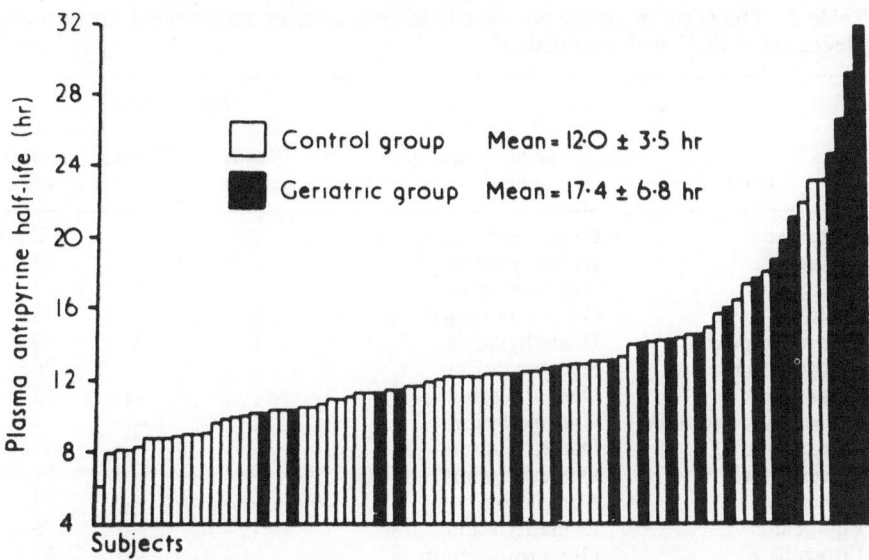

Figure 2 Individual plasma antipyrine half-life values in 61 normal young adults and 19 geriatric patients (O'Malley *et al.*[68], with permission)

siderable overlap between young and old (Figure 2). Secondly, in the studies of Vestal *et al.*[69], it was concluded that cigarette smoking in younger patients may be a more important determinant of the apparent age-related difference in elimination than is age itself.

Changes with age of the elimination kinetics of 19 additional drugs are detailed in Table 7; it can be observed that there is no really consistent pattern. However, the clearance of antipyrine, chlormethiazole, phenylbutazone, quinine, propranolol and chlordiazepoxide are reduced in the elderly. While these changes will result in lower steady state plasma levels of the drug only in the case of antipyrine has a concomitant increase of plasma half-life been demonstrated. Thus, it would seem that while the steady state level of some drugs increase in the elderly accumulation would not be a greater problem in the old compared with the young.

From a practical point of view the most difficult data to interpret is that which shows a prolonged half-life (aspirin, diazepam, desmethylimipramine, lignocaine, nortripyline, paracetamol) in the absence of a decrease in plasma clearance. With many of these drugs there is a fall in apparent volume of distribution. This probably results in unaltered steady state levels but the time taken

Table 7 The effect of ageing on the elimination of some metabolised drugs (after Stevenson *et al.*,[75] with permission)

Drug	Major route of metabolism	Plasma half-life	Plasma clearance	reference
		Effect in old age		
Acetanilide	Hydroxylation	↑	—	72
Acetanilide	Hydroxylation	→	→	73
Antipyrine	Hydroxylation	↑	↓	71,74
Aspirin	Glycine conjugation	↑	→	75
Chlordiazepoxide	Demethylation	↓	↓	50
Chlormethiazole	Hydroxylation	→	↓	76
Diazepam	Demethylation	↑	→	55
Desmethylimipramine	Hydroxylation	↑	—	77
Imipramine	Demethylation	→	—	77
Indomethacin	Demethylation	→	—	51
Isoniazid	Acetylation	→	—	72
Lignocaine	Demethylation	↑	→	76
Lorazepam	Glucuronidation	→	→	56
Nitrazepam	Reduction	→	→	38
Nortriptyline	Hydroxylation	↑	→	78
Paracetamol	Glucuronide and sulphate conjugation	↑	→	79
Phenylbutazone	Hydroxylation	→	↓	74
Phenytoin	Hydroxylation		↑	58
Propranolol	Hydroxylation	—	↓	80
Quinine	Hydroxylation	→	↓	75
Warfarin	Hydroxylation	→	→	62

to achieve steady state and duration of action might well be prolonged.

It is obvious from the disparate changes observed that a generalization as to alterations in drug metabolism with old age cannot be made. Indeed it is obvious that many pharmacodynamic studies must be carried out in association with kinetic studies before we can identify the precise significance of many of the documented kinetic alterations.

Renal elimination

For many drugs the kidney is the main or exclusive route of elimination. For others the kidney may be a secondary though important route of elimination. It is apparent, therefore, that alterations in renal function commensurate with age are likely to have an important bearing on the elimination of many drugs and hence the intensity and duration of pharmacological effects.

In the early 1950s Davies and Shock[81] examined the effect of the age on glomerular filtration rate as measured by inulin clearance, and found that in those over the age of 30 years there is a negative correlation between these two variables such that glomerular filtration rate falls by approximately 1 ml/min per 1.73 m^2 per year. Similarly, Millar *et al.*,[82] examined tubular function using maximum tubular reabsorptive capacity for glucose and found that it falls with advancing years. Finally, Shock in 1952[83] examined renal blood flow using PAH clearance and again the clearance of this substance falls by about 1% per year in the age range 20 – 80.

As glomerular filtration rate, effective renal plasma flow and tubular function all diminish with age it comes as little surprise to find that where the rates of elimination of drugs handled by the kidney were examined there was an association between advancing age and diminished drug elimination.

The elimination rate of the following drugs has been compared in the young and the elderly and found to be lower in the older age group: practolol[53], benzylpenicillin[84,85], phenobarbitone[86], digoxin[27,87], propicillin[31], kanamycin[81] and sulphamethizole[28]. Because of the predictability with which impaired renal function is reflected in impaired clearance of renally eliminated drugs (Figure 3) – one may reasonably expect that the elimination of other renally eliminated drugs is also diminished as a function of old age.

PHARMACODYNAMICS: DRUG RESPONSE

There is relatively limited information available on drug responses in the elderly and in only a few cases have comparative studies of drug action in young and old been made. Strangely, elderly patients are frequently excluded from clinical trials. A brief review of some of the drugs that have been studied in both the elderly and the young follows below.

Drugs acting on the central nervous system
Elderly patients seem to be particularly sensitive to central nervous system depressant effect of drugs. This apparent increase in sensitivity may be due to reduced elimination, altered distribution or to an increase in central nervous system sensitivity. Progressive loss of neurones from the cerebral cortex and reduction in cerebral flow with advancing age are other factors which may contribute to an altered response.

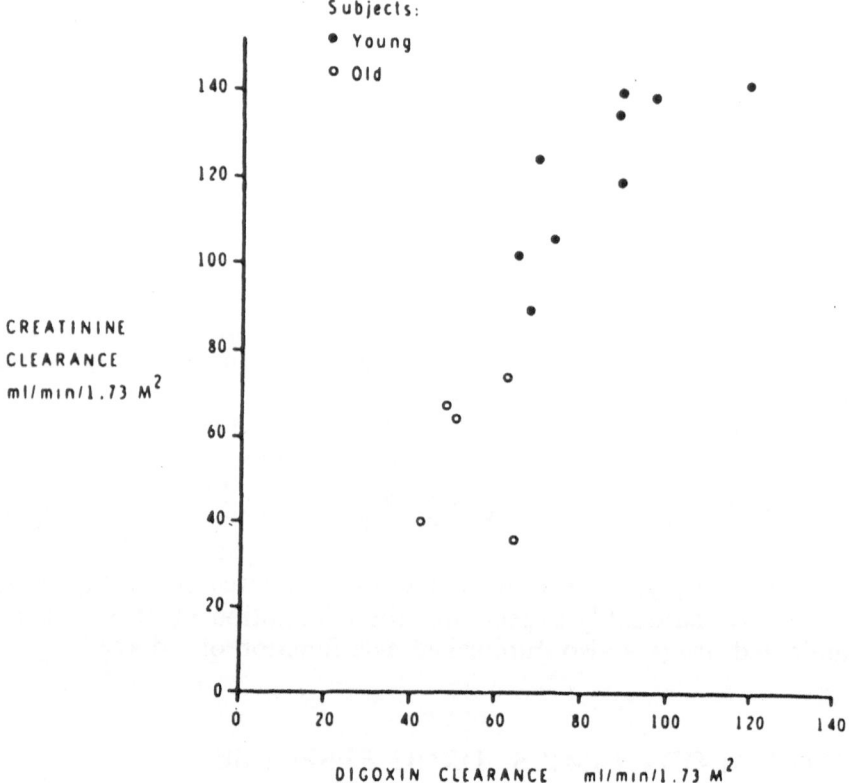

Figure 3   Relationship between creatinine clearance and digoxin clearance in old and young subjects (Ewy et al.,[87], with permission)

Narcotic analgesics

Adverse reactions to pethidine include hypotension, nausea and confusion and they appear to occur more frequently and with greater severity in the elderly[35]. This difference could be due to higher serum levels or to increased sensitivity to the drug in the elderly after a standard dose of the drug. Chan and colleagues[35] demonstrated consistently higher plasma levels and lower red cell binding of pethidine in the elderly. Differences in distribution and a decrease in renal clearance in the elderly may be important factors here.

There is evidence to suggest that the disposition of morphine may alter as a function of age. Berkowitz et al.,[89] showed that within 2 min of an intravenous injection, plasma morphine levels in patients over 50 years were almost twice those obtained in patients under 50 years. A decrease in volume of distribution is probably the most important cause of these high plasma levels and may well contribute to an increase in response. Indeed older patients are apparently more sensitive to morphine[29,90].

Barbiturates
Barbiturates are frequently said to have a prolonged action and an exaggerated response in the elderly[91] but we are not aware of a definitive study which shows this. Traeger *et al.*,[86] showed the half-life of phenobarbitone to be increased in subjects over 70 years. This change could be related to reduced renal excretion with age. In another study[92] elderly subjects were shown to convert a smaller proportion of amylobarbitone sodium to its major metabolite – 3-hydroxy-amylobarbitone – than younger subjects. It was also demonstrated that the mean plasma level of amylobarbitone in the elderly was significantly higher. These changes were attributed to impaired metabolism in the elderly. While elimination of these two babiturates is decreased, there is no conclusive evidence to indicate altered central nervous system sensitivity in the elderly.

Benzodiazepines
Considerable information is accumulating on the pharmacokinetics and pharmacodynamics of the benzodiazepine group of compounds in the elderly.
(a) *Chlordiazepoxide* There are three studies on chlordiazepoxide in the elderly[50,63,93]. A 2–3-fold prolongation of elimination half-life of chlordiazepoxide (9–12 hours to 17–30 hours) in the elderly was reported by Wilkinson[93]. This was due to a proportional decrease in systemic clearance of the drug. The present clinical implications of these studies is not clear as the formation of the active metabolite, desmethylchlordiazepoxide, is reduced.[93] When the presence of an active metabolite is involved, the execution of pharmacokinetic studies in the absence of measuring effect is obviously of limited value and extrapolation to clinical practice is impossible.
(b) *Diazepam* Diazepam has been fairly extensively compared in both the young and old. Although liver disease is by far the most important determinant of diazepam clearance, age is also important[55,94]. The half-life following both intravenous and oral administration showed a striking age dependence ranging from about 20 hours at 20 years to about 90 hours at 80 years[55]. No significant relationship could be discerned between age or cigarette

smoking on the one hand and clearance of diazepam on the other. There was no significant effect of age upon the protein binding of diazepam or desmethyldiazepam. The increase in half-life is attributable to a marked increase in volume of distribution of the drug, rather than age-dependent impairment of drug metabolizing capacity.

Reidenberg et al.,[37] demonstrated that the elderly are more sensitive to the central nervous system depressant effects of diazepam than the young following intravenous premedication with diazepam for elective cardioversion. They individualized the dose required to achieve a degree of central nervous system depression characterized by response to painful stimuli but not to oral command. They found that dose (and resultant plasma levels) varied inversely with age. Thus for a standard response less drug (mg/kg body weight) was required, indicating a possible increase in the central nervous system sensitivity to diazepam in the elderly.

The Boston Collaborative Drug Surveillance Programme[95] demonstrated that undue central nervous system depression with diazepam (or chlordiazepoxide) became more common with increasing age. The drowsiness was clinically significant, as indicated by the fact that in over 80% of the affected patients, therapy was discontinued. Interestingly, they found that excess central nervous system depression complicating treatment was highest in non-smokers and lowest in heavy smokers, suggesting that enhancement of drug metabolism and clearance by enzyme induction protected against the unwanted effect of the drug. Alternatively, cigarette smoking and diazepam may interact at receptor level.

The evidence indicates that elderly patients require lower doses and lower plasma levels of diazepam than younger patients to achieve the same degree of central nervous system depression, and that doses should be lowered accordingly.

(c) *Nitrazepam* It has been generally recommended that nitrazepam should be prescribed at reduced dosage in patients over 65. The main objective evidence for this was provided by Castleden et al.,[38] who compared the effect of a single 10 mg oral dose of nitrazepam with that of placebo in healthy young and old people. The elderly group made significantly more mistakes in psychomotor testing than did the young, despite similar half-lifes and plasma concentration of nitrazepam in the two groups (Figure 4). This difference in response is most likely explained by an increased sensitivity of elderly subjects to the action of nitrazepam. Malpas et al.,[96] have also shown psychomotor impairment on the morning following a single late evening dose of nitrazepam and in addition ob-

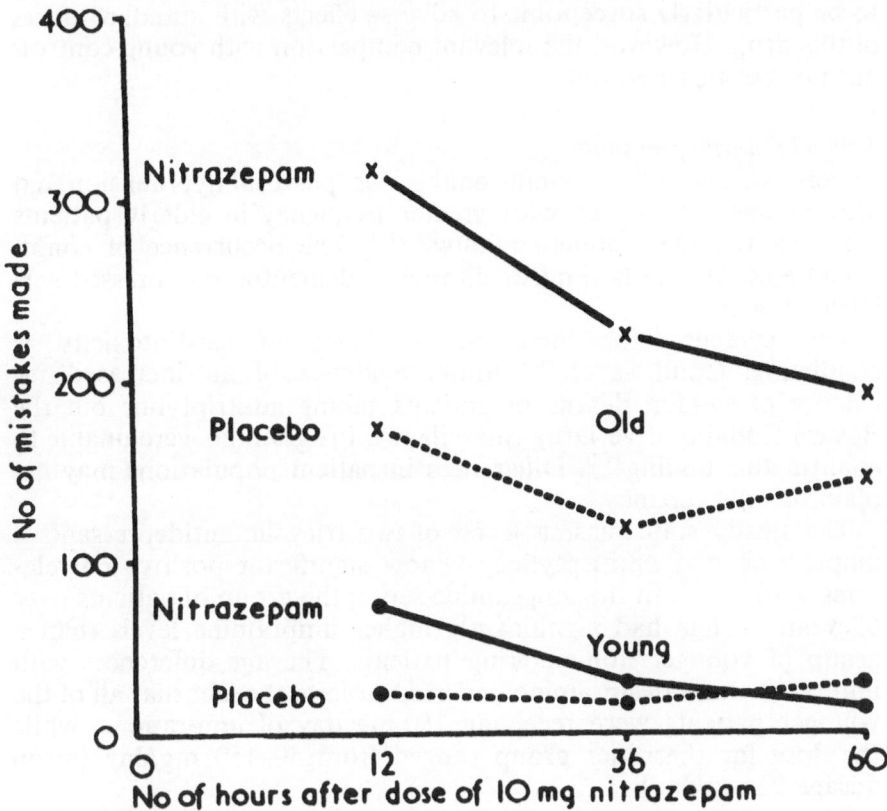

Figure 4 Effect of nitrazepam on performance testing in young and old subjects (Castleden *et al.*,[38], with permission)

served abnormalities for up to 18 hours in the elderly after a single dose.

(d) *Flurazepam* Flurazepam has a long half-life[97] so the onset of problems associated with chronic use may be insidious. The elderly have a higher incidence of unwanted residual drowsiness following flurazepam therapy for insomnia compared with younger patients, especially at doses above 15 mg[98].

Chlormethiazole

Elderly subjects have a prolonged half-life following intravenous administration of chlormethiazole[64]. Also, elderly subjects have higher peak plasma levels following oral administration of chlormethiazole than young people. Plasma red cell binding is significantly reduced in the elderly. Older subjects might reasonably be expected to be particularly susceptible to adverse effects with standard doses of this drug. However, the relevant comparison with young controls has not been carried out.

Tricyclic antidepressants
Adverse effects such as confusional states, postural hypotension and urinary retention occur with greater frequency in elderly patients receiving tricyclic antidepressants[99,100]. The occurrence of confusional episodes is often misdiagnosed as dementia in depressed geriatric patients.

The evidence for increased incidence of cardiotoxicity is conflicting. Coull *et al.*,[101] found evidence of an increased incidence of sudden deaths in patients taking amitriptyline but the Boston Collaborative Drug Surveillance Programme were unable to confirm this finding[100]. Differences in patient populations may explain this discrepancy.

The steady state plasma levels of two tricyclic antidepressants – imipramine and amitriptyline – show significant positive correlations with age[77]. In the imipramine series, the group of patients over 65 years of age had significantly higher imipramine levels than a group of younger non-smoking patients. The age differences with imipramine and desipramine occurred despite the fact that all of the younger patients were receiving 150 mg day of imipramine, while the dose for the older group ranged from 50–150 mg/day (mean dosage 92 mg/day).

Thus on pharmacokinetic grounds and possibly for pharmacodynamic reasons it seems appropriate to reduce the dose of tricyclic antidepressants by approximately 50–70% of the recommended adult dosage. Thus imipramine should be started at 25 mg/day at bedtime, with progressive increments every 4–7 days until a maximum of 100 mg/day is achieved (less if side-effects occur).

Antipsychotic drugs
Antipsychotic drugs have prominent sedative, cardiovascular and anticholinergic side-effects[102]. Parkinsonism and choreiform movements occur with phenothiazine therapy five times more frequently in the aged than in the young[103].

Anticoagulants
Elderly patients are more prone to bleeding episodes whilst on treatment with heparin[104]. No such evidence exists for oral anticoagulants but in a retrospective epidemiological study, O'Malley *et al.*[105]

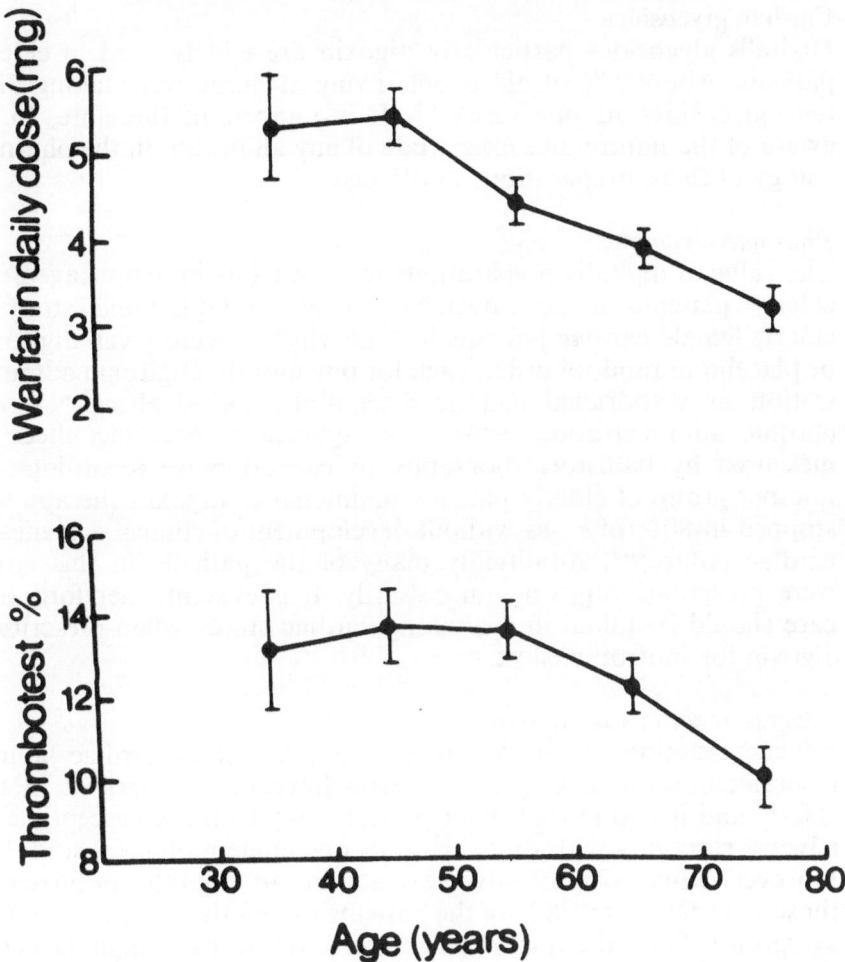

Figure 5   Mean ± SEM daily dose of warfarin and Thrombotest values for 177 patients. The anticoagulant effect increases with increasing age despite decreasing dose (O'Malley *et al.*[105], with permission)

demonstrated a greater degree of anticoagulation in patients over 70 years of age than in younger patients, even though the former received a smaller daily dose of warfarin (see Figure 5). The more marked effect of warfarin in the elderly was further assessed by Shepherd *et al.*[62] who found no age-dependent pharmacokinetic differences, but concluded that the elderly were more sensitive to the action of warfarin, whereby it inhibits vitamin K-dependent clotting factor synthesis.

Cardiac glycosides

Digitalis glycosides particularly digoxin are widely used in elderly patients. About 5% of old people living at home were taking digitalis glycosides in one series[106]. It is important, therefore, to be aware of the nature and magnitude of any alteration in the pharmacology of these preparations in old age.

Pharmacodynamics

The value of digitalis preparations when used as inotropic agents in elderly patients is controversial. In one double-blind study[107] elderly female cardiac patients in sinus rhythm were given digitoxin or placebo in random order, each for one month. Digitoxin administration or withdrawal had no discernible clinical effect. Nor did chronic administration cause any significant inotropic effect as measured by ballistocardiography or carotid pulse recordings. In another group of elderly patients maintenance digoxin therapy was stopped in 80% of cases without development of clinical evidence of cardiac failure[108]. Admittedly many of the patients in this study were prescribed digoxin unnecessarily. It is evident, therefore, that care should be taken in evaluating cardiac status when prescribing digoxin for inotropic effect.

Adverse reactions to digoxin

Adverse reactions including arrhythmias, refractory cardiac failure, mental confusion and gynaecomastia have been described in the elderly and it is said that older patients may be more susceptible to adverse reactions with digoxin[109]. In one epidemiological study[110], however, while 82% of adverse reactions to digitalis occurred in those over 60 years, 78% of the patients taking the drug were in this age group. Thus, the majority of adverse reactions to digitalis occur in older subjects roughly in proportion to their rate of consumption of these drugs (see page 4). Similar studies in which plasma digoxin concentrations were measured produced conflicting results. In one study the mean age of both toxic and non-toxic groups of patients was similar[111] while in the other[112] the mean age of the toxic group (66 years) was slightly but significantly higher than that in the non-toxic group (59 years). More importantly, in both studies the groups with digitalis toxicity also had evidence of renal impairment as indicated by raised serum creatinine concentrations. If a true excess risk of digitalis toxicity is associated with old age it is therefore more likely to be related to concomitant renal impairment with reduced clearance of digoxin than to increased myocardial sensitivity to the drug.

Prescribing digoxin

Maintenance digoxin dose should be reduced in elderly patients. The best guide to renal status is creatinine clearance. Serum creatinine levels can be normal in older persons in the presence of renal impairment because creatinine production in this age group is diminished. A nomogram which takes age into account can be used to calculate creatinine clearance from serum creatinine[113]. This nomogram was used in combination with a formula which calculates maintenance digoxin requirements[114] in a group of 99 patients aged 40–90 years (average aged 70 years) and steady state plasma digoxin levels achieved were all within the therapeutic range, with only five subjects showing signs of toxicity[115]. Other methods of predicting digoxin requirements have been devised[116–118] which can be applied to digoxin therapy in the elderly. A computer program[119] was used by Whiting *et al.* to aid dosage in a group of 42 elderly subjects already on digoxin. The dose was changed in 26 of these with obvious clinical benefit[119]. However, such prescription aids, although they help to rationalize therapy, do not take into account other variables affecting dose requirements in the elderly[120,121] such as extent of absorption and volume of distribution and other factors which alter myocardial sensitivity such as hypokalaemia.

In conclusion, judicious assessment of indications for digitalis therapy is required when treating geriatric subjects. Digoxin maintenance doses should be reduced in proportion to renal function and prescription aids are helpful in estimating dose. Because of the narrow therapeutic ratio of the drug, therapy should be closely monitored by clinical evaluation, helped by plasma level estimations, if in doubt. Digitalis therapy should be reviewed and stopped if the clinical status of the patient permits.

Beta-adrenoceptor blocking drugs

The pharmacokinetics and pharmacodynamics of beta-adrenoceptor blocking drugs are altered in the elderly. There seems to be a basic difference between the young and the old[122] in the response of the sympathetic nervous system. The finding that the number of beta-adrenoceptors is reduced in lymphocytes from elderly subjects[123] suggests that they may be reduced in sites such as the heart as well.

In 1971 Conway *et al.*[124] demonstrated that propranolol-attenuation of heart rate and cardiac output during exercise was less in older subjects (50–65 years) than in young subjects (20–35 years). This was attributed to a reduction with ageing of sympathetic drive to the heart in response to exercise. More recently Vestal *et al.*[125] have demonstrated diminished heart rate response to iso-prenaline and propranolol in the elderly.

Pharmacokinetics of drugs
Castleden *et al.*[53], demonstrated that practolol was eliminated more slowly in the elderly as a result of diminished renal function. More recently, Castleden and George[80], observed marked elevation of propranolol levels in the elderly (Figure 6). They also suggest that the dose of propranolol needed to achieve a given degree of beta blockade or of antihypertensive action is lower in the elderly than in the young. However, this conclusion is based only on kinetic data and does not take into account the possiblility of altered sensitivity, evidence for which is just beginning to emerge (see above, page 23). An increase in effect is supported by the findings of Greenblatt and Koch-Weser[126] who showed that the adverse reaction rate to pro-pranolol in 97 patients over 60 years of age was more than double that of 90 patients under 50 years of age.

Metoprolol has been found to have the same mean plasma half-life in elderly patients as in young healthy volunteers[127]. In another study[128], older subjects had higher peak values, later peaks, and 24-hour values which were higher than the 12-hour mean values in young subjects.

In summary, the position with regard to beta-adrenoceptor block-ing drugs is confusing. The elderly are less sensitive to propranolol and perhaps other beta-adrenoceptor blocking drugs but reduced elimination may offset this effect. Adverse drug reactions are more common in the elderly but there may be important variables in addition to age[122].

Antihypertensive drugs
It is important to prescribe antihypertensive drugs cautiously in the elderly as many factors complicate their use particularly the blunt-ing of homeostatic responses commensurate with ageing. There is little debate that treatment of severe hypertension in the elderly is necessary. The situation with mild and moderate hypertension is more difficult, however. While hypertension in the elderly of even 'minor' degree is associated with increased morbidity and mortality[129] the benefit to be derived from treatment is not certain. However, limited data from the Veterans Administration Study indi-cate that treatment may be beneficial. Of course inappropriate treat-ment can cause serious complications[130]. The European Working Party on Hypertension in the Elderly study[131]; on the effects of the

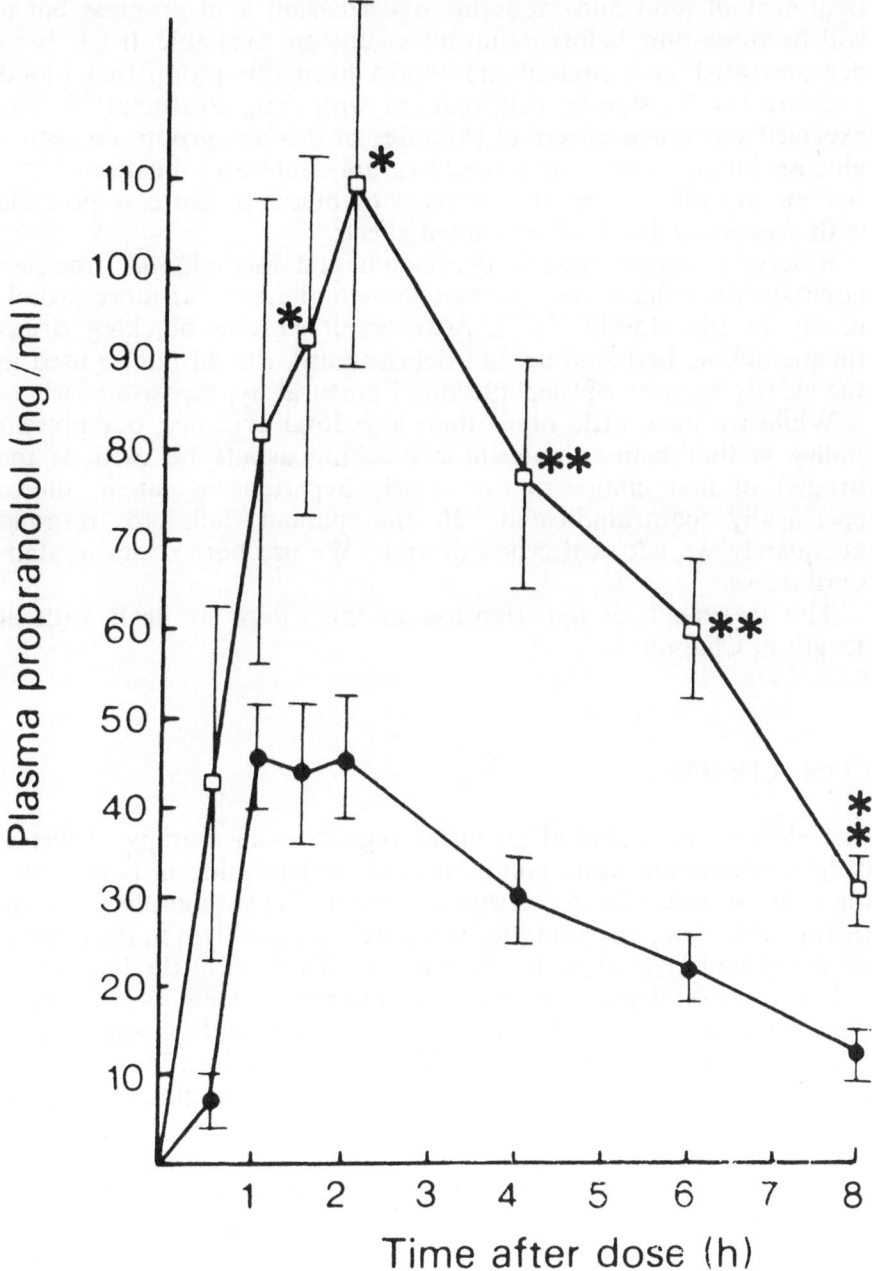

Figure 6   Plasma propranolol concentration in young and old patients following 40 mg taken orally (Castleden and George[80], with permission)

treatment of mild and moderate hypertension is in progress but it will be some time before definitive results are available. It has been demonstrated in a preliminary report from this group that blood pressure can be significantly reduced with drug treatment[132]. The expected unwanted effects of thiazides in this age group are seen – glucose intolerance[133] and raised serum urate and creatinine[132] – but an overall significant reduction of blood pressure is possible with acceptable levels of unwanted effects.

Reserpine causes mental depression and methyldopa produces lassitude, drowsiness and decrease in mental acuity far more prominently in the elderly[134,135]. Adrenergic neurone blocking drugs (guanethidine, bethanidine and debrisoquin), should not be used in the elderly because of their profound postural hypotensive effect.

While we have little other than anecdotal evidence, our present policy is that beta-adrenoceptor blocking agents be used as the drug(s) of first choice in the elderly hypertensive patient unless specifically contraindicated. If the patient fails to respond adequately we add a thiazide diuretic. We use both drugs in standard doses.

The treatment of hypertension in the elderly is dealt with at length in Chapter 4.

CONCLUSIONS

The elderly are a special group as regards drug therapy. Adverse drug reactions are more common in the elderly, due in part to the high rate of prescribing for this age group. While compliance with therapeutic regimens is said to be a particular problem in the elderly we could find little objective evidence of this effect in the literature.

Many physiological changes accompany ageing which may influence drug action. Absorption is not significantly changed. The rate of elimination of metabolized drugs is not uniformly affected by age. Of the four kinetic processes only renal elimination varies predictably with age.

Obviously many more pharmacodynamic studies must be carried out in order to assess possible alterations in responsiveness to drugs in the elderly. The results of these studies will undoubtedly improve our understanding of therapeutic principles to be employed when treating elderly patients. Reliance on pharmacokinetic studies alone will not suffice as the final arbiter must be the response observed in the relevant clinical setting.

References

1 Reidenberg, M. M. (1968). Registry of adverse drug reactions. *J. Am. Med. Assoc.*, **203**, 31

2 Borda, I. T., Slone, D. and Jick, H. (1968). Assessment of adverse reactions within a drug surveillance program. *J. Am. Med. Assoc.*, **205**, 645

3 Reidenberg, M. M. (1967). Adverse drug reactions without drugs. *Lancet*, **ii**, 892

4 Hurwitz, N. (1969). Admissions to hospital due to drugs. *Br. Med. J.*, **1**, 539

5 Caranasos, G. J., Stewart, R. B. and Cluff, E. (1974). Drug-induced illness leading to hospitalisation. *J. Am. Med. Assoc.*, **228**, 713

6 Williamson, J. and Chopin, J. M. (1979). Adverse reactions to prescribed drugs in the elderly – a multicentre investigation. In J. Crooks and I. H. Stevenson (eds.). *Drugs and the Elderly*. (London: Macmillan Press) (In press)

7 Hurwitz, N. (1969). Predisposing factors in adverse reactions to drugs. *Br. Med. J.*, **1**, 536

8 Klein, U., Klein, M., Sturn, H., Rothenbühler, M., Huber, R., Stucki, P., Gikalov, I., Keller, M. and Hoigne, R. (1976). The frequency of adverse drug reactions as dependent upon age, sex and duration of hospitalisation. *Int. J. Clin. Pharmacol.*, **13**, 187

9 Siedl, L. G., Thorton, G. F., Smith, J. W. and Cluff, L. F. (1966). Studies on the epidemiology of adverse drug reactions. *Bull. Johns Hopkins Hosp.*, **119**, 299

10 Porter, A. M. W. (1969). Drug defaulting in a general practice. *Br. Med. J.*, **1**, 218

11 Blackwell, B. (1972). The drug defaulter. *Clin. Pharmacol. Ther.*, **13**, 841

12 Sackett, D. L. (1976). The magnitude of compliance and noncompliance. In D. L. Sackett and R. B. Haynes (eds.). *Compliance with Therapeutic Regimens*, pp. 9–25. (Baltimore: Johns Hopkins University Press)

13 Haynes, R. B. (1976). A critical review of the determinants of patient compliance with therapeutic regimens. In D. L. Sackett and R. B. Haynes (eds.). *Compliance with Therapeutic Regimens*, pp. 26–39. (Baltimore: Johns Hopkins University Press)

14 Haynes, R. B. (1976). Strategies for improving compliance: methodological analysis and review. In D. L. Sackett and R. B. Haynes (eds.). *Compliance with Therapeutic Regimens*, pp. 69–82. (Baltimore: Johns Hopkins University Press)

15 Caron, H. S. and Roth H. P. (1968). Patients' co-operation with a medical regimen. *J. Am. Med. Assoc.*, **203**, 922

16 Wandless, I. and Davie, J. W. (1977). Can drug compliance in the elderly be improved? *Br. Med. J.*, **1**, 359

17 Gibson, I. I. J. M. and O'Hare, M. M. (1968). Prescription of drugs for old people at home. *Gerontol. Clin.*, **10**, 271

18 Baron, J. H. (1963). Studies of basal peak acid output with an augmented histamine test. *Gut*, **4**, 136

19 Richey, D. P. and Bender, A. D. (1977). Pharmacokinetic consequences of ageing. *Ann. Rev. Pharmacol. Toxicol.*, **17**, 49

20 Sherlock, S., Bearn, A. G., Billing, B. H. and Patterson, J. C. S. (1950). Splanchnic blood flow in man by the bromosulphalein method: the relation of peripheral plasma bromosulphalein level to calculated flow. *J. Lab. Clin. Med.*, **35**, 923

21 Warren, P. M., Pepperman, M. A. and Montgomery, R. D. (1978). Age changes in small intestinal mucosa. *Lancet*, **ii**, 849

22 Meyer, J., Sorter, H., Oliver, J. and Necheles, H. (1943). Studies in old age. VII Intestinal absorption in old age. *J. Gastroenterol.*, **1**, 876

23 Sapp, O. L., Seasions, J. T. and Rose, J. W. (1964). Effect of ageing on intestinal absorption of sugars. *Clin. Res.*, **12**, 31

24 Kendall, M. J. (1970). The influence of age on the xylose absorption test. *Gut*, **11**, 498

25 Bender, A. D. (1968). Effect of age on intestinal absorption: Implications for drug absorption in the elderly. *J. Am. Geriatr. Soc.*, **16**, 1331

26 Davidson, C. and Gibson, D. (1973). Clinical significance of positive inotropic action of digoxin in patients with left ventricular disease. *Br. Heart J.*, **35**, 970

27 Cusack, B., Horgan, J., Kelly, J. G., Lavan, J., Noel, J. and O'Malley, K. (1979). Digoxin in the elderly: Pharmacokinetic consequences of old age. *Clin. Pharmacol. Ther.* (In press)

28 Triggs, E. J., Nation, R. L., Long, A. and Ashley, J. J. (1975). Pharmacokinetics in the elderly. *Eur. J. Clin. Pharmacol.*, **8**, 55

29 Kramer, P. A., Chapron, D. J., Beason, J. and Mercik, S. A. (1978). Tetracycline absorption in elderly patients with achlorhydria. *Clin. Pharmacol. Ther.*, **23**, 467

30 Cusack, B., Kelly, J. G., Lavan, J., Noel, J. and O'Malley, K. (1979). Effect of age and smoking on theophylline pharmacokinetics. (In preparation)

31 Simon, C., Malerczyk, V., Müller, U. and Müller, G. (1972). Zur pharmakokinetik von propicillin bei geriatrischen patienten im vergleich zu jüngereen erwachsenen. *Dtsch. Med. Wochenschr.*, **97**, 1999

32 Klotz, U., Avant, G. R., Hoyumpa, A., Schenker, S. and Wilkinson, G. R. (1975). The effects of age and liver disease on the disposition and elimination of diazepam in adult man. *J. Clin. Invest.*, **55**, 347

33 Woodford-Williams, E., Alvarez, A. S., Webster, D., Landless, B. and Dixon, M. P. (1964/65). Serum protein patterns in 'normal' and pathological ageing. *Gerontologia*, **10**, 86

34 Wallace, S., Whiting, B. and Runcie, J. (1976). Factors affecting drug binding in plasma of elderly patients. *Br. J. Clin. Pharmacol.*, **3**, 327

35 Chan, K., Kendall, M. J., Mitchard, M., Wells, W. D. E. and Vickers, M. D. (1975). The effect of ageing on plasma pethidine concentration. *Br. J. Clin. Pharmacol.*, **2**, 297

36 Nation, R. L., Vine, J., Triggs, E. J. and Learoyd, B. (1977). Plasma levels of chlormethiazole and two metabolites after oral administration to young and aged human beings. *Eur. J. Clin. Pharmacol.*, **12**, 137

37 Reidenberg, M. M., Levy, M., Warner, H., Coutinho, C. B., Schwartz, M. A., Yu, G. and Cheripko, J. (1978). Relationship between diazepam dose, plasma level, age and central nervous system depression. *Clin Pharmacol. Ther.*, **23**, 371

38 Castleden, C. M., George, C. F., Marcer, D. and Hallet, C. (1977). Increased sensitivity to nitrazepam in old age. *Br. Med. J.*, **1**, 10

39 Belville, J. W., Forrest, W. H., Miller, E. and Brown, B. W. (1971). Influence of age on pain relief from analgesics. A study of post operative patients. *J. Am. Med. Assoc.*, **217**, 1835

40 Forbes, G. B. and Reina, J. C. (1970). Adult lean body mass declines with age: some longitudinal observations. *Metabolism*, **19**, 653

41 Edelman, I. S. and Leibman, J. (1959). Anatomy of body water and electrolytes. *Am. J. Med.*, **27**, 256

42 Novak, L. P. (1972). Ageing, total body potassium, free fat-mass and cell mass in males and females between 18 and 85. *J. Gerontol.*, **27**, 438

43 Brandfonbrener, M., Landowne, M. and Shock, N. W. (1955). Changes in cardiac output with age. *Circulation,* **12,** 557

44 Hollenberg, N. K., Adams, D. F., Solomon, H. F., Rashid, A., Abrams, H. L., and Merrill, J. P. (1974). Senescence and the renal vasculature in normal man. *Circ. Res.,* **34,** 309

45 Geokas, M. C., and Haverback, B. J. (1969). The ageing gastrointestinal tract. *Am. J. Surg.,* **117,** 881

46 Dandona, P., James, I. M., Newbury, P. A., Woollard, M. L. and Beckett, A. G. (1978). Cerebral blood flow in diabetes mellitus: evidence of abnormal cerebrovascular reactivity. *Br. Med. J.,* **2,** 325

47 Rowe, J. W., Andres, R., Tobin, J. D., Norris, A. H. and Shock, N. W. (1976). The effect of age on creatinine clearance in man: a cross-sectional and longitudinal study. *J. Gerontol.,* **31,** 155

48 Castleden, C. M., Volans, C. N. and Raymond, K. (1977). The effect of ageing on drug absorption from the gut. *Age Ageing,* **6,** 138

49 Salem, S. A. M. and Stevenson, I. H. (1977). Absorption kinetics of aspirin and quinine in elderly subjects. *Br. J. Clin. Pharmacol.,* **4,** 397p

50 Shader, R. I., Greenblatt, D. J., Harmatz, J. S., Franke, R. I. and Koch-Weser, J. (1977). Absorption and disposition of chlordiazepoxide in young and elderly male volunteers. *J. Clin. Pharmacol.,* **17,** 709

51 Traeger, A., Kunze, M., Stein, G. and Ankermann, H. (1973). Zur pharmako-kinetik von indomethacin bei alten menschen. *Z. Alternsforsch.,* **27,** 151

52 Melander, A., Bodin, N.-O., Danielson, K., Gustafsson, B., Haglund, G. and Westerlund, D. (1978). Absorption and elimination of d-propoxyphene, acetyl salicylic acid and phenazone in a combination tablet (Doleron): Comparison between young and elderly subjects. *Acta Med. Scand.,* **203,** 121

53 Castleden, C. M., Kaye, C. M. and Parsons, R. L. (1975). The effects of age on plasma levels of propranolol and practolol in man. *Br. J. Clin. Pharmacol.,* **2,** 303

54 Hayes, M. J., Sprackling, M. M. and Langman, M. J. S. (1977). Changes in the plasma clearance and protein binding of carbenoxolone with age and their possible relationship with adverse drug effects. *Gut,* **18,** 1054

55 Klotz, U. and Miller-Seyditz, P. (1979). Altered elimination of desmethyl-diazepam in the elderly. *Br. J. Clin. Pharmacol.,* **7,** 119

54 Kraus, J. W., Desmond, P. V., Marshal, J. P., Johnson, B. S., Schenker, S. and Wilkinson, G. R. (1978). Effects of ageing and liver disease on disposition of lorazepam. *Clin. Pharmacol. Ther.,* **24,** 411

57 Bender, A., Post, A., Meier, J. P., Higson, J. F. and Reichard, G. Jr. (1975). Plasma protein binding of drugs as a function of age in adult human subjects. *J. Pharm. Sci.,* **64,** 1171

58 Hayes, M. J., Langman, M. J. S. and Short, A. H. (1975). Changes in drug metabolism with increasing age. 2. Phenytoin clearance and protein binding. *Br. J. Clin. Pharmacol.,* **2,** 73

59 Ochs, H. R., Greenblatt, D. J., Woo, E. and Smith, T. W. (1978). Reduced quinidine clearance in elderly persons. *Am. J. Cardiol.,* **42,** 481

60 Miller, A. K., Adir, J. and Vestal, R. E. (1977). Effect of age on the pharmacokinetics of tolbutamide in man. *Pharmacologist,* **19,** 128

61 Hayes, M. J., Langman, M. J. S. and Short, A. H. (1975). Changes in drug metabolism with increasing age. 1. Warfarin binding and plasma proteins. *Br. J. Clin. Pharmacol.,* **2,** 69

62 Shepherd, A. M. M., Hewick, D. S., Moreland, T. A. and Stevenson, I. H. (1977). Age as a determinant of sensitivity to warfarin. *Br. J. Clin. Pharmacol.,* **4,** 315

63 Roberts, R. K., Wilkinson, G. R., Branch, R. A. and Schenker, S. (1978). Effect of age and parenchymal liver disease on the disposition and elimination of chlordiazepoxide (Librium). *Gastroenterology*, **75,** 479
64 Nation, R. L., Learoyd, B., Barber, J. and Triggs, E. J. (1976). The pharmacokinetics of chlormethiazole following intravenous administration in the aged. *Eur. J. Clin. Pharmacol.*, **10,** 407
65 Vestal, R. E., Mc Guire, E. A., Tobin, J. D., Andres, R., Norris, A. H. and Mezey, E. (1977). Ageing and ethanol metabolism. *Clin. Pharmacol. Ther.*, **21,** 343
66 Nation, R. L., Triggs, E. J. and Selig, M. (1977). Lignocaine kinetics in cardiac patients and aged subjects. *Br. J. Clin. Pharmacol.*, **4,** 439
67 Shull, H. J., Wilkinson, G. R., Johnson, R. and Schenker, S. (1976). Normal disposition of oxazepam in acute viral hepatitis and cirrhosis. *Ann. Intern. Med.*, **84,** 420
68 O'Malley, K., Crooks, J., Duke, E. and Stevenson, I. H. (1971). Effect of age and sex on human drug metabolism *Br. Med. J.*, **3,** 607
69 Vestal, R. E., Norris, A. H., Tobin, J. D., Cohen, B. H., Shock, N. W. and Andres, R. (1975). Antipyrine metabolism in man: Influence of age, alcohol, caffeine and smoking. *Clin. Pharmacol. Ther.*, **18,** 425
70 Liddell, D. E., Williams, F. J. M. and Briant, R. H. (1975). Phenazone (antipyrine) metabolism and distribution in young and elderly adults. *Clin. Exper. Pharmacol. Physiol.* **2,** 481
71 Swift, C. G., Homeida, M., Halliwell, M. and Roberts, C. J. (1978). Antipyrine disposition and liver size in the elderly. *Eur. J. Clin. Pharmacol.*, **14,** 149
72 Farah, F., Taylor, W., Rawlins, M. D. and James, O. (1977). Hepatic drug acetylation and oxidation-effects of ageing in man. *Br. Med. J.*, **3,** 155
73 Playfer, J. R., Baty, J. D., Lamb, T., Powell, C. and Price-Evan, D. A. (1978). Age related differences in the disposition of acetanilide. *Br. J. Clin. Pharmacol.*, **6,** 529
74 Crooks, J., O'Malley, K. and Stevenson, I. H. (1976). Pharmacokinetics in the elderly. *Clin. Pharmacokin.* **1,** 280
75 Stevenson, I. H., Salem, S. A. and Shepherd, A. M. (1979). Studies on drug absorption and metabolism in the elderly. In J. Crooks and Stevenson, I. H. (eds.). *Drugs and the Elderly.* (London: Macmillan Press). (In press)
76 Triggs, E. J. (1979). Pharmacokinetics of lignocaine and chlormethiazole in the elderly: With some preliminary observations on other drugs. In J. Crooks and I. H. Stevenson (eds.). *Drugs and the Elderly.* (London: Macmillan Press). (In press)
77 Nies, A., Robinson, D. S., Friedman, M. J., Green, R., Cooper, T. B., Ravaris, C. L. and Ives, J. O. (1977). Relationship between age and tricyclic antidepressant plasma levels. *Am. J. Psychol.* **134,** 790
78 Braithwaite, R., Montgomery, S. and Dawling, S. (1979). Age, depression and tricyclic antidepressant levels. In J. Crooks and I. H. Stevenson (eds.). *Drugs and the Elderly.* (London: Macmillan Press). (In press)
79 Briant, R. H., Dorrington, R. E., Cleal, J. and Williams, F. M. (1976). The rate of acetaminophen metabolism in the elderly and the young. *J. Am. Geriatr. Soc.*, **24,** 359
80 Castleden, C. M. and George, C. F. (1979). The effect of ageing on the hepatic clearance of propanolol. *Br. J. Clin. Pharmacol.*, **7,** 49
81 Davies, D. F. and Shock, N. W. (1950). Age changes in glomerular filtration rate, effective renal plasma flow and tubular excretory capacity in adult males. *J. Clin. Invest.*, **29,** 496

82 Miller, J. H., McDonald, R. K. and Shock, N. W. (1952). Age changes in the maximal rate of renal tubular reabsorption of glucose. *J. Gerontol.*, **7,** 196
83 Shock, N. W. (1952). Age changes in renal function. In Lansing, A. I. (ed.) *Cowdrey's Problems of Ageing*, pp. 614–630. (Baltimore: Williams and Wilkins)
84 Molholm-Hansen, J., Kampmann, J. and Laursen, H. (1970). Renal excretion of drugs in the elderly. *Lancet*, **i,** 1170
85 Leikola, E. and Vartia, K. O. (1957). On penicillin levels in young and geriatric subjects. *J. Gerontol.*, **12,** 48
86 Traeger, A., Kiesewetter, R. and Kunze, M. (1974). Zur pharmakokinetik von phenobarbital bei; erwachsenen und greisen. *Dtsch. Ges. Wesen.*, **29,** 1040
87 Ewy, G. A., Kapadia, G. G., Yao, L., Lullin, M. and Marcus, F. I. (1969). Digoxin metabolism in the elderly. *Circulation*, **39,** 449
88 Kristensen, M., Molholm-Hansen, J., Kampmann, J., Lumholtz, B. and Siersbaek-Nielson, K. (1974). Drug elimination and renal function. *J. Clin. Pharmacol.*, **14,** 307
89 Berkowitz, B. A., Ngai, S. H., Yang, J. C., Hempstead, J and Spector, S. (1975). The disposition of morphine in surgical patients. *Clin. Pharmacol. Ther.*, **17,** 629
90 Salter, W. and White, M. L. (1949). Morphine sensitivity. *Anaesthesiology*, **10,** 553
91 Bender, A. D. (1964). Pharmacological aspects of ageing. A survey of increasing age on drug activity in adults. *J. Am. Geriatr. Soc.*, **12,** 114
92 Irvine, R. E. Grove, J. Toseland, P. A. and Trounce, J. R. (1974). The effect of age on the hydroxylation of amylobarbitone sodium in man. *Br. J. Clin. Pharmacol.*, **1,** 42
93 Wilkinson, G. R. (1979). The effect of ageing on the disposition of benzodiazepines in man. In J. Crooks and I. H. Stevenson (eds.). *Drugs and the Elderly.* (London: Macmillan Press). (In press)
94 Greenblatt, D. J., Harmatz, J. S. and Shader, R. I. (1978). Factors influencing diazepam pharmacokinetics: age, sex and liver disease *Int. J. Clin. Pharmacol. Biopharm.*, **16,** 177
95 Boston Collaborative Drug Surveillance Programme (1973). Clinical depression of the CNS due to diazepam and chlordiazepoxide in relation to cigarette smoking and age. *N. Engl. J. Med.*, **288,** 277
96 Malpas, A., Rowan, A. J., Joyce, C. R. B. and Scott, D. F. (1970). Persistent behavioural and EEG changes after single dose of nitrazepam and amylobarbitone sodium. *Br. Med. J.*, **2,** 762
97 Greenblatt, D. J., Shader, R. I. and Koch-Weser, J. (1975). Flurazepam hydrochloride, a benzodiazepine hypnotic. *Ann. Intern. Med.* **83,** 237
98 Greenblatt, D. J., Allen, M. D. and Shader, R. I. (1977). Toxicity of high dose flurazepam in the elderly. *Clin. Pharmacol. Ther.*, **21,** 355
99 Muller, O. F., Goodman, N. and Bellet, S. (1961). The hypotensive effect of imipramine hydrochloride in patients with cardiovascular disease. *Clin. Pharmacol. Ther.*, **2,** 300
100 Boston Collaborative Drug Surveillance Programme. (1972). Adverse reactions to tricyclic antidepressant drugs. *Lancet*, **i,** 529
101 Coull, D. G., Crooks, J., Dingwall-Fordyce, I., Scott, A. M. and Weir, R. D. (1970). Amitriptyline and cardiac disease: Risk of sudden death identified by monitoring system. *Lancet*, **ii,** 590
102 Goodman, L. S. and Gilman, A. (1975). *Pharmacological Basis of Therapeutics.* 5th ed, 1704p. (New York: Macmillan Press)
103 Saltzman, C., Shader, R. I. and Vander Kolk, B. A., (1976). Clinical psychopharmacology and the elderly patient. *NY State J. Med.*, **76,** 71

104 Jick, H., Slone, D., Borda, I. T. and Shapiro, S. (1968). Efficacy and toxicity of heparin in relation to age and sex. *N. Engl. J. Med.*, **279**, 284

105 O'Malley, K., Stevenson, I. H., Ward, C. A., Wood, A. J. and Crooks. J. (1977). Determinants of anticoagulant control in patients receiving warfarin. *Br. J. Clin. Pharmacol.*, **4**, 309

106 Caird, F. I. (1972). Metabolism of digoxin in relation to therapy in the elderly. *Gerontol. Clin.*, **16**, 68

107 Starr, I. and Luchi, R. J. (1969). Blind study on the action of digitoxin in elderly women. *Am. Heart J.*, **78**, 740

108 Dall, J. L. C. (1970). Maintenance digoxin in elderly patients. *Br. Med. J.*, **2**, 705

109 Dall, J. L. C. (1965). Digitalis intoxication in elderly patients. *Lancet*, i, 194

110 Hurwitz, N. and Wade, O. L. (1969). Intensive hospital monitoring of adverse reactions to drugs. *Brit. Med. J.*, **1**, 531

111 Beller, G. A., Smith, T. W., Abelmann, W. H., Haber, E. and Hood, W. B. (1971). Digitalis intoxication, a prospective clinical study with serum level correlations. *N. Engl. J. Med.*, **284**, 989

112 Smith, T. W. and Haber, E. (1970). Digoxin intoxication: The relationship of clinical presentation to serum digoxin concentration. *J. Clin. Invest.*, **49**, 2377

113 Kampmann, J., Siersbaek-Nielsen, K., Kristensen, M. and Molholm-Hansen, J. (1974). Rapid evaluation of creatinine clearance. *Acta Med. Scand.*, **196**, 517

114 Jelliffe, R. W. (1968). An improved method of digoxin therapy. *Ann. Intern. Med.*, **69**, 703

115 Christiansen, N. J. B., Kølendorf, K., Siersbaek-Nielsen, K. and Mølholm-Hansen, J. (1973). Serum digoxin values following a dosage regimen based on body weight, sex, age and renal function. *Acta Med. Scand.*, **194**, 257

116 Nicholson, P. W., Dobbs, S. M., McGill, A. P. J., Rodgers, E. M. and Slater, E. (1978). A score for prescribing digoxin. *Br. Heart J.*, **40**, 177

117 Jelliffe, R. W. and Brooker, G. (1974). A nomogram for digoxin therapy. *Am. Heart J.*, **57**, 63

118 Mawer, G. E. (1976). Computer assisted prescribing of drugs. *Clin. Pharmacokin.*, **1**, 67

119 Whiting, B., Wandless, I., Sumner, D. J. and Goldberg, A. (1978). Computer assisted review of digoxin therapy in the elderly. *Br. Heart J.*, **40**, 8

120 Simonson, W. and Stennett, D. J. (1978). Estimation of serum digoxin levels in geriatric patients. *Am. J. Hosp. Pharm.*, **35**, 943

121 Aronson, J. K. (1978). Monitoring digoxin therapy: *III* How useful are the nomograms? *Brit. J. Clin. Pharmacol.*, **5**, 55

122 Vestal, R. E. (1978). Drug use in the elderly. A review of problems and special considerations. *Drugs*, **16**, 358

123 Shocken, D. and Roth, G. (1977). Reduced beta adrenergic receptor concentrations in ageing man. *Nature (London)*, **267**, 856

124 Conway, J., Wheeler, R. and Sannerstedt, R. (1971). Sympathetic nervous activity during exercise in relation to age. *Cardiovasc. Res.*, **5**, 577

125 Vestal, R. E., Wood, A. J. J. and Shand, D. G. (1978). Reduced β adrenoceptor sensitivity in the elderly. (Abst.) *Clin. Res.*, **26**, 488A

126 Greenblatt, D. J. and Koch-Weser, J. (1973). Adverse reactions to propranolol in hospitalised medical patients: A report from the Boston Collaborative Drug Surveillance Programme. *Am. Heart J.*, **86**, 478

127 Lundborg, P. and Steen, B. (1976). Plasma levels and effect on heart rate and blood pressure of metoprolol after acute oral administration in 12 geriatric patients. *Acta Med. Scand.*, **200**, 397

128 Kendall, M. J., Brown, D. and Yates, R. A. (1977). Plasma metoprolol concentrations in young, old and hypertensive subjects. *Br. J. Clin. Pharmacol.*, **4,** 497

129 Kannel, W. B. and Gordon, T. (1978). Evaluation of cardiovascular risk in the elderly: The Framingham Study. *Bull. N. Y. Acad. Med.*, **54,** 573

130 Jackson, G., Pierscianowski, T. A., Mahon, W. and Condon. J. (1976). Inappropriate antihypertensive therapy in the elderly. *Lancet*, **ii,** 1317

131 Amery, A. and De Schaepdryver, A. (1973). European working party on high blood pressure in elderly (EWPHE). Organisation of a double-blind multicentre trial on antihypertensive therapy in elderly patients. *Clin. Sci. Mol. Med.*, **45,** 71s

132 Amery, A., Berthaux, P., Birkenhäger, W., Boel, A., Brixko, P., Bulpitt, C., Clement, D., Deruyterre M., De Schaepdryver, A., Dollery, C., Fagard, R., Forette, F., Henry, J. F., Hellemans, J., Laaser, U., Lund-Johansen, P., MacFarlane, J., Maling, T., Mutsers, A., Nissinen, A., Ohm, O. I., Pelemans, J., Suchkettkaye, A. I., Tuomilehto, J. and Willems, J. (1978). Antihypertensive therapy in patients above age 60. Third interim report of the European working party on high blood pressure in elderly (EWPHE). *Acta Cardiol.*, **33,** 113

133 Amery, A., Berthaux, P., Bulpitt, C., Deruyterre, M., De Schaepdryver, A., Dollery, C., Fagard, R., Forette, F., Hellemans, J., Lund-Johansen, P., Mutsers, A. and Tuomilehto, J. (1978). Glucose intolerance during diuretic therapy. Results of trial by the European working party on hypertension in the elderly. *Lancet*, **i,** 681

134 Lindeman, R. D., Bouthilet, G. N., Ashley, W. R. and Morris J. R. (1963). Effect of hydrochlorothiazide-reserpine therapy on cerebral function in elderly hypertensives. *J. Am. Geriatr. Soc.*, **2,** 597

135 Davison, W., (1972). Unwanted drug effects in the elderly. In L. Meyler and H. P. Peck (eds.). *Drug Induced Diseases*, 4th ed, 617p. (Amsterdam: Exerpta Medica)

General references

Triggs, E. J. and Nation, R. L. (1975). Pharmacokinetics in the aged: A review. *J. Pharmacokin. Biopharm.*, **6,** 387

Lamy, P. P. and Kitler, M. E. (1971). Drugs and the geriatric patient. *J. Am. Geriatr. Soc.*, **19,** 23

O'Malley, K., Judge, T. and Crooks, J. (1979). Geriatric clinical pharmacology and therapeutics: In G. S. Avery (ed.). *Drug Treatment*, 2nd Ed, pp. 123–142 (Sydney: Adis Press)

Lamy, P. P. and Vestal, R. E. (1976). Drug prescribing for the elderly. *Hosp. Prac.*, **9,** 111

2

Antibiotic practice in elderly patients

P. J. Sanderson and M. J. Denham

INTRODUCTION

Antibiotics are widely prescribed to all age groups[1], and although the degree of compliance of drug taking by older people may not be as good as the doctor would wish, unfortunately the incidence of reactions is still high[2,3]. Continual advances in antibiotic therapy are being made. Previously accepted regimens are being altered or modified and new drugs continue to be introduced. Consequently the properties of antibiotics and their use in different clinical situations should be appreciated in order to obtain the best response. Although some antimicrobial agents are not derived from living organisms and are therefore not properly called antibiotics, they all have the common purpose of eliminating bacterial pathogens and the terms antimicrobial agent and antibiotic will be used in this chapter without distinction.

ANTIBIOTIC PRACTICE

Importance of bacteriological investigation

There is now a large array of antibiotics and each group of these drugs, and indeed some individual agents, have sufficiently different antibiotic spectra and properties to give them particular roles in treating infection. There is no single agent that can attack the majority of pathogenic bacteria; on the other hand, certain agents are 'drugs of choice' for certain bacteria. It is vital therefore to obtain as much evidence as possible as to the source and nature of the infec-

35

tion to be treated, and to form an impression of the type of organism causing the disease. Specimens of pus, urine, sputum, and specimens of biopsy tissue from liver, bone, bone marrow and joint fluid, for example, must be sent to the laboratory before treatment is begun. Inappropriate antibiotics may destroy bacteria in blood or urine without eliminating the focus of infection. Isolation of the organism will allow determination of antibiotic sensitivities and so give precision to the antibiotic regimen. Antibiotic therapy without the aid of bacteriology is largely guesswork however informed the guess may be.

In elderly patients the signs and symptoms of infection may be difficult to obtain; a poor history and multiple pathology may obscure the clinical picture. It is always valuable to obtain blood cultures if the presence of infection is questioned. In one study bacteraemia was found with pneumococcal pneumonia in 7% of patients between the ages of 12 to 49 years, but in 20% of patients more than 50 years of age[4]. The incidence of bacteraemia was increased in patients with pre-existing disease of the respiratory tract, cardiovascular system or malignancy. Two sets of blood cultures taken at least 1 hour apart should be taken before therapy is started and these should be repeated the next day if therapy is withheld.

In difficulty or doubt consultation with a microbiologist may help clarify problems of diagnosis, appropriate specimens, antibiotic therapy and cross-infection hazards. Bactericidal antibiotics are preferred to bacteriostatic drugs in elderly patients, since they may suffer from other conditions in addition to the infection being treated, such as anaemia, chronic infection elsewhere, immunosuppression or malignancy which may reduce their ability to eliminate infection. Bactericidal antibiotics (Table 1) are independent of the patient's defences against infection. However, it has been known from early experiments with benzylpenicillin that some organisms in cultures of *Staphylococcus aureus* remain alive during exposure to the antibiotic, and it is thought that these 'persisters' may regrow in

Table 1 Antibiotic action

Bactericidal	Bacteriostatic
Penicillin-type drugs	Erythromycin (in usual doses)
Cephalosporins	Sulphonamides
Aminoglycosides	Co-trimoxazole
Fucidin	Clindamycin
	Tetracyclines
	Chloramphenicol

patients following excretion of the antibiotic[5]. Recently, 'tolerant' strains of *Staphylococcus aureus*, which are characterized by a high proportion of individual organisms that cease to reproduce but resist the killing effect of pencillins, have been isolated from patients[6]. The existence of both 'persisters' and of 'tolerant' strains of staphylococci emphasizes the value of using two antibiotics acting in different ways in order to bring about a bactericidal effect when dealing with serious staphylococcal infection.

Routes of administration
Some antimicrobial agents, such as chloramphenicol, some sulphonamides, fucidin and metronidazole are absorbed well from the intestinal tract. In the case of other antibiotics derivatives have been found that are better absorbed from the gut than the original compound, and these should always be used, for example phenoxymethyl-penicillin for benzylpenicillin, flucloxacillin for cloxacillin, amoxycillin or talampicillin for ampicillin and clindamycin for lincomycin. It is advisable to give the drug at least half an hour before food. The intramuscular (i.m.) and intravenous (i.v.) routes will ensure that the entire dose is absorbed, and are consequently more efficient than the oral route. Intramuscular injection will usually provide a satisfactory serum peak concentration of the drug when given in the recommended dose. Nevertheless, there is often a decline of serum concentration to less than the minimal inhibitory concentration (mic) of the infecting organism before the next dose is due.

The i.v. route allows administration of the drug by bolus injection over a 5 min interval or by infusion over 1 hour. Infusions for a longer time, and continuous infusions, may not give satisfactory serum levels (that is, sufficiently above the mic of the infecting organisms). A bolus injection will give a high peak which rapidly falls during the first half an hour or so during the 'phase of distribution' of the drug in the body; serum levels then become more stable, though still declining, during the 'phase of equilibration'. Consequently, blood concentrations measured within the first half hour of a bolus injection can be misleadingly high.

Antibiotics are, usually, compatible with saline but there are several important exceptions[7], and a pharmacist or the manufacturer's 'insert' literature should be consulted in cases of doubt. Antibiotics (or other drugs) must not be added to amino acid solutions, lipid mixtures, mannitol solutions, blood or blood products. Penicillin-type antibiotics must be added only to sodium chloride 0·9% solution and used immediately after preparation. Antibiotics should not be mixed with each other, or with other drugs. Carbenicillin should be prepared for infusion with the diluent provided in the drug pack and erythromycin lactobionate with 5% dextrose. A useful and effective procedure is to give an antibiotic by syringe and needle through the tubing or a side port of a giving set over a period of 5 min; provided that none of the incompatible materials mentioned above have been infused previously the tubing may be cleared first by an injection of saline.

Frequency of dosage
It is not known whether it is better to maintain antibiotics in blood and body tissues at concentrations that are constantly above the mic of the infecting organism, or whether concentrations should be allowed to fall between doses ('seesaw' serum profile) so that nongrowing organisms or 'persisters' can grow out and again become susceptible to the action of penicillin-type drugs (where growth of the organism is required for drug action). It seems possible that regrowth of the infecting organism may lead to recrudescence of the infection and, in any case, the body defences will themselves eventually remove 'persisters'. These latter arguments mean that antibiotic regimens require short intervals between doses and administration should be arranged on a 6 hourly interval, particularly for penicillin-type drugs which tend to be excreted more rapidly than others. When antibiotic administration is imperative to the patient's care it is valuable to set up an infusion in a peripheral vein using a steel needle, to avoid the recurring discomfort of multiple intramuscular injections. The infusion site should be covered with a dressing but otherwise handled as little as possible. The infusion line can be maintained by a slow infusion of saline dextrose, which is often a useful means of ensuring adequate hydration in an elderly patient with infection. Where peripheral veins are not available in life-threatening situations, a central infusion line may be necessary to ensure proper administration of antibiotics.

Dosage of antibiotics
Elderly patients have three characteristics that affect the quantity of antibiotic they should receive:

(1) They tend to have lower body weight than younger patients upon whom 'normal' dosage is based;
(2) They may have reduced renal and liver function; and
(3) They are frequently prescribed more than one drug.

The serum urea or creatinine concentration and the creatinine clearance test may not reflect the degree of renal dysfunction that is often present in older patients. Their reduced muscle mass produces less creatinine than younger patients, and together with some defective tubular exchange elderly patients may maintain an apparently normal excretion rate of serum urea and creatinine in the presence of a glomerular filtration rate as low as 60 ml/min. As an example of reduced excretion of an antibiotic in the presence of normal urea and creatinine values, it was found that the serum half-life of amoxycillin in four elderly female patients (2·7 hours) was more than twice that in younger volunteers (1·05 hours)[8]. All penicillin-type antibiotics, cephalosporins, aminoglycosides and colistin are excreted through the kidney, and it is worth remembering that sick, elderly patients may have greater impairment of renal function than healthy individuals of similar age[9]. Markedly delayed renal excretion of mecillinam (a new penicillin-type antibiotic) has been found in elderly patients also[10]; indeed the serum half-life of this compound was 3·97 hours in a group of six patients over the age of 65 with apparently normal renal function compared to 0·88 hours in young subjects. Other drugs are metabolized, or partially metabolized, in the liver; but even here some of the unaltered drug, together with its breakdown products, are excreted by the kidney. Liver function may also be reduced in elderly patients; it has been found that the half-life of phenylbutazone and antipyrine is lengthened in older patients.

It must not be forgotten however that the antibiotic dose must be sufficient to ensure adequate concentration of the drug at the site of infection. The laboratory report may indicate sensitivity of an organism to a particular antibiotic but an adequate dose is necessary for the drug to reach the infecting organism. Despite the slower excretion of some drugs by elderly patients it is wise to use doses on the higher side of those recommended. This is particularly the case in infections of the renal tract, where slow excretion by the kidney may justify larger doses in order to obtain satisfactory urine concentrations[10]. High doses can be used for 48 hours, and perhaps then or later the oral route substituted. An initial loading dose will be widely distributed in the body, and will not by itself lead to toxic side-effects because of accumulation, even in the presence of renal failure. In any case, antibiotic prescriptions should always be reviewed actively and at recognized intervals of 48 hours, 5 days and 10 days.

Interaction of antibiotics with other drugs

Elderly patients may be given drugs for more than one condition and the possibility of drug interaction in them is increased. Antibiotics may affect the activity of other drugs by (1) displacement from serum protein carrier sites, (2) interaction with liver enzymes and (3) competition for tubular secretion in the kidney[11].

Anticoagulants
It is advisable to check the prothrombin time of a patient on war-farin when starting a course of antibiotics. Sulphonamides, co-trimoxazole and naladixic acid compete with warfarin for serum protein carrier sites, while chloramphenicol, sulphonamides and cotrimoxazole decrease breakdown of the drug by liver enzymes. These antibiotics will increase the patient's sensitivity to warfarin and stopping antibiotic therapy will decrease his response to the anticoagulant. Griseofulvin may increase liver breakdown of warfarin, and broad spectrum antibiotics reduce vitamin K produc-tion by intestinal bacteria.

Oral hypoglycaemics
Sulphonamides, co-trimoxazole and chloramphenicol may decrease liver breakdown of tolbutamide. Sulphonamides and co-trimoxazole compete with the sulphonylureas for carrier sites on serum proteins and for renal tubular excretion.

Antacids
These may reduce the absorption of penicillin-type antibiotics and of sulphonamides, tetracyclines and nitrofurantoin.

Frusemide
This and other K^+-losing diuretics will lead to nephrotoxicity if given with cephaloridine and cephalothin. This interaction is less likely with the newer cephalosporins. However it is probably wise to avoid these diuretics when prescribing aminoglycosides.

Use of antibiotics in renal failure
Penicillin-type antibiotics, and those drugs excreted mainly in the liver (metronidazole, erythromycin, clindamycin, chloramphenicol and fucidin) require no adjustment in dosage in moderate degrees of renal failure, such as creatinine clearance (50–80 ml/min) (Table 2). High doses of sulphonamides, co-trimoxazole and cephalosporins should be avoided[12,13]. Aminoglycoside dosage should be con-trolled by serum assay of the drug, and colistin and vancomycin should be avoided in this, as in other degrees of renal failure. Tetracyclines (except doxycycline), nitrofurantoin and methenamine mandelate require a reduced dose, probably to about half normal doses. For patients with a creatinine clearance of 10–50 ml/min

Table 2 Antibiotic dose interval in renal failure[a] (interval in hours)

		Creatinine clearance		
	Normal	50–80 ml/min	10–50 ml/min	<10 ml/min
Penicillin-type drugs				
Benzylpenicillin	4 or 6	6	6	12
Cloxacillin	6	6	6	12
Ampicillin	6	6	6	12
Carbenicillin	6	6	6	12
Erythromycin	6	6	6	12
Sulphadimine	6	6	12	24
Co-trimoxazole	12	12	24	48
Tetracyclines[b]	6	avoid	avoid	avoid
Doxycycline	24	24	24	48
Clindamycin	6	6	6	12
Fusidic acid	8	8	8	12
Cephaloridine	6	12	avoid	avoid
Cephazolin	6	6	12	24
Cephalexin	6	6	12	24
Chloramphenicol	6	6	12	avoid
Gentamicin[c]	6	6–12	12–24	48

[a] partly from Bennett *et al.*[14] and Sharpstone[13]
[b] nephrotoxic (see text)
[c] assay of serum concentrations advisable

Note: Colistin, methenamine mandelate, nitrofurantoin and vancomycin require severe reduction in dosage in the presence of any degree of renal failure (see text).

severe reduction in dose or avoidance of tetracycline, colistin, methenamine mandelate, chloramphenicol and nitrofurantoin will be required, with some reduction in sulphonamides, co-trimoxazole and the other cephalosporins.

In severe renal failure (creatinine clearance <10 ml/min) the usual tetracyclines, methenamine mandelate and nitrofurantoin should not be prescribed, while the doses of other antibiotics excreted by the kidney will need to be greatly reduced and monitored by serum and urine assay, if possible. It is probable that doxycycline can be prescribed in reduced doses in these circumstances. However, at a creatinine clearance of <10 ml/min, it is important to recognize that penicillin-type antibiotics will continue to be excreted to some extent provided urine output is maintained; as a rough guide, doses of these antibiotics should be halved. Some reduction in dosage of those antibiotics excreted in the liver will be required at this degree of renal dysfunction. Tables have been published to give guidance on doses of antibiotics with differing degrees of renal failure[13-15].

PROPERTIES AND USES OF ANTIBIOTICS

Penicillin-type antibiotics

Penicillin-type antibiotics possess the β-lactam nucleus in their molecule but differ in their side-chain structure. Benzylpenicillin is a safe drug with a short serum half-life of only 25 min[16]. In life-threatening infections such as septicaemia, meningitis or endocarditis, high doses must be given at frequent intervals. This drug will inhibit the growth of β-haemolytic streptococci, clostridia and *Neisseria meningitidis*, and sensitive strains of staphylococci and pneumococci, at a lower concentration than any other antibiotic. The appropriate oral form of penicillin is phenoxymethyl-penicillin, but intestinal absorption of this drug is often relatively poor. Cloxacillin and flucloxacillin resist the β-lactamase enzymes produced by organisms resistant to benzylpenicillin and ampicillin. They should therefore be used in the first instance against staphylococci, until the sensitivity of the patient's strain is known. They are usually safe drugs of narrow spectrum and may be used in high doses with few side-effects.

Amoxycillin and talampicillin are esters of ampicillin with improved oral absorption and should be used in place of ampicillin for this route. Talampicillin is converted to ampicillin in the gut wall, but amoxycillin is absorbed from the gut and is active in the body without change to the molecule. Amoxycillin penetrates into sputum in higher amounts than ampicillin[17] and has been shown to protect laboratory animals from experimental infections more quickly and at relatively lower dosage levels[18]. Both ampicillin and amoxycillin are broad spectrum, being active against a wide range of Gram-positive and Gram-negative bacilli including those of the body's normal flora. These drugs are inactivated by the β-lactamases produced by most strains of staphylococci and many Gram-negative bacilli, particularly *Klebsiella* spp. and *Enterobacter* spp., and are inactive against some anaerobic cocci and all *Bacteroides* spp. Ampicillin and its esters are the drugs of choice for infection with *Haemophilus influenzae* (sinusitis, bronchitis, postoperative pnueumonia), and are usually more active than other agents against *Streptococcus faecalis*. Carbenicillin is a broad spectrum penicillin-type antibiotic usually active against *Pseudomonas* spp. and other resistant aerobic Gram-negative bacilli. It should be reserved for patients with serious undiagnosed infections and for those known to be infected with resistant organisms or *Pseudomonas* spp. In the latter case, high doses must be used (30–40 g/day). This drug is usually presented as a sodium salt and high doses may lead to sodium ion overload (5 g carbenicillin is equivalent to 27 mEq Na^+). In addition, hypokalaemia may result from the ionic attraction of potassium ions to the carbenicillin molecule in renal tubules. More rarely, high doses may lead to a prolonged bleeding time and other disturbances of blood coagulation. In combination with gentamicin this drug may show synergy against *Pseudomonas* spp.[19,20]; indeed, this pair of antibiotics shows wide activity against many organisms (except to *Streptococcus faecalis* and *Bacteroides* spp.) and is a useful combination of antibiotics for severe infection in susceptible patients before bacterial diagnosis has been made[21].

Penicillin-type antibiotics are generally safe antibiotics with a wide therapeutic margin. They are associated with allergic-type reactions manifested usually as an urticurial skin rash. Much less often an anaphylactoid reaction may occur; this event is more common following i.v. or i.m. administration, although the reaction may also occur with the oral route. Anaphylaxis may occur after any number of previous doses or courses of drugs. When a penicillin-type drug is given by bolus i.v. injection for the first time to a patient, it is wise for a medically qualified person to be present. Occasionally serum sickness and exfoliative dermatitis is seen with penicillin-type drugs.

A macular skin rash is quite frequently seen with ampicillin and it is questioned whether this always represents a true allergy to the other penicillin-type antibiotics. In a patient suffering from a disease in which benzylpenicillin is the drug of choice, such as *Streptococcus viridans* endocarditis or gas gangrene, a history of ampicillin rash does not prevent the use of the antibiotic but requires cover with antihistamines or steroids. More remote side-effects of penicillin-type antibiotics result from high serum concentrations. Epileptiform fits may occur with high serum concentrations of benzylpenicillin (although some of the early cases may have been due to impurities of manufacture). Hypernatraemia and hypokalaemia, and a bleeding tendency may occur with high dosage of carbenicillin (30–40 g/day). Interstitial nephritis has been reported with methicillin and ampicillin[22].

Cephalosporins
Cephalosporins and the closely similar cephamycins act on the bacterial cell wall in a fashion similar to that of the penicillin-type

antibiotics. Side-chains may be added to the molecular nucleus and several varieties of these drugs are, and will become, available. However, Gram-negative bacilli are able to produce β-lactamases which destroy these drugs, especially those drugs which have been available for some years. Cephaloridine and cephalothin are potentially nephrotoxic if given with loop diuretics or gentamicin and have been superseded in clinical use by the newer but more expensive cephalosporins (cited below) which have a wider spectrum of activity and are probably safer. Nevertheless, the combination of even these later cephalosporins with gentamicin may jeopardize renal function and it is wise to avoid their combination if possible or to monitor renal function frequently. Cephazolin gives a high serum concentration although it is extensively protein-bound; cefoxitin (a cephamycin) has a wider spectrum of activity by resisting the β-lactamases of many Gram-negative bacilli and is active against *Bacteroides* spp.; cefuroxime possesses a wide spectrum of activity and is particularly active against *Haemophilus influenzae* but less active against *Bacteroides* spp. The latest available cephalosporin, cefotaxime, is more active in terms of bacterial mics[23] than any of the above drugs of this type, and if clinically useful at lower doses seems likely to avoid nephrotoxicity[24]. Cephalexin and cephradine are oral cephalosporins and provide satisfactory blood concentrations by this route. A newer oral form of this type of drug is cephaclor; it possesses lower mics to *Streptococcus pneumoniae*, *Haemophilus influenzae* and several other bacteria than its predecessors. All of these drugs provide a broader spectrum of bactericidal activity than ampicillin or the tetracyclines; they may therefore have a role in chest infection acquired in hospital where broad spectrum activity, including *Streptococcus pneumoniae* and *Haemophilus influenzae*, is required. They must compete with the acceptable combination of a penicillin with an aminoglycoside in septicaemia and other serious infections. Clinical use of the newer cephalosporins may or may not lead to increasing bacterial resistance to them. They and the cephamycins are said to be less nephrotoxic than their predecessors but experience with these drugs is incomplete. They may require higher than recommended doses for good therapeutic effect.

Mecillinam and pivmecillinam
Mecillinam is an amidinopenicillin which has recently become available. The spectrum of activity is wide amongst Gram-negative bacilli, but it is less active against Gram-positive organisms. An ester, pivmecillinam, is available for oral use. In view of this drug's limited spectrum of activity it may have a role in urinary tract

infection[25], where Gram-negative bacilli are the most common pathogens, and it may have less effect on the normal flora of the gut, mouth and vagina, so avoiding some of the complications found with other antibiotics.

Aminoglycosides
Aminoglycosides include the following antibiotics available in this country: streptomycin, kanamycin, gentamicin, tobramycin and amikacin. Newer drugs within this group may become available in the future. These antibiotics are broad spectrum and bactericidal and are valuable in serious undiagnosed infection and in treating bacteria resistant to other antibiotics[26]. Streptomycin should be reserved for tuberculosis since its role in bacterial infection, like that of kanamycin, has been superseded by gentamicin which has wider activity.

Tobramycin is more active than gentamicin, usually against *Pseudomonas* spp., but should not be used except for this organism since its spectrum is otherwise identical to gentamicin. Amikacin has, however, a wider spectrum than these drugs but should be reserved for infections with organisms resistant to gentamicin. Gentamicin is the recommended aminoglycoside at the present time[27], but it is possible that resistance will increase amongst the aerobic Gram-negative bacilli which form its main target. It should be remembered that gentamicin is inactive against most species of Gram-positive cocci (except *Staphylococcus aureus*) and anaerobic bacteria.

The aminoglycosides are nephrotoxic and ototoxic, and since the therapeutic range of the gentamicin type drugs is narrow it is wise to monitor serum concentrations of gentamicin and tobramycin. When aminoglycosides are given with cephaloridine or cephalothin some degree of nephrotoxicity is probable.

Erythromycin and clindamycin
Erythromycin and clindamycin are active against staphylococci and streptococci. Erythromycin is also active against *Haemophilus* spp., *Mycoplasma pneumonia*, *Coxiella burnetti* and *Chlamydia psittaci* and at the present time is the antibiotic of choice for Legionnaire's disease[28]. Clindamycin possesses broad-spectrum activity against anaerobic organisms but is associated with pseudomembraneous colitis. These drugs should normally be used in patients allergic to the penicillins or for the specific organisms mentioned above. Clindamycin has been more frequently associated with pseudomembraneous colitis that any other antibiotic but the condition may also occur with ampicillin, penicillin, co-trimoxazole and erythromycin[29].

Co-trimoxazole and cotrimazine

Co-trimoxazole is a combination of sulphamethoxazole and trimethoprim[30]. A similar, but new combination of sulphadiazine and trimethoprim has been named cotrimazine. These drug pairs are synergistic against a wide spectrum of organisms including Gram-positive and Gram-negative bacteria but they are less active against pneumococci, streptococci and staphylococci than the appropriate penicillin or erythromycin. Anaerobic organisms are often resistant to these combinations, including many strains of *Bacteroides* spp. Synergy between a sulphonamide and trimethoprim depends upon a specific ratio of their concentrations, defined by the degree of sensitivity of the organism to each drug. Their relative concentrations in the different body tissues may not always be appropriate for synergy due to differences in tissue penetration. It is claimed that cotrimazine may provide more appropriate concentrations of sulphadiazine for synergy in the urinary tract.

Few side-effects have been reported with co-trimoxazole but it should be remembered that its mode of action may potentiate a folate deficiency state, culminating in bone marrow depression with leucopenia, anaemia and thrombocytopenia. Consequently it is probably wise not to use the drug in patients with megaloblastic haemopoiesis[31]. Other side-effects include gastro-intestinal irritation and rashes due to the sulphamethoxazole component of the drug.

Tetracyclines

Tetracyclines, chloramphenicol and colistin, have a small role in elderly patients. Resistance to tetracyclines is fairly common amongst streptococci, staphylococci and Gram-negative bacilli, although these drugs are appropriate for psittacosis and infections with *Coxiella burnetti* and mycoplasmas. Side-effects of tetracyclines include gastrointestinal irritation and possible superinfection with *Candida* spp. in the gut, vagina and mouth. These drugs increase breakdown of aminoacids and consequently may make worse or precipitate renal dysfunction[32]. However, doxycycline seems to be free of this side-effect. It is important to avoid high doses and long-term courses of the usual tetracyclines in elderly patients, and to remember the relative advantages of better absorption and less toxicity of doxycycline compared to the other tetracyclines. Chloramphenicol is bacteriostatic, depresses bone marrow function and very rarely induces aplastic anaemia. There is evidence that the metabolic breakdown products of this drug produced in the liver and excreted by the kidney are also toxic to the bone marrow. Colistin has broad spectrum activity, including *Pseudomonas* spp., but is potentially toxic to bone marrow, liver and kidney. It should be used only if gentamicin is inappropriate.

Other antibiotics in current use

Fucidin is a valuable antibiotic for serious staphylococcal infection. It should always be used in combination with cloxacillin or erythromycin, or possibly clindamycin, since bacteria develop resistance to it rapidly. There are few side-effects, but doses should be reduced in liver dysfunction.

Vancomycin should be held in reserve for bacteria resistant to antibiotics already described. It has wide bactericidal activity against staphylococci, streptococci and clostridia but not against aerobic Gram-negative bacilli. It is ototoxic and nephrotoxic. It has been used successfully in the treatment of pseudomembraneous colitis[33] and in some cases of *Streptococcus faecalis* endocarditis.

Metronidazole is bactericidal to obligate anaerobic bacteria. It penetrates body tissues well and is absorbed from the gastrointestinal tract by either the oral or rectal route. It has an important place[34,35] in infection originating from the bacterial flora of the bowel, vagina or upper respiratory tract. It is used therefore in postoperative infection of the abdominal cavity after intestinal or gynaecological surgery, and in postoperative infection of the lung following thoracic surgery. It should be used in lung abscess and empyema, where anaerobic organisms are frequently involved, and as part of the antibiotic regimen in the treatment of brain abscess. Metronidazole is the drug of choice for any infection involving anaerobic organisms, now that clindamycin has become clearly associated with pseudomembraneous colitis.

Rifampicin is widely active, and bactericidal in action. It should normally be reserved for tuberculosis but may need to be used for infections with rare organisms resistant to many other antibiotics including the aminoglycosides.

INFECTIONS OF THE RESPIRATORY TRACT

Infections of the upper respiratory tract

Sore throat is most often due to virus infection, but roughly a third of the total cases is caused by haemolytic streptococci, usually of Lancefield's group A (*Streptococcus pyogenes*). This organism should be treated with phenoxymethyl-penicillin orally for fourteen days, or benzylpenicillin i/m for 48 hours followed by the oral penicillin. Alternative antibiotics are erythromycin or cephalexin, as some 40% of strains of *Streptococcus pyogenes* are resistant to tetracyclines. Other bacterial causes of a sore throat are rare; *Staphylococcus aureus*, *Streptococcus pneumoniae*, *Haemophilus influenzae* infection may follow primary viral infection or local lesion. *Corynebacterium diphtheriae* infection may follow contact with a case of diphtheriae. Erythromycin should be used both for treatment and prophylaxis.

Sinusitis
Sinusitis is usually caused by *Streptococcus pyogenes*, *Streptococcus pneumoniae* or *Haemophilus influenzae*. The appropriate antibiotic is therefore amoxycillin or erythromycin in adequate doses by mouth. Otitis externa may be caused by a wide number of pathogens including *Staphylococcus aureus*, haemolytic streptococci, and *Pseudomonas* spp. Local cleaning and topical application of chloramphenicol or neomycin may be sufficient treatment. In severe infection, flucloxacillin orally will treat *Staphylococcus aureus* and *Streptococcus pyogenes*, which are often the pathogenic organisms in such circumstances, although these bacteria may be overgrown on culture of a superficial ear swab by *Proteus* spp. or pseudomonas organisms. Otitis media in the acute form is usually due to the organisms mentioned above and may be treated by amoxycillin, erythromycin or cephalexin. Chronic otitis media will probably respond to antibiotics poorly. Laryngitis is usually a viral infection, but *Haemophilus influenzae* may cause an acute epiglottitis[36] and tracheitis in adults.

Conjunctivitis
Conjunctivitis may be due to a wide variety of organisms in elderly patients, particularly if acquired in hospital, but *Staphylococcus aureus* or streptococci are most common pathogens. Antibiotic therapy should be guided by bacteriological investigation. If antibiotics are used topically an ointment is probably more satisfactory than eye-drops. Inspection of the eye should be undertaken regularly, in order to anticipate infection of the orbital tissues or the interior of the eye.

Bronchitis
Acute bronchitis in a previously normal patient is usually initiated by a viral infection. *Haemophilus influenzae* and *Streptococcus pneumoniae* may cause, however, both a primary or secondary infection in acute bronchitis[37,38]. In chronic bronchitis the role of infective agents in the progress of the disease remains debatable, but it is well

established that the bacterial species already mentioned are constantly associated with exacerbations. These organisms are best treated with adequate doses of amoxycillin or co-trimoxazole. Penetration of antibiotics into alveolar secretions is probably poor, and dosage should therefore be regularly spaced at 6 hourly intervals. Some 5–40% of *Streptococcus pneumoniae* strains are resistant to tetracyclines, while cephalexin and cephradine are less active against these organisms than amoxycillin or cotrimoxazole.

Bronchopneumonia
Bronchopneumonia, when contracted in the community by elderly patients, is usually associated with *Streptococcus pneumoniae* and *Haemophilus influenzae*[39]. Again, amoxycillin (orally) or ampicillin (i.m. or i.v.) or cotrimoxazole are appropriate for these organisms in this situation. Use should be made of the i.v. or i.m. routes in patients who are acutely ill. Cloxacillin must be used for *Staphylococcus aureus* pneumonia which often results in a destructive infection of lung tissue with abscess formation. Combination of cloxacillin with fucidin, or erythromycin is required in these circumstances and treatment must be given parenterally.

Pneumonias
Pneumonia due to *Klebsiella* spp. and other Gram-negative bacilli such as *Enterobacter* spp., *Escherichia coli*, or more rarely, *Proteus* spp., requires i.m. treatment with gentamicin or possibly cephazolin or cefoxitin. In treating pneumonias with these drugs care must be taken to ensure adequate dosage; it has been shown that a peak serum concentration of 8 μg/ml gentamicin is required for adequate therapy of lung infection[40].

Classic lobar pneumonia is almost always caused by *Streptococcus pneumoniae* and in severe infections with this organism benzylpenicillin i.m. or i.v. is the drug of choice, because the mic of this antibiotic against the organism is less than that of any other drug.

An elderly patient admitted from the community with a severe pneumonia requires antibiotics active against *Streptococcus pneumoniae*, *Haemophilus influenzae*, as well as *Staphylococcus aureus* and perhaps aerobic Gram-negative bacilli and *Bacteroides* spp. It is difficult to encompass all these organisms, even with a regimen of two antibiotics, and the appropriate drugs will depend on the history of the patient and the clinical signs. An immediate Gram film of purulent sputum may indicate whether a predominant organism is a Gram-positive coccus or a Gram-negative bacillus. A history of bronchitis requires ampicillin, (preferably amoxycillin or talampicillin). Flucloxacillin (orally) or cloxacillin (i.m.) should be used if there is a possibility of *Staphylococcus aureus* infection, such as a rapid onset of a severe pneumonia; a pneumonia secondary to viral infection (particularly influenza); signs of neglect; or signs of early abscess formation on chest X-ray. A lobar pneumonia requires benzylpenicillin (by i.m. route). A history of aspiration, alcoholism or recent admission to hospital may indicate infection with *Klebsiella* spp. or other Gram-negative bacillus, and gentamicin should be given. A patient on broad spectrum antibiotics, who has recently been given assisted respiration in an intensive therapy unit, should be considered as a candidate for pseudomonas pneumonia and treated with both carbenicillin and gentamicin. A clinical picture suggestive of *Mycoplasma* spp., *Coxiella* spp. or *Psittacosis* spp. requires erythromycin, and this antibiotic should be used when a patient is allergic to penicillins. Previous lung abscess or empyema, a recent chest operation, or a prolonged history of lung infection may indicate *Bacteriodes* spp. infection. Doses of drugs should be high for the first 48 hours and then reduced, or changed if necessary, on review of the antibiotic regimen.

A pneumonia acquired in hospital may result from infection with a wider range of organisms, particularly Gram-negative bacilli such as *Enterobacter* spp., *Escherichia* or *Pseudomonas* spp. These organisms may cause infection from sources within the patient, who has become colonized with them perhaps as a result of broad-spectrum antibiotic treatment, or from sources in the hospital. However, it has been shown that postoperative pneumonias are most frequently associated with *Haemophilus influenzae* and *Streptococcus pneumoniae*, presumably from the patient's own respiratory tract flora[41]. The drugs discussed previously for these organisms remain appropriate in this circumstance, but in order to cover the wider spectrum of organisms that may be involved in an hospital acquired infection it is probably better to begin therapy with co-trimoxazole or cephalexin if oral therapy is thought to be adequate. However, an elderly patient who acquires a serious pneumonia with changes visible on chest X-ray, after more than 48 hours in hospital, requires a combination of amoxycillin/ampicillin and gentamicin or intravenous co-trimoxazole. One of the newer cephalosporins (cefoxitin, cefuroxime) might be suitable in this situation, by the same route, if there is a high incidence of antibiotic resistance amongst Gram-negative bacilli isolated from other sources in the hospital.

Anaerobic bacteria, particularly *Bacteroides* spp. and anaerobic cocci also cause pneumonias[42]. They may initiate infection following operations in which the chest has been opened, such as pneumonectomy or oesophagectomy, following aspiration, and may secondarily infect pneumonic lung tissue. The drug of choice for anaerobic infection in the lung, as elsewhere, is metronidazole. It is probably unnecessary to add this drug to the regimen for acute pneumonias acquired in the community or in hospital, but a history of aspiration, lung infection after chest operation, an unresolved pneumonia, abscess formation or a foul sputum, are indications for its use.

Lung abscess, empyema and *bronchiectasis* are difficult to treat with antibiotics alone. Prolonged antibiotic therapy with high doses of appropriate agents may, however, allow resolution of lung abscess, and in the authors' experience multiple lung abscesses caused by *Bacteroides* spp. following a postoperative pneumonia were resolved by metronidazole. However, surgical drainage of abscesses and empyemas, together with antibiotics, probably leads to a more rapid cure. In these conditions it is important to include metronidazole in the therapeutic regimen because of the important role of anaerobes[43]. Infection in bronchiectasis may be contained and often improved by antibiotics, but is liable to recur so long as the structural defect is present. Organisms leading to exacerbation of infection in bronchiectasis are usually *Staphylococcus aureus*, Gram-negative bacilli, including *Klebsiella* spp. and *Pseudomonas* spp., and anaerobes. Antibiotic therapy should be controlled by bacteriological examination of sputum which, in this condition, is more reliable than in the pneumonias.

Pneumonias are also caused by *Mycoplasma pneumoniae, Chlamydia psittaci,* and *Coxiella burnetti.* Mycoplasma pneumonia is endemic but a consistent pattern of 4 year epidemics has been found in several countries[44]. Up to 40% of pneumonias have been ascribed to this agent in certain communities but a rate of 10% seems to be more usual. Infection occurs at any time of the year but more often in autumn or winter. Psittacosis and coxiella pneumonia are less common and the former typically follows an exposure to psittacine or ornithine birds which usually, but not always, show evidence of illness. Coxiella pneumonia follows exposure to infected cattle and therefore usually occurs in rural communities. These pneumonias have an incubation period of some two to three weeks and may begin with a general illness of malaise and headache some days before chest symptoms appear. There is usually a cough, particularly in mycoplasma pneumonia, and chest X-ray examination shows a patchy area of consolidation in the hilar or lower lobe regions. Each of these infections responds to erythromycin and the tetracyclines;

there is some evidence that the former drug is more effective in mycoplasma pneumonia[45]. These agents are bacteriostatic rather than bactericidal and clinical improvement is not always associated with complete elimination of the organism[46], treatment should probably, therefore, continue for some weeks.

Legionnaire's disease is a severe pneumonia caused by a Gram-negative bacillus which has been isolated from the cooling water of air-conditioning systems[47,48]. The incubation period is some 7–12 days and there may be evidence of systemic illness in that liver enzyme changes and renal dysfunction often occur. Patients may require assisted ventilation in an intensive care unit. Antibiotics of choice are erythromycin and rifampicin.

Unfortunately antibiotic therapy in lung infection must frequently proceed without benefit of bacteriological guidance, since sputum is notoriously unreliable as a bacteriological specimen. It may be difficult for the patient to raise alveolar exudate from the site of infection, and in any case sputum is always contaminated by bacteria present in the throat and mouth. Contaminating organisms may grow to significant numbers by the time the sputum reaches the laboratory. Repeat specimens may give an indication of the consistency of an isolate but in a seriously ill patient attempts should be made to obtain a more reliable specimen by transtracheal aspiration or tissue biopsy (by fibreoptic bronchoscopy or needle biopsy). In addition, it is advisable to obtain a sample of serum as soon as a pneumonia due to a non-bacterial agent or Legionnaire's disease is suspected; a second specimen should follow within 10 days.

Cystitis

This infection must be distinguished, particularly in elderly patients, from the urethral syndrome which gives rise to similar symptoms. The urethral syndrome may occur in vaginitis, after gynaecological surgery, in urethritis and prostatitis. A properly collected midstream specimen of urine is a reliable specimen if not delayed before culture, and antibiotic therapy should be guided by the bacteriology results. Where treatment for cystitis must be started without the help of bacteriology, co-trimoxazole or amoxycillin should be used. A 10 day course of treatment is required and, at an interval after the end of treatment, the urine should again be cultured to check for sterility. It is possible that treatment with penicillin-type antibiotics may lead to the survival of cell wall-deficient bacteria in the relatively hyperosmolar environment of urine. It has not been possible to assess the relevance of this somewhat theoretical problem because of the difficulty of culturing such deficient bacteria in the laboratory. If this event is suspected, further therapy should consist of an antibiotic which acts on bacterial metabolism, such as cotrimoxazole, nitrofurantoin or erythromycin[49]. Repeated infection in either sex requires investigation for renal infection, stone or tumour. In elderly female patients an atrophic vulva or patulous urethra may predispose to cystitis and justify long-term low dose treatment with cotrimoxazole or amoxycillin.

Pyelonephritis
Both acute and chronic pyelonephritis are usually caused by Gram-negative bacilli, such as *Escherichia coli*, *Proteus* spp., *Klebsiella* spp. and *Pseudomonas* spp. Several midstream urine cultures, blood cultures, and cultures of renal pelvic urine and biopsy tissue when available, should be examined in the laboratory. Antibiotic treatment must be guided by the results of bacteriological investigation, but if therapy must begin before results are available, co-trimoxazole, carbenicillin or gentamicin may be used parenterally, while cotrimoxazole and cephalexin can be used orally. An oral form of carbenicillin (carfecillin) may be used for urinary tract infection with *Pseudomonas* spp., but since absorption from the intestinal tract is poor, doses on the higher side of those recommended must be given. Long-term therapy in chronic pylenephritis is safely undertaken with co-trimoxazole (one or two tablets per day); but nitrofurantoin may be dangerous in the presence of impaired renal function and long-term therapy with this drug in elderly patients may lead to pulmonary fibrosis and peripheral neuropathy. Long-term low dose therapy with an appropriate penicillin-type antibiotic or cephalosporin is acceptable.

Long-term catheterization
An elderly patient with a permanent urinary catheter will probably have an infected bladder. Indeed, it is difficult to avoid infection even with strict adherence to a closed drainage system, which is essential, for several reasons:

(1) infection is encouraged by the permanent pool of urine held in the bladder below the catheter outlet;

(2) retrograde spread of organisms from contaminated urine in the drainage bag;

(3) contamination of the lumen of the catheter by breaking the closed system when collecting a urine specimen or performing a bladder washout; and

(4) spread of organisms between the catheter and urethra into the bladder.

Nevertheless, lower renal tract infection is often well tolerated in elderly patients, and the use of antibiotics in this situation may result in infection with resistant organisms. More dangerous anti-biotics will then have to be used for treatment of exacerbations of cystitis or renal infection. It is good practice for patients to be given antibiotics when (a) there is actual clinical evidence of local infec-tion, such as fever, leucocytosis, loin pain or urethral pus; (b) there is evidence of infection in the kidney; and (c) to provide antibiotic cover for a change of catheter. The last is undertaken by giving the appropriate antibiotic 1 hour before catheterization and for two doses afterwards at 8 hourly intervals.

There may be some value in long-term therapy with methenamine mandelate for patients with a permanent catheter. The urine must be maintained at an acid pH, perhaps by daily dosage with vitamin C, and the urine should be regularly tested for acidity. It has been shown that bladder irrigation with neomycin and polymyxin is of no value in preventing or treating infection and may predispose to infection with more resistant organisms[50]. Bladder washouts require nursing time and entail opening and handling of the bladder drain-age system. It is perhaps better to ignore this approach, except in the treatment of candida cystitis.

Little can be done to prevent urethral passage of bacteria but a local antiseptic aerosol spray, such as 'Rotersept spray' or 'Dispray', is readily applied to the urethral opening and the surface of the catheter adjacent to the urethra. It is also worthwhile adding an antiseptic to the urine collection bag. Despite the difficulties of antibiotic control of cystitis in patients with a permanent catheter, it is good practice to be aware of the organisms present in the urinary tract. Specimens of urine should be taken by syringe and needle from the lumen of the catheter and sent to the laboratory at weekly or fortnightly intervals.

SEPTICAEMIA

Although the incidence of bacteraemia rises with age[51-53] the diag-nosis may be easily missed because there are few symptoms or signs[54]. A high index of suspicion is required, as the only clue may be unexplained confusion or non-specific malaise. The value of taking blood cultures in patients with a known source of infection but without overt evidence of septicaemia is stressed; specimens must be taken before therapy is begun since inappropriate or inadequate antibiotics may eliminate a bacteraemia temporarily with no effect on the source of infection.

It will usually take 48 hours for the laboratory to establish the nature of the organism causing a septicaemia. In order to use appropriate antimicrobial agents before bacteriological results are available, it is best to obtain some indication of the organism involved from clinical evidence. This can be done often by locating the likely origin of infection and by observing the course of the illness. Infection of the urinary tract, and surgical operation or instrumentation on some part of the urinary tract particularly in the presence of infection are potent causes of Gram-negative bacilli in the bloodstream. Similarly, operations on the large bowel, peritonitis, and abdominal abscess are sources of Gram-negative bacilli and of anaerobes. *Bacteroides* spp. may cause a severe septicaemia following operations on the gut or female genital tract, and should not be excluded from antibiotic cover when the potential source of a septicaemia includes these sites. The biliary tract, in infection or after operation, may allow Gram-negative bacilli, haemolytic streptococci (particularly groups D and F) and anaerobes to enter the bloodstream. Pneumonia is frequently associated with a *Streptococcus pneumoniae* septicaemia and less often with septicaemias of *Staphylococcus aureus*, Gram-negative bacilli and anaerobes. Spreading cellulitis and skin infection act as a source of haemolytic streptococci (particularly group A, very occasionally groups C and G) and *Staphylococcus aureus*. Inflamed sacral pressure sores may rarely lead to septicaemia with a wide range of organisms originating from the nearby bowel flora. *Staphylococcus aureus* may enter the bloodstream from osteomyelitic lesions, burns, postoperative wound infection and septic drip sites; less often haemolytic streptococci, anaerobes and Gram-negative bacilli originate in these lesions. Of special relevance to elderly patients is gas gangrene after above-knee amputation; the source of infection is the skin of the perineum or thigh which often carries spores of *Clostridium welchii* deposited from the bowel flora. Spores are eliminated by adequate skin preparation with a compress of povidone iodine or with systemic benzylpenicillin at the time of operation[55,56].

A rapidly developing illness accompanied by symtoms of shock and circulatory collapse tends to indicate a Gram-negative bacillus. Again, it must be emphasized that these symptoms may well be muted in the elderly. When the signs of septicaemia develop over some hours a Gram-positive coccus is more likely although *Streptococcus pyogenes* and *Staphylococcus aureus* may cause a rapidly developing illness, but usually unaccompanied by the 'shock syndrome'.

The immediate choice of antibiotics in septicaemia, before blood culture results are obtained, is governed by the nature of the organism as determined by the source of infection. A septicaemia resulting from a source of infection which may contain an aerobic Gram-negative bacillus should be treated by appropriate doses of gentamicin, so as to obtain a peak serum concentration of 5–8 μg/ml with a trough concentration of 2–3 μg/ml[40]. These concentrations usually require a dose of 6 mg/kg(day), and this dose is unlikely to be toxic even to very old patients (with apparently normal renal function) over a period of 48 hours, after which the regimen should be reviewed. Serum concentrations should be monitored by the laboratory since, unlike the penicillins, cephalosporins or metronidazole, the narrow therapeutic range of aminoglycosides makes it more difficult to achieve the appropriate serum concentrations, and there is still a tendency to underprescribe this drug. Where Gram-negative bacilli show resistance to gentamicin, amikacin should be used in a dose of 500 mg 8 hourly for the initial 48 hours, before review of the regimen.

Septicaemia likely to be caused by *Staphylococcus aureus* should be treated by cloxacillin i.m. or i.v. in a dose of 2–4 g/day, given in 6 hourly intervals. If the organism proves sensitive to benzylpenicillin this antibiotic should be substituted or added to the regimen, if the clinical response has been slow. *Streptococcus pneumoniae*, haemolytic streptococci, and *Clostridium welchii* must be treated with 2 mega units of benzylpenicillin 2 hourly or 4 hourly. *Streptococcus faecalis* septicaemia should be treated with ampicillin i.m. or i.v. Anaerobes require metronidazole, 500 mg 6 hourly i.v. for the first 48 hours, and then 1 g suppositories 8 hourly if the patient's progress has been satisfactory. If *Pseudomonas* spp. is suspected, or has been found in blood cultures, then carbenicillin (10 g 8 hourly by infusion over 1 hour) should be combined with gentamicin or amikacin. Where the probable source of septicaemia indicates that several organisms may have invaded the bloodstream, combinations of antibiotics need to be used. For example, a septicaemia from infection in the intestinal tract should be treated with gentamicin and metronidazole; septicaemia from the biliary tract or after operations involving the chest should be treated with this combination as well as with a penicillin. A pneumonia leading to septicaemia should be treated with cloxacillin and/or benzylpenicillin with or without metronidazole.

ENDOCARDITIS

The incidence of endocarditis increases with age[57], but because of the paucity of physical signs and the more insidious nature of the disease in the elderly, there is often delay in diagnosis[58]. Frequently there is no obvious source of infection, although recent dental extraction, in spite of known dangers in patients with heart murmurs, still causes a few cases. The incidence of the pathological conditions which predispose to endocarditis is also changing, in the elderly as in other age groups. While rheumatic heart disease remains an important cause of endocarditis, cardiac operations, prosthetic valves, congenital malformations, arteriosclerotic damage and less frequently, pacemaker leads are now found more frequently as antecedents to endocarditis. Endocarditis begins with bacterial invasion of sterile thrombotic vegetations which originate at sites of damage and on the 'sink' side of a pressure leak.

The organisms most commonly involved are *Streptococcus viridans*, *Streptococcus faecalis* and non-haemolytic streptococci in rheumatic lesions; with *Staphylococcus epidermidis* and *Candida* spp. occurring in prosthetic valves and following cardiac surgery. A rapidly progressive endocarditis can be caused by *Staphylococcus aureus*, *Streptococcus* group A and *Neisseria gonorrhoeae*. Less frequently brucellosis, Gram-negative bacilli, (which may have an increased incidence in elderly patients) and anaerobes have been associated with endocarditis. Endocarditis has also been described with psittacosis and *Coxiella burnetti* infection, with or without an associated myocarditis.

The conventional nomenclature of *Streptococcus viridans* and *Streptococcus faecalis* includes several distinct species (for example, *Streptococcus sanguis*, *Streptococcus mitior*, *Streptococcus bovis* and others). It is helpful if the laboratory can identify the species of a *Streptococcus viridans* or *Streptococcus faecalis*, as this may be useful for future reference should infection recur. The laboratory will report the antibiotic sensitivities of the organism by the usual techniques and it is also important to determine the mic (minimal inhibitory concentration) and mbc (minimal bactericidal concentration) of the organism to the antibiotics used in therapy. It is also helpful to retain a culture of the strain.

Streptococcus viridans-type organisms are treated by high and frequent i.v. doses of benzylpenicillin (20 mega units/day) combined with gentamicin (6 mg/(kg day)). A more rapid rate of elimination of this organism from cardiac vegetations in a rabbit model of endocarditis has been repeatedly demonstrated[59,60] with this combination, compared to benzylpenicillin used alone.

These drugs and the route of administration should be maintained for at least 2 weeks and usually 6 weeks, depending on the patient's response. *Streptococcus faecalis* is usually treated with ampicillin, but it is useful to compare the mic and mbc of this organism to both ampicillin and benzylpenicillin and the drug with the lower values should be used with gentamicin as described above. *Staphylococcus aureus* should be treated by benzylpenicillin (if sensitive) or by cloxacillin, and again, experimental work has demonstrated the advantage of using these drugs with gentamicin for this organism[61]. The sensitivities of *Staphylococcus epidermidis* are less easy to predict, but combined therapy of a penicillin or erythromycin with gentamicin is probably valuable. *Candida* spp. should be treated by amphotericin B (test dose, followed by 25 mg/alternate days progressing to 50 mg/alternate days) and 5-fluorocytosine (200 mg/(kg day)). *Streptococcus pyogenes* (Lancefield's group A) and *Neisseria gonorrhoeae* are treated by high and frequent doses of benzylpenicillin. Brucellosis endocarditis requires combination therapy with two of the following antibiotics: tetracyclines, co-trimoxazoles or gentamicin.

There is less experience in the treatment of endocarditis due to Gram-negative bacilli although these organisms may be relatively more common as a cause of endocarditis in the elderly. Accurate antibiotic therapy will in any case be dependent upon laboratory investigation of the isolated organisms. As initial therapy, a broad-spectrum cephalosporin or gentamicin should be used in high dosage. If resistant organisms have been found in the hospital environment, then amikacin will provide a wider spectrum of activity. Metronidazole or clindamycin are the drugs of choice for anaerobes, perhaps together with benzylpenicillin in the case of anaerobic cocci.

In all cases of endocarditis it is essential to assay blood concentrations of the antibiotics used for therapy. This should be done on the second or third day of therapy and again at intervals thereafter, depending on the previous results and changes made to the antibiotic regimen. Two blood specimens are usually required, one at the end of the interval between doses, immediately before giving the antibiotic (trough concentration), and another 1 hour after the antibiotic dose (peak concentration). The peak concentration will confirm that adequate amounts of drugs are being given and the trough concentration will demonstrate adequate excretion or, conversely, accumulation of the drug. It is vital therefore to relate serum concentrations (and specimens of blood sent to the laboratory) to the time-interval from the previous dose of antibiotic. A less elaborate but very useful test of the efficacy of antibiotic therapy, which can be carried out rapidly in any laboratory, is performed by measuring the antibacterial activity of the patient's serum by simple dilution. This test demonstrates the bacteriostatic and bactericidal titre of the patient's serum against his own organism.

After adequate duration of therapy by the i.v. or i.m. route, antibiotics should be continued by the oral route using the appropriate oral form of antibiotic. A few days after the start of oral therapy serum concentrations should be measured to ensure adequate absorption of the drug. Oral therapy should continue for some weeks or months depending on the speed of response of the patient and the severity of the disease.

If the patient undergoes cardiac surgery either before or after infection has been eliminated antibiotic cover will be required for the operation. The first dose of antibiotic prophylaxis should be given 1 hour before operation by the i.m. or i.v. route, and continued for some days afterwards. It is probably wise to use the antibiotic that brought about clinical cure in the patient, together with a second antibiotic chosen to provide cover against (1) *Staphylococcus aureus* and *Staphylococcus epidermidis* which may be required from exogenous sources during the operation, and (2) a wider spectrum of organisms, including those from the patient's own flora. Cloxacillin and gentamicin, or a cephalosporin, would be appropriate choices[62].

Meningitis

The organisms that most frequently cause meningitis in elderly patients are *Streptococcus pneumoniae*, and less frequently *Neisseria meningitidis*, and *Haemophilus influenzae*[63]. The incidence of *Streptococcus pneumoniae* meningitis is higher in elderly patients than in younger age groups (except children and adolescents) and the disease has a poorer outcome than in these age groups. Treatment must be started without delay preferably as soon as lumbar puncture has been performed. *Streptococcus pneumoniae* and *Neisseria meningitidis* meningitis are treated by high and frequent doses of benzylpenicillin i.m. or i.v. (18 mega units/day/in 4 hourly doses). Some doubt still surrounds the value of giving intrathecal benzylpenicillin; if this route is used the dose should not be greater than 20 000 units. Some strains of *Neisseria meningitidis* are now resistant to sulphonamides, the incidence varying among the different antigenic groups of the organism. The overall rate of resistance is about 15% in this country and rather higher in North America.

Sulphonamides are therefore no longer used in treating meningitis caused by this organism. In any case, clinical response to benzylpenicillin alone appears to be as rapid as with the combination. Although there is no evidence at present that *Neisseria meningitidis* shows increased resistance to benzylpenicillin, it should be remembered that fully resistant strains of *Neisseria gonorrhoeae* have been isolated in the Far East, Africa and Western countries. It is possible that the mechanism of resistance found in *Neisseria gonorrhoeae* could also accur in *Neisseria meningitidis* and the laboratory must test the sensitivity of this organism to benzylpenicillin whenever it is a significant isolate.

Strains of *Streptococcus pneumoniae* isolated in South Africa have been described which are resistant to benzylpenicillin and to many other antibiotics. These strains have not, at the time of writing, been isolated elsewhere. However, in South Africa these strains were found in carriers in eight out of 28 hospitals surveyed, largely in children although also in staff. Community spread occurred in contacts of hospitalized patients[64]. It is essential, again, that all significant isolates of *Streptococcus pneumoniae* isolated in any part of the world are tested by the laboratory for sensitivity to benzylpenicillin.

Haemophilus influenzae meningitis should be treated by ampicillin or chloramphenicol. Some 2–5% of these organisms are resistant to ampicillin in this country and it may be wise to begin therapy with chloramphenicol, since there is a very low incidence of resistance to this antibiotic[65]. Chloramphenicol should be given in a dose of 1 g 6 hourly by intravenous injection; this drug is less well absorbed when given by intramuscular injection than by the oral or i.v. routes.

In elderly patients Gram-negative bacilli, *Staphylococcus aureus*, *Listeria* spp., occur more frequently as causes of meningitis than in younger age groups, except neonates. The appropriate treatment for Gram-negative bacilli follows bacteriological sensitivity testing. *Staphylococcus aureus* should be treated by cloxacillin, perhaps in combination with fucidin, erythromycin or clindamycin. If the patient is sensitive to penicillin-type antibiotics, erythromycin in combination with fucidin or clindamycin may be used. *Listeria* meningitis is treated with high doses of ampicillin or benzylpenicillin, or one of these antibiotics in combination with gentamicin[66,67]; in an elderly patient such a combination may help to induce a more rapid clinical response. Less often, erythromycin has been used with a penicillin. Organisms more rarely found as a cause of meningitis are haemolytic streptococci, *Salmonella* spp., and *Pseudomonas* spp.

Haemolytic streptococci require benzylpenicillin, and pseudomonas meningitis a combination of carbenicillin with gentamicin. Salmonella meningitis will probably respond best to chloramphenicol.

A Gram stain of cerebrospinal fluid deposit in bacterial meningitis will usually indicate the nature of the causative organism and so help orientate antibiotic therapy. However, if the Gram film is unhelpful and the more common organisms mentioned above require to be covered, perhaps the best antibiotic combination to start treatment is a penicillin-type drug with chloramphenicol. The former will usually be benzylpenicillin, but if cover for *Staphylococcus aureus* is necessary cloxacillin should be used.

Intracranial abscess

Many types of organisms may cause intracranial abscess according to the source of infection[68]. Frontal lobe abscesses originating from infection in the facial sinuses usually yield haemolytic streptococci (particularly *Streptococcus milleri*) and anaerobes, (particularly *Bacteroides fragilis* or *Bacteroides melaninogenicus*) and organisms typical of dental abscess[69]. Temporal lobe abscess originating from middle ear infection yield anaerobes as well as *Streptococcus pneumoniae* and *Haemophilus influenzae*. A mixed culture of different organisms is characteristically found in abscesses developing from local sites of infection. Cerebral abscess resulting from endocarditis yields the corresponding organism, and intracranial abscess resulting from trauma often yields *Staphylococcus aureus*. Metastatic abscesses are caused by the organisms found at the site of infection.

Antibiotic treatment may need to begin before bacteriological results are available, but as soon as intracranial abscess is suspected a specialist surgical opinion should be sought as it is unlikely that antibiotics alone will resolve the condition. The antibiotic regimen adopted should include metronidazole because of the high incidence of anaerobic organisms in intracranial abscesses originating from local sites of infection and other sources[70]. In view of the frequency of streptococci in these lesions, both from local sources of infection and from endocarditis, the antibiotic regimen should include benzylpenicillin. Finally, in order to provide wide cover against other organisms it may be good practice to include chloramphenicol or gentamicin with the above agents[71].

As soon as bacteriological results are available the antibiotics must be reorientated towards the causative organism. If *Staphylococcus. aureus* is found, cloxacillin with fucidin or erythromycin or clindamycin should be used. Indeed, if there has been a source of infection such as trauma, osteomyelitis or septicaemia due to this organism, treatment should include cloxacillin from the beginning. Similarly, if the source of infection appears to be from the sinuses or middle ear then gentamicin is less important. However, if the source of infection remains obscure every attempt should be made to determine the causative organisms by aspiration of the abscess or by biopsy during intracranial operation.

INFECTIONS OF THE INTESTINAL AND BILIARY TRACTS: ABDOMINAL CAVITY

Food poisoning

Clostridium welchii and *Staphylococcus aureus* are the commonest organisms involved in this condition and cause food poisoning by the production of an extracellular toxin that is formed in the food before ingestion. *Bacillus cereus* may also form a toxin and lead to vomiting and diarrhoea within a few hours of ingesting contaminated, lightly fried rice. *Salmonellae* and *Vibrio parahaemolyticus* cause food poisoning by multiplication within the intestinal tract. Although the time of onset of illness after ingestion will vary according to the cause of illness, the symptoms of food poisoning usually pass within 48 hours and antibiotic therapy is not indicated. It has been shown that salmonella excretion in the faeces may persist for a longer time in those patients given antibiotics. Occasionally an elderly patient may show signs of systemic infection such as septicaemia or metastatic infection, particularly if the patient is immunodeficient. Antibiotic therapy should then be undertaken with one of the following drugs, ampicillin or amoxycillin, co-trimoxazole, or chloramphenicol, since they will be active against *Salmonellae*. It is unlikely that those organisms producing a toxic effect will multiply and cause infection in the body.

Enteric fever is caused by *Salmonella typhi*, and *Salmonella paratyphi* A, B or C. As mentioned above, other salmonella organisms may occasionally spread beyond the intestinal tract, but this occurrence should be distinguished from the classic enteric fevers caused by *Salmonella typhi* or *Salmonella paratyphi*. Enteric fever requires therapy with chloramphenicol, ampicillin or co-trimoxazole. Although the first drug is bacteriostatic and has serious side-effects it remains a popular choice in enteric fever; adequate doses of amoxycillin i.m. or i.v., or of co-trimoxazole i.v., will probably give a similar clinical response. A history of travel abroad, particularly to the Indian subcontinent, or contact with an infected person, together with appropriate symptomatology and clinical signs, should be sufficient evidence to institute treatment. Chloramphenicol-resistant strains of *Salmonella typhi* have been reported in recent years from Mexico, South America and the Far East, but these strains have been found less frequently in the immediate past.

Cholera
This continues to spread from the Far East to the Middle East and has occured in North Africa, Portugal and Italy; a small outbreak was also described in 1978 in Louisiana, USA. It may be wise to exclude this illness in elderly patients returning from a cruise or a trip to the Mediteranean littoral, by making a special request to the laboratory. Treatment requires correction of fluid and salt balance and tetracyclines should be added to the regimen in order to shorten the course of illness and reduce the large number of organisms in the gut and excreta. Patients colonized with enteric organisms, other *Salmonellae* and cholera organisms must be isolated and their excreta (both faeces and urine) handled with gloves during disposal. Hands must be washed after each procedure involving potential contamination with excreta.

Cholecystitis and cholangitis
A wide variety of bacteria cause these infections, originating both from the flora of the intestinal tract and from organisms that survive passage through the stomach from the upper respiratory tract. In order to provide as wide a cover as possible, including anaerobes, an antibiotic regimen should include metronidazole with ampicillin or co-trimoxazole. It is possible that cefoxitin would also be an efficient antibiotic in this situation. It has been shown that it is probably more satisfactory to use antibiotics that attain high serum levels than choosing those that are excreted in larger amounts in normal bile[71]; in the presence of infection biliary excretion of antibiotics is severely reduced.

Enterocolitis and pseudomembraneous colitis
Infection of the intestinal tract may occur with *Staphylococcus aureus*, *Pseudomonas* spp., and *Candida* spp., usually in patients treated with wide-spectrum antibiotics and resulting in devastating fluid loss. Antibiotic therapy should be appropriate to the organisms seen in a Gram film or obtained by culture of faecal material. Therapy should be both parenteral and by the oral route.

Pseudomembraneous colitis occurs in patients previously treated with antibiotics, particularly clindamycin, and may begin up to 4 weeks following antibiotic therapy. It is now thought that the infection is due to *Clostridium difficile*. Vancomycin in a dose of 500 mg i.v. given 6 hourly has been used successfully in treatment of this condition[33]. It is possible that this organism would also respond to metronidazole, although this drug may be too rapidly and completely absorbed from the gut for good effect.

Peritonitis
The organisms involved in peritonitis are those of the bowel flora. The infection is therefore a mixed one of Gram-negative bacilli, frequently including *Pseudomonas*, anaerobes and often *Streptococcus faecalis*. A combination of gentamicin with metronidazole provides wide cover against the organism mentioned except for *Streptococcus faecalis*. However, surgery will probably be required in order to obtain drainage and prevent accumulation of pus with abscess formation. Exudate obtained at operation should be sent for Gram film and culture, and antibiotics adjusted to the organisms found. Antibiotics will aid in the prevention of direct metastatic spread of infection, abscess formation and septicaemia.

Diverticular disease
Antibiotics have a role in the medical management of diverticular disease. In addition to a high residue diet, phthalylsulphathiazole, neomycin or co-trimoxazole may be given. If perforation occurs then the treatment mentioned earlier should be given.

Subphrenic, abdominal and pelvic abscess
As subphrenic and abdominal abscesses are usually caused by organisms of the bowel flora, appropriate antibiotics will be those mentioned above. However, surgical intervention will normally be required and every attempt should be made to obtain a sample of pus by needle aspiration or operation. Antibiotic therapy should then be reorientated according to the bacteriological results. Pelvic abscesses may originate from the female gentital tract and frequently contain anaerobes[72], often together with haemolytic and microaerophilic streptococci. Metronidazole and benzylpenicillin are antibiotics of choice for pus or abscesses in this site, before bacteriological results are available.

Liver abscess
A wide range of organisms may be responsible for liver abscesses, again, particularly those of the bowel flora. As a cautionary note, it is always wise to exclude the possibility of an amoebic abscess par-

ticularly if the patient is on steroids; serological tests are available to make this diagnosis. Antibiotic therapy of bacterial causes of liver abscess will include metronidazole, and a penicillin (benzylpenicillin or ampicillin) and gentamicin. It is possible that a cephalosporin could replace the penicillin and gentamicin combination. However, more accurate therapy would follow culture of a needle biopsy of the abscess. The duration of therapy is governed by the speed of resolution of the abscess and this can be monitored by ultrasound imaging. Antibiotics may be required for some weeks and should continue until the abscess is no longer detectable, since recrudescence of infection tends to occur if therapy is too short.

INFECTIONS OF THE SKIN AND SOFT TISSUES

Infected dermatitis and eczema

Bacteriological investigation should be made in these conditions and antibiotic therapy, if required, guided by the results of sensitivity tests. The agents used topically should not be those that can be used systemically, for example, neomycin should be used in place of gentamicin. Chloramphenicol and chlortetracycline (which have restricted use systemically) will provide broad-spectrum cover without being absorbed from surface lesions. An increase in the rate of recovery of *Staphylococcus aureus* strains which were resistant to gentamicin was found in a dermatology unit using this antibiotic topically[73]. Gentamicin should be used topically only for pseudomonas infection of the conjunctivae and eye.

Burns

Many organisms may infect burns; perhaps the most frequent and dangerous are *Staphylococcus aureus*, haemolytic streptococci, *Clostridium welchii* and *Pseudomonas* spp. In extensive burns systemic spread of infection and septicaemia may occur. Antibiotic therapy should be guided by bacteriological investigation and prevention of infection should be attempted by appropriate isolation techniques. Antiseptic agents, such as silver sulphadiazine and povidone iodine, can be successfully used to prevent infection. However, these agents, like antibiotics, may be absorbed in extensive burns and continued use of povidone iodine has led to acidosis. If systemic therapy is required a suitable regimen is benzylpenicillin with gentamicin. If *Staphylococcus aureus* is known to be causing infection cloxacillin should be substituted for benzylpenicillin, until the sensitivities of the strain are known.

Erysipelas

This is usually caused by *Streptococcus pyogenes* and requires 48 hour treatment with parenteral benzylpenicillin followed by phenoxymethyl-penicillin orally if response has occured. If the patient is allergic to penicillin, erythromycin or cephalosporin should be given i.m. followed by oral forms of these drugs (cephalexin or cephaclor).

Paronychia

This may be caused by a variety of bacteria, as well as by *Candida* spp. and *Herpes simplex*. Systemic antibiotic therapy is not usually indicated unless there is spread of infection to soft tissues or bone.

Cellulitis

This is usually caused by *Streptococcus pyogenes*, that is, Lancefield's group A, though other groups may sometimes be involved. *Staphylococcus aureus* may also occur, more often in hospital patients. Antibiotic therapy requires systemic benzylpenicillin or cloxacillin according to the organism.

Infected infusion sites

Staphylococcus aureus is usually the pathogen in this condition having been introduced during the procedure or during the infusion by handling of the site with contaminated fingers and hands. Almost any organism may cause infection if deposited at the site in this way. Treatment will usually require local cleansing, and antibiotic therapy is unnecessary unless there is evidence of spread of infection, either locally or systemically, such as cellulitis, lymphangitis or lymphadenitis, in which case cloxacillin i.m. or flucloxacillin orally should be used until bacteriological results are available. If several patients have been found with infected infusion sites epidemiological investigation should be undertaken by the control of infection staff.

Pressure sores

A large variety of organisms may be found in these ulcers at any one time, usually colonizing the surface of the sore rather than causing infection. Progress of the lesion is due more to oedema or poor arterial blood supply than to damage from bacterial contamination. Although the bacteria colonizing the lesion should be monitored by regular swabs, it is unlikely that antibiotic therapy will have any effect on their numbers or lead to improvement in the lesion. Pressure sores should be kept clean and treated with local antiseptics such as chloramine or eusol. Occasionally there may be evidence of local infection, with surrounding soft tissue infection and cellulitis or deep infective necrosis of tissue. More rarely, systemic infection may follow. In these situations antibiotic therapy must be guided by knowledge of the organisms present.

Wound infections
Wounds resulting from road traffic accidents may become infected with a variety of organisms, most commonly *Staphylococcus aureus*. Antibiotic therapy will be guided by the clinical evidence of infection and the results of bacteriology; protection against tetanus must be given routinely. In traumatic wounds of the lower limb the possibility of gas gangrene should be remembered, and frequently other anaerobic organisms may also be present in traumatic wounds at this site.

The most common organism causing *postoperative wound infection* is *Staphylococcus aureus*; many other organisms may also cause infection and their type will largely depend upon the site of operation; for instance, if the intestinal tract has been opened the wound may be infected with Gram-negative bacilli and anaerobes. Antibiotic therapy will not be required for small stitch abscesses and minor infection; deep infection and surrounding inflammation, however, may require therapy which should be guided by the results of bacteriological investigation. Cleaning of the wound and drainage of pus are required more often than antibiotics.

It is good practice to monitor the incidence of postoperative sepsis and if this increases, or if there appears to be several cases due to one organism, the control of infection staff should be informed.

INFECTIONS OF THE BONES AND JOINTS

The incidence of osteomyelitis increases with age[74]. The site of attack in the adult is usually the flat bones of the pelvis and the spine. The disease tends to be gradual in onset, slow in course and confusing in clinical pattern[75]. A common presenting symptom is low back pain, a not uncommon complaint in the elderly.

The disease is most frequently due to *Staphylococcus aureus*; other organisms include haemolytic and non-haemolytic streptococci, *Haemophilus influenzae*, Gram-negative bacilli including *Pseudomonas* and salmonella, as well as anaerobic organisms. Antibiotic therapy must be guided by the results of bacteriological investigation and every attempt should be made to obtain an adequate specimen for culture. A swab taken from the mouth of a sinus at the skin surface may well yield organisms of the skin flora only; it is vital to obtain pus known to be coming from the source of infection or, better, to obtain material from the site of the lesion in the bone itself. Previous osteomyelitis with *Staphylococcus aureus* may indicate current infection with the same organism. Antibiotic therapy for *Staphylococcus aureus* in osteomyelitis is cloxacillin i.m. and fucidin i.v. or orally; these drugs must be continued for 6 weeks and further treatment with flucloxacillin and fucidin given orally for 3 months. Erythromycin can be used when patients are allergic to penicillin. Appropriate antibiotics for other organisms must be guided by the results of sensitivity tests, and should continue for 6 weeks parenterally, followed by oral therapy. A combination of antibiotics may be required, particularly for *Pseudomonas* spp. where carbenicillin and gentamicin form the regimen. In all acute cases except those which have responded to early antibiotic therapy, surgical intervention will benefit the patient by substantiating the diagnosis, providing biopsy tissue for culture and by releasing purulent material if present.

Contaminated compound fractures should be protected from infection by flucloxacillin orally 500 mg 6 hourly (given as soon as possible after swabs have been taken, in the Accident and Emergency Department) and continued until the skin lesions have healed.

Joint infection is, again, usually caused by *Staphylococcus aureus*, or streptococci and in the elderly produces muted symptoms. Frequently the patient presents with confusion or loss of mobility rather than complaining of an acutely painful joint. A Gram film of joint fluid will aid the initial choice of antibiotics, and this can be modified in the light of the results of culture.

INFECTIONS WITH FUNGI

Candida spp

Infection with this organism may occur at superficial sites, such as in an atrophic vagina, paronychia, in the mouth and ear. Infection of the urinary tract with this organism in the presence of a permanent catheter is common. Deep tissue infection is much more rare, but it may occur in the intestinal tract and lung in immunocompromised patients. Septicaemia caused by candida may also occur, from deep tissue infection, pyelonephritis or cardiac operation. In both superficial and deep infection invasion by the organism may have been encouraged by the use of antibiotics. Stopping these drugs may allow restitution of the normal flora with removal of the candida infection in superficial sites. In vaginitis, nystatin or miconazole suppositories can be used, and in severe paronychia infection long-term local miconazole or amphotericin therapy is appropriate. Infection in the mouth can be treated by amphoteracin lozenges which are allowed to dissolve slowly on the tongue, or by nystatin mouth washes, and fungicidal ointments can be used in the ear. Nystatin bladder washouts may be attempted in catheterized patients, although this procedure is usually unsuccessful and time-consuming, but may reduce the number of yeasts present.

Deep tissue infection with *Candida* spp. requires amphotericin B (in doses described previously) together with 5-fluorocytosine. These drugs should also be used together for candida septicaemia, and in all cases current antibiotic therapy should be stopped, if possible. Miconazole is also active systemically against candida and experience with this drug is being obtained at the present time. However, it is too early to know whether this drug will be as effective as amphotericin and 5-fluorocytosine used in combination.

Aspergillus
Lung tissue may become infected with this fungus secondarily to old tuberculosis or previous bacterial infection. An aspergillus fungus ball may develop in a tuberculous cavity or infection may occur as a spreading mycelial invasion of the smaller bronchii. If treatment is required amphotericin should be used, since clinical experience with miconazole is insufficient at the present time to assess its role. *Aspergillus* spp. may cause a persistent infection of the ear which is difficult to treat, and advice from a specialist surgeon should be sought. Infection elsewhere with this organism is rare.

Cryptococcus neoformans
Invasion of the body with this organism begins in the lung; it may or may not be detected at this site. In immunodeficient patients, particularly, spread may then occur to the meninges. The signs of meningeal infection develop slowly over several days or some weeks. Treatment must be undertaken by a combination of amphotericin B and 5-fluorocytosine, since the organism may rapidly develop resistance to 5-fluorocytosine and the best results are obtained by combination therapy[76].

Infection with other fungi are very rare in patients indigenous to this country who have not travelled abroad. Histoplasmosis and coccidioidomycosis occur in patients who have been to the western United States, while blastomycosis occurs in patients from Central and South America and Africa. Sporotrichosis is rare in this country, while infection with *Mucor* and *Phycomyces* occurs rarely in debilitated or immunocompromised patients. All of these fungi are treated with amphotericin B.

FUTURE DEVELOPMENTS IN ANTIBIOTIC THERAPY

It seems probable that new modes of action by antibiotics are now less likely to be discovered[77]. New developments therefore in antibiotic therapy seem likely to follow in directions which increase the value of the major types of antibiotics already available, that is, a wider spectrum and more efficient activity against bacteria and better means of delivery of antibiotics to the site of infection. The development of drugs with better activity against fungi and viruses than those available is still needed. The large number of antibiotics now available and the seemingly endless development of new varieties may lead to a false sense of security. Many new antibiotics are a variation on a previous drug, often with improved properties but with a similar action on bacteria as their predecessors.

Wider spectrum and more efficient activity
Many bacteria produce extracellular enzymes that destroy antibiotics; for example, most strains of *Staphylococcus aureus* and many Gram-negative bacilli produce β-lactamases that act against penicillin-type drugs, while some Gram-negative bacilli produce enzymes able to destroy aminoglycosides. Less often, bacteria are protected by the impermeability of their membranes to antibiotics and in a few instances bacteria develop metabolic pathways or cell structures that avoid antibiotic action. The isoxazolyl penicillins (such as cloxacillin and flucloxacillin) resist β-lactamases, but these penicillins remain inactive against aerobic Gram-negative bacilli. Consequently a β-lactamase resistant, bactericidal, penicillin-like drug active against Gram-positive and Gram-negative bacteria would find a prominent place in the antibiotic armamentarium and this has led to the massive development of the cephalosporins which fulfil this role. However, clinical practice will have to determine whether the latest examples of these drugs, cefoxitin, cefuroxime or cefotaxime, will be clinically successful and if so for how long, since there are bacteria which produce β-lactamases able to destroy each of these drugs and they may increase with greater use of the antibiotics. Research in this direction has led to the discovery of clavulanic acid which also possesses a β-lactam molecule that can be joined to certain penicillin-type drugs. The clavulanic moiety preferentially

reacts with any β-lactamases present, allowing the penicillin to remain active. It will be interesting to see whether a commercially viable combination of clavulanic acid with a penicillin type will become available. Similarly, amongst the aminoglycosides, the newer drugs are less sensitive to the enzymes that attack gentamicin, and perhaps future antibiotics of this type (including amikacin, sisomicin and others) will have a broader spectrum of activity than gentamicin against aerobic Gram-negative bacilli.

Once antibiotics have reached the site of infection they must still penetrate bacterial cells. It has been shown that exposure of streptococci to penicillins allows better penetration of streptomycin[78,79], and the value of this combination in treating streptococcal endocarditis has been demonstrated. Further research into the means by which antibiotics penetrate bacteria may lead to more efficient drugs.

Antibiotics with low mics to organisms are at an advantage compared to antibiotics requiring higher concentrations to destroy bacteria, since less drug will be needed to penetrate to the site of infection and the lower doses required will eliminate side-effects. A recently described cephalosporin (cefotaxime) seems to have very low mics and mbcs to a wide variety of Gram-negative bacilli at least *in vitro*[23] and clinical experience with this drug may or may not show the value of this seemingly efficient cephalosporin in clinical practice. Antibiotics with activity against a wide range of Gram-positive cocci and aerobic Gram-negative bacilli as well as anaerobes would have a considerable advantage, because at present a combination of antibiotics is required for a mixed infection with these common organisms. Cefoxitin has wide activity against these groups of bacteria. Clinical experience with this antibiotic may demonstrate whether there is clinical need for such broad spectrum aerobic and anaerobic cover, as well as showing whether those species able to resist this drug at the present time become more common. Further, an antibiotic active against *Pseudomonas* spp. and other resistant Gram-negative bacilli (*Serratia* spp., *Alcaligenes* spp.) would also have considerable advantage since, again, combinations of antibiotics would be avoided when dealing with undiagnosed infection that may include *Pseudomonas* spp.

Delivery of antibiotics to site of infection
Research continues into the means by which antibiotics may be better absorbed from the intestinal tract and subsequently transported to the site of infection. Also, antibiotics able to penetrate the many different compartments of the body in substantial concentra-

tion are required, particularly those able to penetrate the blood – brain barrier. Although the greatly increased blood supply brought about by inflammation may deliver antibiotics to most sites of infection, it would be reassuring to know that the antibiotic was still able to penetrate when inflammation subsided.

Improved oral absorption has been found by the use of 'prodrugs', such as talampicillin. This ester of ampicillin, unlike ampicillin itself, is almost entirely absorbed from the intestine and rapidly converted to ampicillin in the gut wall. Similarly carfecillin, an ester of carbenicillin, is absorbed from the gut in sufficient quantity for therapy of infection in the urinary tract where the drug is concentrated for excretion. Indeed, the ability to use many drugs by the oral route which must be given intramuscularly or intravenously at the present time would be a humane development. Perhaps it will be possible to develop 'prodrugs', which penetrate body compartments well and become active only at the site of inflammation. Research has suggested[80] that antibiotics can be delivered to sites of infection by liposomes. Antibiotics have been incorporated into artificially produced liposomes which were then injected into recipient animals. The liposomes were phagocytosed by polymorphs and subsequently delivered to various organs. It is thought that carriage of drugs to sites of infection may be more efficient by this means than by using naked drugs, and some specificity of delivery could be introduced by immunoglobulin attachment onto the carrier cells.

The factors that control the distribution of antibiotics in the different body compartments are largely unknown. Fucidin has been shown to achieve good concentrations in body compartments and this is said to be due to the lipid solubility of the compound. It is not unreasonable to hope that antibiotic molecules might be constructed with lipophilic or other moieties that lead to better penetration of the body tissues.

The means of administering antibiotics is also under investigation and the use of the efficient and convenient i.v. route is now fairly commonplace. The development of simple and reliable infusion pumps may lead to a thorough comparison of intermittent doses (which produce 'seesaw' serum concentrations) with continuous infusions which can provide an adequate and stable antibiotics serum concentration[16].

Preservation of the usefulness of antibiotics requires that they are used with precision, but the profusion of antibiotics on the market helps to make this difficult. Guidance from microbiologists and pharmacologists must continue to be available. Antibiotic prophylaxis in some kinds of surgery has been shown to reduce wound sepsis[81], but the evidence that only three, or even only one dose[82], are sufficient for prophylactic effect still requires wider publicity. More clinical trials are needed on the length of time antibiotic treatment is required in different conditions. The relative value and dangers of high doses of antibiotics over short periods of time also merits investigation.

The increasing incidence of immunocompromised patients makes the development of efficient drugs against fungi more imperative. Similarly, the development of drugs against viruses has proven to be difficult and slow. There is still room for further research work with interferon against virus diseases, but the difficulty of obtaining relatively huge doses of this material is a deterrent. Antiviral agents such as amantadine and ribovarin still require clinical trials to determine their usefulness in practice.

References

1 Skegg, D. C. G., Doll, R. and Perry, J. (1977). Use of medicines in general practice. *Br. Med. J.* **2**, 1561

2 Hurwitz, N. and Wade, O. L. (1969). Intensive hospital monitoring of adverse reactions to drugs. *Br. Med. J.* **1**, 531

3 Williamson, J. and Chopin, J. M. (1979). Adverse reactions to prescribed drugs in the elderly – a multicentre investigation. In Crooks, J. and Stevenson, I. M. (eds.) *Drugs and the Elderly* (London: Macmillan)

4 Austrian, R. (1968). Current status of bacterial pneumonia with especial reference to pneumococcal infection. *J. Clin. Pathol.* (Supplement), **21**, 93

5 Bigger, J. W. (1944). Treatment of staphylococcal infections with penicillin by intermittent sterilisation. *Lancet*, **ii**, 497

6 Sabath, L. D., Laverdiere, M., Wheeler, N., Blazevic, D. and Wilkinson, B. J. (1977). A new type of penicillin resistance of *Staphylococcus aureus*. *Lancet*, **i**, 443

7 Brodlie, P., Henney, C. and Wood, A. J. J. (1974). Problems of administering drugs by continuous infusion. *Br. Med. J.*, **1**, 383

8 Ball, P., Banford, T., Gilbert, J., Johnson, T. and Mitchard, M. (1978b). Prolonged serum elimination half-life of amoxycillin in the elderly. *J. Antimicrob. Chemother.*, **4**, 385

9 Denham, M. J., Hodkinson, H. M. and Fisher, M. (1975). Glomerular filtration rate in sick elderly inpatients. *Age Ageing*, **4**: 32

10 Ball, A. P., Viswan, A. K., Mitchard, M. and Wise, R. (1978a). Plasma concentrations and excretion of mecillinam after oral administration of pivmecillinam in elderly patients. *J. Antimicrob. Chemother.*, **4**, 241

11 Kabins, S. A. (1972). Interactions among antibiotics and other drugs. *J. Am. Med. Assoc.*, **219**, 206

12 Editorial (1971). Antibacterial agents in renal failure. *Lancet* **i**, 621

13 Sharpstone, P. (1977). Diseases of the urinary system. Prescribing for patients with renal failure. *Br. Med. J.*, **2**, 36

14 Bennett, W. M., Singer, I. and Coggins, C. M. (1970). A practical guide to drug usage in adult patients with impaired renal function. *J. Am. Med. Assoc.*, **214**, 1468

15 Gingell, J. C. and Waterworth, P. M. (1968). Dose of gentamicin in patients with normal renal function and renal impairment. *Br. Med. J.*, **1**, 191
16 Wootton, R. and Sanderson, P. J. (1979). The use of impulse analysis for predicting antibiotic doses. *J. Antimicrob. Chemother.*, (In press)
17 May, J. R. and Ingold, A. (1972). Amoxycillin in the treatment of chronic non-tuberculous bronchial infections. *Br. J. Dis. Chest*, **66**, 185
18 Comber, K. R., Osborne, C. D. and Sutherland, R. (1975). Comparative effects of amoxycillin and ampicillin in the treatment of experimental mouse infections. *Antimicrob. Agents Chemother.*, **7**, 179
19 Brumfitt, W., Percival, A. and Leigh, D. A. (1967). Clinical and laboratory studies with carbenicillin. A new penicillin active against *Pseudomonas pyocyanea*. *Lancet*, **1**, 1289
20 Klastersky, J., Cappel, R. and Daneau, D. (1973). Therapy with carbenicillin and gentamicin for patients with cancer and severe infections caused by Gramnegative rods. *Cancer*, **31**, 331
21 Bodey, G. P., Middleman, E., Umsawasdi, T. and Rodrigquez, V. (1971). Intravenous gentamicin therapy for infections in patients with cancer. *J. Infect. Dis.* (Supplement), **124**, 174
22 Editorial (1978a). Antibiotic damage to damaged kidneys. *Lancet* **ii**, 558
23 Hamilton-Miller, J. M. T., Brumfitt, W. and Reynolds, A. V. (1978). Cefotazime (HR 756) a new cephalosporin with exceptional broad spectrum activity *in vitro*. *J. Antimicrob. Chemother.*, **4**, 437
24 Heymes, R., Lutz, A. and Schrinner, E. (1977). Experimental evaluation of HR 756 a new cephalosporin derivative: pre-clinical study. *Infection*, **5**, 259
25 Araas, I., Skarsten, K. W. and Neess, H. C. (1977). Pivmecillinam in the treatment of post-operative bacteruria in gynaecological patients. A double-blind comparison with pivmecillinam and pivampicillin. *J. Antimicrob. Chemother.*, **3**, 227
26 Noone, P. (1978). Use of antibiotics: aminoglycosides. *Br. Med. J.*, **2**, 549
27 Reeves, D. S. (1974). Gentamicin therapy. *Br. J. Hos. Med.*, **11**, 837
28 Report: Morbidity and Mortality Weekly Report (1977), **26**, No 18, 151
29 Roddis, M. J. (1978). Antibiotic-associated colitis: A retrospective study of fifteen cases. *Age Ageing*, **7**, 182
30 Reeves, D. S., Bint, A. J. and Bullock, D. W. (1978). Use of antibiotics: sulphonamides, cotrimoxazole and tetracyclines. *Br. Med. J.*, **2**, 410
31 Chanarin, I. and England, J. M. (1972). Toxicity of trimethoprim – sulphamethoxazole in patients with megaloblastic haemopoiesis. *Br. Med. J.*, **1**, 651
32 Phillips, M. E., Eastwood, J. B., Curtis, J. R., Gower, P. E. and de Wardener, H. E. (1974). Tetracycline poisoning in renal failure. *Br. Med. J.*, **1**, 149
33 Keighley, M. R. B., Burdon, D. W., Arabi, Y., Alexander-Williams, J., Thompson, H., Youngs, D., Johnson, M., Bentley, S., George, R. H. and Mogg, G. A. G. (1978). Randomised control trial of vancomycin for pseudomembranous colitis and post-operative diarrhoea. *Br. Med. J.*, **ii**, 1667
34 Roe, F. J. C. (1977). Metronidazole: review of uses and toxicity. *J. Antimicrob. Chemother.*, **3**, 205
35 Eykyn, S. J. and Phillips, I. (1976). Metronidazole and anaerobic sepsis. *Br. Med. J.*, **2**, 1418
36 Rainer, E. H. (1971). Acute epiglottitis in adults. *J. Laryngol. and Otol.*, **85**, 493
37 May, J. R. (1968). *Chemotherapy of Chronic Bronchitis*. (London: English Universities Press)
38 Burns, M. W. (1972). The pattern of bacterial infection in bronchial diseases in Australia. A serological and bacteriological survey. *Med. J. Aust.*, **2**, 697

39 Garb, J. L., Brown, R. B., Garb, J. R. and Tuthill, R. W. (1978). Differences in etiology of pneumonias in nursing home and community patients. *J. Am. Med. Assoc.*, **246,** 2169

40 Noone, P., Parsons, T. M. C., Pattison, J. R., Slack, R. C. B., Garfield-Davies, D. and Hughers, K. (1974). Experience in monitoring gentamicin therapy during treatment of serious Gram-negative sepsis. *Br. Med. J.*, **1,** 477

41 Wilkinson, P. J., Ball, A. J., Doran, J., Gillespie, W. A. and Orton, V. (1977). Routine laboratory assessment of post-operative chest infection: a prospective study. *J. Clin. Pathol.*, **30,** 417

42 Bartlett, J. G., Gorback, S. L. and Finegold, S. M. (1974a). The bacteriology of aspiration pneumonia. *Am. J. Med.*, **56,** 202

43 Bartlett, J. G., Gorback, S. L., Thadepalli, H. and Finegold, S. M. (1974b). Bacteriology of empyema. *Lancet*, i, 338

44 Noah, N. D. (1974). *Mycoplasma pneumoniae* infection in the United Kingdom 1967–73. *Br. Med. J.*, **2,** 544

45 Watson, G. I. (1977). The treatment of *Mycoplasma pneumoniae* infections. *Scot. Med. J.*, **22,** 361

46 Foy, H. M., Ochs, H., Davis, S. D., Kenny, G. E. and Luce, R. R. (1973). *Mycoplasma pneumoniae* infections in patients with immunodeficiency syndromes: Report of four cases. *J. Infect. Dis.*, **126,** 388

47 Report: Morbidity and Mortality Weekly Report (1978a), **27,** No 1, 1

48 Glick, T. H., Gregg, M. B. and Berman, B. (1978). Pontiac fever: an epidemic of unknown aetiology in a health department. *Am. J. Epidemiol.*, **107,** 149

49 Asscher, A. W. (1977). Diseases of the urinary system: Urinary tract infections. *Br. Med. J.*, **1,** 1332

50 Warren, J. W., Platt, R., Thomas, R. J., Rosner, B. and Kass, E. H. (1978). Antibiotic irrigation and catheter-associated urinary tract infections. *N. Engl. J. Med.*, **299,** 570

51 Schirger, A., Martin, W. J. and Nichols, D. R. (1956). Streptococcal bacteraemia without endocarditis: clinical observations. *Ann. Intern. Med.*, **45,** 1001

52 MacHenry, M. C., Martin, W. J. and Wellman, W. E. (1962). Bacteraemia due to Gram-negative bacilli. *Ann. Intern. Med.*, **56,** 207

53 Jansson, E. (1971). A ten year study of bacteraemia. *Scand. J. Infect. Dis.*, **3,** 151

54 Denham, M. J. and Goodwin, G. S. (1977). The value of blood cultures in geriatric practice. *Age Ageing*, **6,** 85

55 Drewett, S. E., Payne, D. J. H., Tuke, W. and Verdon, P. E. (1972). Skin distribution of *Clostridium welchii*: use of iodophor as a sporicidal agent. *Lancet*, i, 1172

56 Parker, M. T. (1969). Post-operative Clostridial infections in Britain. *Brit. Med. J.*, **3,** 671

57 Finland, M. and Barnes, M. W. (1970). Changing aetiology of bacterial endocarditis in the antibiotic era. *Ann. Intern. Med.*, **72,** 341

58 Anderson, H. J. and Staffurth, J. S. (1955). Subacute bacterial endocarditis in the elderly. *Lancet*, ii, 1055

59 Durack, D. T., Palletier, L. L. and Petersdorf, R. G. (1974). Chemotherapy of experimental streptococcal endocarditis. *J. Clin. Invest.*, **53,** 829

60 Sande, M. A. and Irvin, R. G. (1974). Penicillin–aminoglycoside synergy in experimental *Streptococcus viridans* endocarditis. *J. Infect. Dis.*, **129,** 572

61 Sande, M. A. and Johnson, M. L. (1975). Antimicrobial therapy of experimental endocarditis caused by *Staphylococcus aureus*. *J. Infect. Dis.*, **131,** 367

62 Editorial (1977). Preventing endocarditis. *Br. Med. J.*, **2,** 1564

63 Lambert, H. P. (1978). Use of antibiotics: meningitis. *Br. Med. J.*, **2,** 259

64 Report: Morbidity and Mortality Weekly Report (1978b), **27,** No 39, 368
65 Williams, J. D. and Andrews, J. (1974). Sensitivity of *Haemophilus influenzae* to antibiotics. *Br. Med. J.,* **1,** 134
66 Moellering, R. C., Medoff, G. and Leech, I. (1972). Antibiotic synergism against *Listeria monocytogenes. Antimicrob. Agents Chemother.,* **1,** 30
67 Watson, G. W., Fuller, T. J., Elms, J. and Kluge, R. M. (1978). Listeria cerebritis. *Arch. Intern. Med.,* **138,** 83
68 De Louvois, J., Gortvai, P. and Hurley, R. (1977). Bacteriology of abscesses of the central nervous system: a multicentre prospective study. *Br. Med. J.,* **2,** 981
69 Ingham, H. R., High, A. S., Kalbag, R. M., Sengupta, R. P., Tharagonnet, D. and Selkon, J. B. (1978). Abscesses of the frontal lobe of the brain secondary to covert dental sepsis. *Lancet,* **ii,** 497
70 Editorial (1978b). Chemotherapy of brain abscess. *Lancet,* **ii,** 1081
71 Keighley, M. R. B. (1977). Micro-organisms in the bile: a preventable cause of sepsis after biliary surgery. *Ann. Roy. Coll. Surg.,* **59,** 328
72 Ledger, W. J., Sweet, R. L. and Headington, J. T. (1971). Bacteroides species as a cause of severe infections in obstetric and gynaecologic patients. *Surg. Gynaecol. Obstet.,* **133,** 837
73 Wyatt, T. D., Ferguson, W. P., Wilson, T. S. and McCormick, E. (1977). Gentamicin resistant *Staphylococcus aureus* association with the use of topical gentamicin. *J. Antimicrob. Chemother.,* **3,** 213
74 Waldvogel, F. A., Medoff, G. and Swartz, M. N. (1970). Osteomyelitis: A review of clinical features, therapeutic considerations and unusual aspects. *N. Engl. J. Med.,* **282,** 262
75 Stone, D. B. and Bonfiglio, M. (1963). Pyogenic vertebral osteomyelitis. *Arch. Intern. Med.,* **112,** 491
76 Cartwright, R. Y. (1978). Use of antibiotics: antifungals. *Br. Med. J.,* **2,** 108
77 Lowbury, E. J. L. and Ayliffe, G. A. J. (1974). *Drug Resistance in Antimicrobia Chemotherapy.* (Springfield, IU.: Thomas)
78 Plotz, P. H. and Davis, B. D. (1962). Synergism between streptomycin and penicillin: a proposed mechanism. *Science,* **135,** 1067
79 Moellering, R. C. and Weinberg, A. N. (1971). Studies on antibiotic synergism against enterococci. *J. Clin. Invest.,* **50,** 2580
80 Fendler, J. H. and Romero, A. (1977). Liposomes as drug carriers. *Life Sci.,* **20,** 1109
81 Stokes, E. J., Waterworth, P. M., Franks, V., Watson, B. and Clarke, C. C. (1974). Short term routine antibiotic prophylaxis in surgery. *Br. J. Surg.,* **61,** 739
82 Griffiths, D. A., Shorey, B. A., Simpson, R. A., Speller, D. C. E. and Williams, N. B. (1976). Single dose pre-operative antibiotic prophylaxis in gastro-intestinal surgery. *Lancet,* **ii,** 325

Review articles

Garrod, L. P., Lambert, H. P. and O'Grady, F. (1974). *Antibiotics and Chemotherapy.* (Edinburgh: Livingstone)
Smith, H. (1977). *Antibiotics in Clinical Practice.* (London: Pitman Medical)
Noone, P. (1977). *A Clinician's Guide to Antibiotic Therapy.* (Oxford: Blackwell Scientific Publications)
Bint, A. J. (1978). A guide to new antibiotics. *Br. J. Hosp. Med.,* **19,** 335
Ingham, H. R., Selkon, J. P. and Hale, J. H. (1975). The antibacterial activity of metronidazole. *J. Antimicrob. Chemother.,* **1,** 355
Garrod, L. P. (1972). Causes of failure in antibiotic treatment. *Br. Med. J.,* **2,** 473

3

Treatment of cardiovascular disease in the elderly

R. W. Stout

CARDIOVASCULAR DISEASE IN OLD AGE

Heart disease is the commonest cause of death in all age groups and becomes increasingly common with advancing age. It is also the commonest cause of serious illness in the older age groups. The pattern of heart disease in old age differs somewhat from that in younger people[1]. Ischaemic heart disease becomes relatively more important and rheumatic heart disease less so, as the latter is principally a disease of young adults and is usually not consistent with survival into advanced old age. Rheumatic fever and rheumatic heart disease are also becoming less common in the community as a whole and hence rheumatic heart disease in old age will become even less common. On the other hand the advent of successful surgical treatment for rheumatic heart disease will increase the survival of patients with this condition and treated rheumatic heart disease may therefore soon be found in older patients. Of congenital heart disease only the bicuspid aortic valve commonly causes problems in old age although again successful surgical treatment may soon allow prolonged survival of patients with other types of congenital heart disease. The bicuspid aortic valve often produces no symptoms for the first four to five decades of life but as calcification occurs the symptoms and signs of aortic valve disease become increasingly prominent. Pulmonary heart disease can occur at any age but is less common in old age as severe respiratory disease resulting in right-sided cardiac failure is a disease of middle-age and usually does not result in survival into the oldest ages. Congestive and hypertrophic

77

cardiomyopathies[2] are usually described in young and middle-aged adults but have been found in older people[3]. However the true prevalence of these conditions in old age is difficult to assess as diagnosis requires extensive investigation. It is likely that at least some cases of congestive cardiomyopathy are misdiagnosed as ischaemic heart disease and in the oldest age groups cardiac amyloidosis becomes increasingly common, but clinical diagnosis is difficult[4].

Treatment of heart disease in older patients often differs little from that in younger people. Any differences are usually not fundamental but rather differences of degree. Patterns of disease in different age groups merge into one another. Descriptions of heart disease and its treatment in old age are therefore frequently incomplete, and often comparison with younger age groups have not been made. Thus some of the suggestions regarding treatment in old age are not based on good factual information but on clinical impressions or extrapolation of data which may not be entirely valid.

This review will concentrate on aspects of the treatment of cardiovascular disease which are relevant to older patients and about which there has been recent new information or controversy. Old age is arbitrarily defined as 75 years or older. Treatment of cardiovascular disease in old age has been the subject of a number of comprehensive recent reviews[5, 6], and the reader is referred to them for further details and references.

THE AGEING HUMAN HEART

Although much is known about cardiac disease in old age, there is less information about age changes in the normal human heart unrelated to disease. It is, of course, difficult to separate ageing effects from the effects of disease particularly when atherosclerosis of coronary arteries is virtually universal in older age groups. Age changes in the heart have been reviewed by Burch[7]. The heart remains normal in size or may decrease slightly in association with a general reduction in body size, when the heart tends to reduce relatively less in size than the rest of the body. In wasting conditions, the heart decreases both in size and in fat mass. The colour of the myocardium tends to darken due to an increase in concentration of lipofuscin in the myocardium with age. The endocardium becomes thicker due to fibrosis, the left side of the heart being affected more than the right. The valves also become fibrotic with thickening and rigidity of the valve leaflets. Again the left side of the heart is more affected than the right. Calcium may be deposited in the valve leaflets and cusps and may involve the rings of the mitral and aortic valves. Usually these changes are not severe enough to produce haemodynamic changes, although occasionally aortic valve stenosis or regurgitation or mitral regurgitation may occur. Mitral stenosis due to the ageing process alone is extremely rare. Microscopically there is an increase in collagen and elastic fibres throughout the ageing heart. This chiefly involves the endocardium but it also occurs in the myocardium and the conducting tissue.

Physiological changes also occur with age. There is an inverse relationship between cardiac output and age and the ability of the heart to increase its performance in response to exercise diminishes. Myocardial reserve is reduced. Experimentally, ageing has been found to be associated with increased passive stiffness and decreased speed of contraction of the ventricular myocardium without changes in strength[8]. Peripheral vascular resistance is increased in older people and systolic blood pressure also increases. The heart becomes more irritable and arrhythmias become more common. This may of course be due to ischaemia as well as to the effects of age itself.

The ECG in elderly people may be different from that in younger people without there being clear evidence of disease. The most frequent change is alteration in the configuration of the ST segment and the T wave. The ST segment tends to become isoelectric or flattened and the T wave usually assumes a lower configuration in leads 1, V5 and V6. A prolonged PR interval, prolongation of the QRS complex and left axis deviation have also been described. However, because of the high incidence of heart disease in older people it is difficult to be certain that these abnormalities are due to age rather than disease.

In treating the elderly patient with heart disease the physician must always remember that the problem with the heart is almost certainly only one of several problems with which the elderly patient has to contend and that these problems may interact. Associated illnesses must be managed along with the treatment of the heart disease itself. The relationship of treatment of one symptom to management of others must also be borne in mind.

DRUG THERAPY IN OLD AGE

Recently there has been increased interest in the handling of drugs in older people and a number of reviews have discussed this topic[9-13]. Information on pharmacokinetics in old age is starting to accumulate but there are still large gaps in our knowledge.

In the handling of orally administered drugs a number of factors are important:

(1) The absorption of the drug from the gastrointestinal tract. Although changes in gastrointestinal function occur in older subjects, age itself does not appear to influence the rate of drug absorption. For example, it has been reported that the absorption of digoxin is unaltered in elderly subjects compared to younger patients[14].

(2) The distribution of the drug in the body. This depends on, among other things, the body composition, binding to plasma proteins, the apparent volume of distribution of the drug, and regional blood flow and tissue permeability. There is some evidence that changes in body composition in older subjects alter the handling of ethanol[15] but there is little evidence on its effect on other drugs. It appears that the binding capacity of plasma proteins is unaltered in old age but that plasma protein levels may be reduced in ill elderly people, and hence the binding of certain drugs including warfarin[16] and phenytoin[17] may thereby be reduced. There is little evidence that the apparent volume of distribution changes in older subjects, and regional blood flow and tissue permeability may be affected by disease rather than age itself.

(3) The metabolism of the drug in the liver. Clearance of drugs by the liver appears to be reduced in old age and there is evidence that both drug acetylation and oxidation are reduced in older subjects[18]. In addition, induction of drug metabolism in the liver is reduced in elderly subjects[19].

(4) Probably the most marked change with regard to handling of drugs occurs in the ability of the kidney to excrete the drug or the product of drug metabolism. The glomerular filtration rate and renal plasma flow both decrease with age in the absence of overt renal disease and hence drugs which are excreted by the kidney are excreted less efficiently in old age[20].

(5) The sensitivity of the tissues to the drugs may be altered in old age. This is a difficult variable to measure but evidence has recently been published of increased sensitivity to nitrazepam in elderly patients[21].

The other major variable with regard to drug handling is disease. Despite the fact that drugs are normally given to people who are ill, the influence of disease on the handling of drugs has been little studied. Most studies of pharmacokinetics have been carried out in healthy normal volunteers.

However, a recent study[22] has shown that in patients with cardiac failure the pharmacokinetics of the drug aminopyrine, which is metabolized by the liver, are greatly altered. While the absorption of the drug was unaltered, the half-life was prolonged, the metabolic clearance rate reduced, and the apparent volume of distribution increased. Thus elimination of the drug was reduced, with the possibility of prolonged pharmacological effects and possible toxicity if the dose and dosage interval were not appropriately adjusted. Drugs which are metabolized in this way include the benzodiazapines, phenobarbitone, phenytoin, theophylline, tolbutamide and warfarin. Thus the presence of cardiac failure will affect the handling of drugs which may be given concomitantly for other conditions. Whether the presence of cardiac failure affects the handling of drugs used in its own treatment is unknown. The influence of disease and age will often be additive and hence the use of drugs in elderly subjects may well be subject to much more variation than is currently appreciated.

CARDIAC FAILURE

Left ventricular failure and congestive cardiac failure are the commonest presentations of cardiac disease in old age. The most frequent cause is ischaemic heart disease, often presenting without the typical symptoms and signs[23]. The underlying disorder in cardiac failure is a decrement in cardiac function resulting in a decrease in forward flow from the right or left ventricles and venous congestion in either or both of the pulmonary or systemic circulations. As a result of compensatory mechanisms which may be inappropriate fluid retention occurs, hypervolaemia results and oedema develops in the lungs or the peripheries. The rationale of treatment of cardiac failure is to improve the cardiac output and decrease the fluid retention. Digoxin is the drug which is used to improve cardiac output while diuretics are used to reverse fluid retention. These drugs are described in turn, and the treatment of cardiac failure is then discussed.

Digoxin
Digitalis and its derivatives have been used in therapeutics for many years. Their beneficial effects were apparent long before the mode of action was known, and there has for a long time been controversy over the exact action of digitalis on the heart. The actions and uses of digitalis have been the subject of a recent comprehensive review[24]. Digitalis has both a positive inotropic effect increasing the force of myocardial contraction and resulting in an increased car-

diac output, and a chronotropic effect resulting in slowing of the heart chiefly by impeding conduction between atria and ventricles through the specialized conducting tissue. The main action of digitalis is probably its ability to increase the force of myocardial contraction. The result of this is an increase in cardiac output, a decrease in heart size and venous pressure, and the heart performs more work at a given filling pressure. This inotropic effect is most apparent in the diseased heart and is more difficult to demonstrate in a normal heart. The effect of digitalis in slowing the heart rate is most marked in patients with atrial fibrillation. The reduction in cardiac rate which occurs in patients with cardiac failure, sinus rhythm, and a compensatory tachycardia may be secondary to the improvement of the circulation rather than being due to a primary therapeutic action of the drug. Digitalis does not appear to have a direct diuretic effect but may indirectly increase urinary output by improving cardiac output and hence renal blood flow.

Digoxin is rapidly absorbed by mouth but may also be given intramuscularly or intravenously. Intramuscular injection is painful and may result in muscle necrosis with a release of muscle enzymes which may cause confusion in the diagnosis of myocardial infarction[25]; intramuscular administration is therefore not recommended. About 60–85% of digoxin is absorbed from the gastrointestinal tract. It is rapidly distributed to the tissues and protein binding is minimal [26]. Its onset of action occurs between 15 and 30 min after intravenous administration, the peak effect being 1–5 hours. The normal plasma concentration is 0·8–1·6 ng/ml and the plasma half-life is 36 hours. Concentrations of more than 3 ng/ml are usually toxic. About 70% of the administered dose of digoxin is excreted unchanged by the kidney. Thus renal impairment, whether as a result of age or disease, impairs renal excretion of digoxin resulting in higher blood levels. Hence digoxin toxicity is more common in older subjects[27] and in those with renal disease, and the dose in these subjects has to be reduced. In the elderly, the same dose of digoxin results in a higher blood concentration and a longer half-life. This is due to the smaller body size and diminished urinary excretion of digoxin in old age[28]. Digoxin can be measured in the circulation by sensitive radioimmunoassays and the development of this technique has provided a large amount of new information in the pharmacokinetics of the drug. The therapeutic index of digoxin is low, levels which cause therapeutic effects being only a little lower than those causing toxic effects. Although it is often stated that the elderly heart is more sensitive to digoxin than the heart of younger subjects, it is not clear whether this is a true increase in cardiac sensitivity or whether it is due to the higher blood levels which may occur in older subjects given fixed doses of digoxin.

Toxic effects of digoxin are common and may be fatal. Among the earliest effects of overdose are gastrointestinal symptoms of anorexia, nausea and vomiting; abdominal discomfort and diarrhoea may also occur. The most serious toxic effects of digoxin occur in the heart. In general digitalis slows atrioventricular conduction and increases the irritability of the ventricular myocardium[24]. Almost every type of arrhythmia may occur as a complication of digitalis therapy, and an increasing severity of congestive cardiac failure may result from digitalis intoxication. The most serious and most common arrhythmias are ventricular in origin, the characteristic being coupled extra systoles producing pulsus bigeminus. Atrioventricular block either partial or complete may also occur; atrial tachycardia with atrioventricular block is an important arrhythmia produced by digoxin. Other toxic effects of digoxin include headache, fatigue, malaise and mental symptons including disorientation and confusion. Vision may be blurred, and colour vision can be disturbed. Digitalis intoxication can usually be diagnosed clinically and the diagnosis confirmed by measurement of digoxin levels in the blood, although an overlap in values in patients with and without toxicity has been reported[29]. Treatment of digitalis intoxication is by stopping the drug and administering potassium chloride to raise plasma potassium concentrations to the upper range of normal. Antiarrhythmic drugs may be used, beta-adrenoreceptor blocking agents probably being the most useful.

The advent of sensitive methods of measuring digitalis concentrations revealed that different commercial preparations of digoxin gave great variations on plasma concentrations of the drug. This seemed to be due to the physical characteristics of the tablets and changes in their dissolution rates. As a result there is a new description in the British Pharmacopoeia and digoxin tablets have to meet new standards. Nevertheless, it is worthwhile confining prescribing to one brand of digoxin so that its dose and the avoidance of toxic effects can become familiar. The use of other drugs especially those with actions on the gastrointestinal tract may also effect the bioavailability[30,31] or absorption[32] of digoxin.

Recently pharmacokinetic principles have been used to design a therapeutic regime for the use of digoxin in elderly patients[33]. It is suggested that in older patients with normal renal function (serum urea less than 12 mmol/l and creatinine less than 175 μmol/l) a starting dose of 0·5 mg should be given orally followed by a daily dose of 0·25 mg. If the renal function is impaired, then the maintainance dose should be 0·125 mg/day. It is the maintenance dose that determines the likelihood of toxic effects from digoxin.

There is some controversy as to the place of digoxin in the treatment of cardiac failure as modern potent diuretics often remove all signs and symptoms of fluid retention on their own[34]. With the present state of knowledge it is not possible to make definite statements about the relative values of digoxin and diuretics and no long-term trials have taken place comparing the use of digoxin and diuretics on the health and survival of patients with cardiac failure. Thus problems with toxic effects, convenience and patient acceptability are factors which must be taken into consideration. Digoxin is a relatively safe drug if used properly and in correct dose. Unpredictable events may occur, of course, and the patient on correct dose may develop renal impairment and hence toxic effects. Digoxin is easy to take, needs only be taken once daily and in the absence of toxic effects produces no uncomfortable or inconvenient symptoms. Although perhaps the more beneficial effects of digoxin are found in patients who have both atrial fibrillation and cardiac failure, the drug is also beneficial when sinus rhythm is present. Digoxin is useful regardless of whether the cardiac failure is left or right-sided or involves both sides of the heart. Atrial fibrillation and atrial flutter without cardiac failure are also treated with digoxin. A recent myocardial infarction is not a contraindication provided the digoxin is used carefully and in normal doses. In patients with angina, who are in early cardiac failure, digoxin may improve the coronary circulation by improving heart action and hence relieve the pain. Digoxin is not effective in heart disease associated with hyperthyroidism unless the thyroid condition is also treated. In partial heart block digoxin may cause complete heart block and it should not be used in patients with ventricular arrhythmia.

It was often taught in the past that once patients were started on digoxin they had to continue to take the drug for the rest of their lives. However, it is now clear that this is not necessarily true and that digoxin can be discontinued, even in older patients, without untoward effects[35,36]. Thus, if a patient has a short episode of cardiac failure or cardiac arrhythmia which is successfully treated with digoxin and the condition remits, it is worthwhile attempting to withdraw the drug under careful supervision. In a large proportion of patients the drug can be successfully withdrawn.

Diuretics
There are a large number of diuretics available[37,38]. These act in different ways and on different parts of the nephron but in general

they cause salt excretion accompanied by water loss. The individual classes of commonly used diuretic drugs will be considered separately and then the unwanted effects and uses will be discussed.

Loop diuretics

These are sometimes called 'high ceiling diuretics' and are the most potent diuretics. They are thought to exert their action on the ascending limb of the loop of Henle inhibiting sodium and chloride reabsorption and hence causing salt and water loss. Potassium and magnesium excretion is also increased. The three drugs in this group are frusemide, ethacrynic acid and bumetanide. These diuretics are usually given orally when they are readily absorbed from the gastrointestinal tract, bound to plasma proteins and rapidly excreted in the urine. They may also be given parenterally. Their onset of action is rapid, within 1 hour of oral dose and 2–10 min of an intravenous injection, and the diuresis is of large volume and of short duration. Unwanted effects are similar to those of the thiazide diuretics. Loop diuretics are most useful in treating patients in the acute stage of cardiac failure, particularly left ventricular failure, when relief of symptoms is usually rapid. These very powerful drugs should be reserved for acute severe cardiac failure and, when this stage has passed, less potent diuretics should be used for maintenance treatment.

Thiazide diuretics

Thiazide diuretics (benzothiadiazides) have been used in medicine for many years. There is a large number of preparations which differ little in action. Thiazides act on the distal convoluted tubule of the nephron preventing sodium reabsorption and hence resulting in a sodium chloride and water diuresis. They are rapidly absorbed from the gastrointestinal tract and are bound to plasma proteins. Potassium and magnesium excretion is also increased. Although the onset of action is rapid it is delayed compared to that of the loop diuretics and the duration of action is much longer. Hence they cause a more gentle but more prolonged diuresis although the total volume of the diuresis may be as great as that with loop diuretics. Thiazides also have a small but significant hypotensive effect. This appears to be mediated on the arterioles and may be related to sodium flux across the cell walls of the smooth muscle of these vessels. The loop diuretics also have a hypotensive effect but this is not correspondingly more potent than that of the thiazide diuretics. The thiazide diuretics are useful in mild or moderate cardiac failure and as maintenance therapy after a short spell of treatment with the loop diuretics.

Spironolactone
This diuretic inhibits the action of aldosterone on the distal convuluted tubule presumably by competing for aldosterone receptor sites. Aldosterone causes sodium retention and potassium excretion. Spironolactone thus results in sodium excretion and potassium retention. It is not a potent diuretic on its own but has an additive effect when combined with loop or thiazide diuretics. This is probably because the other diuretics, by means of their action earlier on the nephron, result in presentation to the distal convuluted tubule of fluid high in sodium. In the presence of spironolactone the sodium is not reabsorbed, hence the diuresis is potentiated. The potassium-retaining effects of spironolactone counteract the potassium-losing effects of the loop and thiazide diuretics. Spironolactone is most useful in conditions where there is a rise in aldosterone secretion, which commonly occurs in oedema due to hepatic disease or the nephrotic syndrome. Hyperaldosteronism does not occur in acute uncomplicated cardiac failure but may in chronic cardiac failure particularly in subjects who have been under intensive diuretic therapy. In these circumstances the diuretic effect of loop and thiazide diuretics is reduced, but the diuresis can be restarted with the help of spironolactone. Potassium supplements should not be used in patients taking spironolactone as hyperkalaemia may result.

Other diuretics
Triamterine is a mild diuretic which acts on the distal convoluted tubule to cause sodium and chloride loss and potassium retention. It is of low potency used on its own but in combination with thiazide diuretics it results in an adequate diuresis and obviates the need for potassium supplements. Amiloride is another diuretic causing mild sodium loss from the distal convoluted tubule and potassium retention. Again it is most often used in combination with thiazide diuretics. Carbonic anhydrase inhibitors, such as acetazolamide, are very mild diuretics and are now used almost solely in the treatment of glaucoma.

Complications of diuretic therapy

Toxic effects
Gastrointestinal disturbances, blood dyscrasias, skin rashes and hepatic dysfunction may occur with all the diuretics. With loop and thiazide diuretics hyperglycaemia and hyperuricaemia may occur. Deafness may be a rare complication of ethacrynic acid, and it

should not be used if a potentially ototoxic antibiotic is used as well. The glomerular filtration rate may be decreased by loop and thiazide diuretics and hepatic failure may be aggravated.

Potassium loss
The most commonly used loop and thiazide diuretics cause potassium excretion. This may result in profound hypokalaemia with symptoms of weakness and ultimately paralysis. With most diuretics the magnitude of potassium loss is unpredictable. If the patient is on digoxin as well as diuretics the hypokalaemia may cause increased cardiac sensitivity to digoxin resulting in dangerous arrhythmias. However, increased sensitivity of the heart to digoxin in the presence of hypokalaemia has recently been questioned[39]. To prevent hypokalaemia potassium supplements are usually given with these diuretics and their use is discussed below. Magnesium depletion may also sensitize the heart to digoxin[26].

Sodium loss
Although most diuretics act by causing sodium excretion it is only recently that the effects of excess sodium loss on the circulatory system have been studied. Sodium loss with its accompanying fluid loss results in hypovolaemia and this can cause postural or sustained hypotension. This is probably more common than was previously realized and indeed it may be that the problems from sodium loss in elderly patients on diuretic therapy may be more serious than the problems from potassium loss. In intensive long-term therapy the diuretic-induced renal loss of sodium chloride may lead to extracellular dehydration with or without hyponatraemia. The condition usually responds to discontinuation of the diuretic agent and the elimination of sodium chloride from the diet. Another complication is chronic dilutional hyponatraemia which is associated with persistent oedema and expanded extracellular volume. It may occur as a result of severe cardiac failure itself but is more often a consequence of diuretic therapy. Treatment is by water restriction and perhaps a short course of a corticosteroid.

Side-effects of diuretics which are particularly important in the elderly
The primary action of diuretics in increasing urinary output causes inconvenient and antisocial side-effects in patients of all ages. These effects may cause particular difficulties in elderly patients. The fact that the patient has to be able to reach a toilet rapidly at the time the diuretics are working may be socially inconvenient in younger

patients and may interfere with work. In older patients impaired mobility, poor eyesight and mental impairment may make it difficult to cope with an increased urinary output. The diuresis stresses the bladder's capacity and stresses the ability of the brain to inhibit bladder emptying. If these factors are already compromised then the increase in urinary output caused by potent diuretics may overcome the impaired bladder control mechanism. Thus, diuretics are an important cause of incontinence in elderly people for two reasons, lack of mobility, and impaired inhibition of bladder emptying. Diuretics may also precipitate acute urinary retention in elderly men with enlarged prostrates who are just able to manage a normal urinary output. Thus the urinary symptoms which are common in elderly patients may be made worse by diuretics and their use has to be more carefully considered in older than in younger patients. It may be more beneficial for a patient to remain continent but to have swollen ankles than to have no oedema and to be incontinent. Postural hypotension resulting from sodium and water loss may also be a cause of considerable problems in the elderly resulting in falls with perhaps injury and disability.

Because mental impairment is relatively common in old age, accurate compliance with a complicated diuretic regime may be a problem. Potassium supplements, usually in the form of large tablets, are often omitted with a consequent risk of hypokalaemia. Occasionally the reverse may occur with the diuretic being omitted while the potassium continues to be taken. If fluid intake is reduced, or excessive loss of fluid from vomiting or diarrhoea occurs, continued administration of a diuretic may cause severe dehydration and hence precipitate or worsen confusion. Patients or their relatives are sometimes so indoctrinated in the importance of adhering to treatment regimes that drugs continue to be taken despite marked changes in the patient's condition.

Potassium supplements
Potassium supplements are frequently given with diuretics to counteract the potassium loss which occurs with most of the more potent diuretic drugs. The potassium is often given separately from the diuretic but preparations in which the diuretic is combined with potassium in one tablet are also available. These, however, have the disadvantage that the dose of potassium cannot be varied independently from the dose of the diuretic. The amount of potassium incorporated in these combined preparations is also relatively small. An alternative is to give the potassium supplement as a separate preparation. This has the disadvantage that the patient often has to

take many large tablets, and that either the diuretic or the potassium may be taken and the other preparation omitted. To be effective the potassium has to be in the form of potassium chloride, though potassium chloride solutions are unpalatable and potassium chloride tablets cause gastrointestinal ulceration. Special preparations of potassium have thus been made, including slow-release potassium chloride and effervescent potassium chloride.

Recently the potassium status of patients on diuretic therapy has been studied by a number of investigators. In patients with hypertension but no cardiac failure, it was found that frusemide had very little effect on total body potassium[40]. No depletion of total body potassium was found in any of the groups on diuretics whether or not they were given potassium supplements. The requirement for potassium supplementation was questioned in such patients although, of course, the situation in patients with cardiac failure may well be different. None of the patients in the study were in the older age groups, the oldest being 69. Total body potassium in relation to fat free mass was studied in 19 elderly patients receiving diuretics and potassium supplements for cardiac failure and in 13 elderly controls [41]. The total body potassium to fat free mass ratio was reduced in the patients, and was negatively correlated with age but not plasma potassium or the dose of potassium supplements. It was suggested that age influences potassium status and that diuretics and cardiac failure have a greater effect on total body potassium in old age than in youth or middle age. However, the independent effects of diuretics and cardiac failure were not studied nor is it clear whether potassium supplements have any influence on the potassium status in these patients. It seems from the evidence available that cardiac failure itself reduces total body potassium, perhaps by the effects of anoxia on cell membranes but it is not clear that diuretics necessarily have an additive effect or that potassium supplements are effective in counteracting the potassium-reducing effects of cardiac failure[42–44].

Not only is there doubt about the effectiveness of potassium supplements in patients on diuretic therapy, but potassium supplements themselves may be responsible for adverse reactions. In the Boston Collaborative Drug Surveillance Program[45], 4921 patients receiving potassium chloride were studied; 30% had cardiovascular disease and 9% had hepatic disease. In 87% the indication for potassium supplements was prophylaxis and in 12% it was electrolyte depletion. 5·8% of the patients had adverse reactions attributed to potassium chloride. Hyperkalaemia was the most common side-effect, occurring in 3·6% of patients; gastrointestinal disturbances occurred in 1·6% The adverse effects of potassium chloride were judged to have contributed to the death of seven patients, to have threatened the lives of a further 21, and to have produced a major or moderate morbidity in another 29. The frequency of hyperkalaemia was significantly related to age, the starting indication and the blood urea. Hyperkalaemia was not reported in any of 170 patients who received potassium-sparing diuretics in the absence of other diuretics or potassium supplements. Of patients receiving potassium-depleting diuretics without potassium supplements or other diuretics, 4·9% developed hypokalaemia but in no case was this life-threatening nor did it lead to a fatal outcome. This study suggested that potassium depletion from diuretic therapy was not a serious hazard, but that potassium supplements may cause dangerous hyperkalaemia.

The evidence available at present does not allow a definite conclusion to be reached on the requirements and hazards of potassium supplements in elderly patients receiving diuretic therapy for cardiac failure. Elderly patients are relatively potassium-depleted compared to younger patients and cardiac failure results in further potassium depletion. The influence of diuretics themselves on total body potassium status is not clear nor is it clear that potassium supplements influence potassium status significantly. Side-effects of potassium supplements are also more common in elderly patients. This may be related to the impairment of renal function which is common in old age. On the other hand detailed studies of potassium status in elderly patients with cardiac failure have not been carried out and the possible detrimental effect of hypokalaemia in patients receiving digitalis must be considered. In practice, therefore, it seems advisable that patients on potent diuretics should be under close supervision, preferably in hospital, and that potassium supplements should be used judiciously in these patients with close monitoring of plasma potassium and blood urea. Patients who do not require hospitalization probably do not need the most potent diuretics, and in these a mild diuretic with potassium supplementation may be adequate, or a combined preparation of a potassium-depleting and a potassium-sparing diuretic, such as a thiazide combined with triamterene or amiloride.

Treatment of cardiac failure

The diagnosis of cardiac failure involves the identification of two factors – the cardiac failure itself and the cause of the failure. In a patient with acute cardiac failure, whether left ventricular failure or congestive cardiac failure, immediate treatment does not depend on the cause. However, if the cause or precipitating factor is reversible, only temporary support for the circulation will be necessary, and once the cause is adequately treated, therapy for cardiac failure can probably be discontinued. Examples of reversible causes and precipitating factors are anaemia, thyrotoxicosis and respiratory tract infection. If the cause of the cardiac failure is an acute myocardial infarction, cardiac performance will often improve with healing of the infarct and long-term maintenance treatment may not be necessary. If the cause is permanent damage to the myocardium from ischaemic or other heart disease, continuing maintenance therapy will be required.

In acute cardiac failure, particularly if pulmonary oedema is present, the first drug of choice is a loop diuretic, frusemide or bumetanide. These drugs are usually given intravenously in these circumstances, although oral administration also results in a very rapid diuresis. Other measures such as bedrest, oxygen, and sedation must be prescribed. Treatment is continued with regular daily oral doses of the chosen diuretic, usually with potassium supplements, and with careful monitoring of plasma potassium and blood urea, until all signs of cardiac failure have disappeared. Treatment is then changed to a milder thiazide diuretic[46], which will often be given in a combined preparation with a potassium-sparing diuretic, such as triamterene or amiloride. The advantage of this type of preparation is that it reduces the number of tablets the patient is taking. This is particularly important in the elderly who are often taking a number of drugs and whose ability to remember the treatment regime may be impaired. It ensures that the correct dose of both drugs is taken and that the diuretic is not taken without any potassium or vice versa. The duration of bedrest depends on the patient's response to the treatment. Sitting in a chair is as restful as lying in bed and is often more comfortable. Prolonged immobility is deleterious to older patients and should be avoided except in prolonged and very severe cardiac failure.

The question as to whether or when to add digoxin to the treatment regime cannot be answered with certainty. It appears that, despite the primary role of cardiac disease in congestive cardiac failure, when oedema is mobilized by diuretic drugs an improvement in myocardial performance occurs. Thus diuretic drugs benefit total cardiac status. In the initial stages of cardiac failure, particularly if the heart is in sinus rhythm, many physicians will treat cardiac failure with diuretics alone. If the response is not adequate, digoxin will be added. On the other hand, the underlying abnormality in cardiac failure is an inadequate cardiac performance and it seems logical to employ the positive inotropic properties of digoxin when the patient's condition is at its worst. If rapid atrial fibrillation is present then digoxin should always be used. Thus, having established that the patient is not already taking digoxin, digitalization should be carried out early in the patient's illness.

If maintenance treatment is required consideration must be given as to whether digoxin or a diuretic is more desirable. This depends on the general condition of the patient, particularly with regard to his mental function and to his urinary system, and on the amount of supervision that can be reliably given. It is probable that in elderly patients maintenance treatment with a small dose of digoxin is preferable to the prolonged use of diuretics. Used properly, digoxin does not cause unpleasant symptoms and toxicity should not be a problem. If maintenance diuretic therapy is used it is important to review regularly the need for its continuation in patients who have recovered from cardiac failure. If the patient is symptom-free, supervised withdrawal of the diuretic may be attempted, and in a proportion of patients withdrawal will be permanent[47]. Similarly, digoxin may be successfully withdrawn from a proportion of patients in sinus rhythm[35,36].

When cardiac failure is secondary to lung disease, cor pulmonale, the principles of treatment are essentially the same. The lung disease, usually an infective exacerbation of chronic obstructive airways disease, is treated with an appropriate antibiotic, bronchodilators and controlled oxygen. Treatment of the lung disease will result in an improvement in cardiac function. The cardiac failure can be helped further by diuretic therapy. Digoxin is often not required in cor pulmonale and may be less effective than in cardiac failure from other causes.

Assessment of treatment
The response to treatment of cardiac failure can be measured by standard clinical methods. Reduction of venous pressure, clearance of pleural effusions and crepitations from the lung bases, decrease in the extent of oedema, and in severe cases, reduction in the length and intensity of a basal systolic murmur and in the intensity of a third heart sound are all evidence of improvement in cardiac performance and reduction in fluid overload. The extent of the diuresis can be measured by charting the fluid intake and output, or less directly but more conveniently by weighing the patient. Repeated chest X-rays will confirm the clearing of pulmonary oedema and of fluid in the pleural space.

Failure to respond

Despite the prescription of optimum treatment, some patients with cardiac failure will not improve. There are a number of reasons why this may occur and steps should be taken to identify and if possible correct these factors.

The first point to be considered is whether the patient is actually taking the drugs prescribed. Theoretically this should not be a problem if the patient is in hospital, although determined patients can overcome the best designed arrangements for the administration of drugs. Outside hospital, failure of compliance is a major problem. Recent studies in Belfast[48] on compliance of patients prescribed digoxin, using plasma drug levels as an indicator of compliance, revealed that 48% of patients admitted as medical emergencies were taking their digoxin improperly, the majority (41%) taking less than the prescribed dose. Similarly, 46% of patients prescribed digoxin by their general practitioners were not taking the prescribed dose. The patient's history of compliance did not relate to the plasma drug levels. Overall, between 40 and 50% of patients prescribed digoxin appear not to take it properly, and around 10% may not take it at all. There is no reason to believe that similar figures do not apply to other drugs. Indeed the unpleasant and antisocial effects of diuretics might be expected to reduce compliance for these drugs even further. In patients outside hospital it is likely that failure to take the prescribed drugs is a major, if not the major, cause of failure to respond to treatment. Methods of improving compliance have been suggested[49] but the value of these is not yet clear. Thus if the patient is not responding as expected, enquiry into compliance should be the first step. Measurement of the plasma digoxin level 6 hours after the last dose may be useful. If the level is below the therapeutic range, either the dose is too low or the patient is not taking the drug as prescribed. If the dose seems to be appropriate for the patient's size, age and renal function, then poor compliance is likely to be the explanation for the low plasma levels. If this is the case, raising the dose will be ineffective if compliance remains poor, and may produce toxic levels if compliance improves.

A second reason for failure to improve is incorrect use of drugs. The dose or preparation of the diuretic may be incorrect. If renal function is impaired, a thiazide diuretic may be ineffective and substituting a loop diuretic may induce a diuresis[46]. If the patient has had longstanding diuretic therapy for cardiac failure secondary hyperaldosteronism may have occurred, and the addition of spironolactone to the regime may result in an improved diuresis. Electrolyte abnormalities, particularly hyponatraemia, may have complicated intensive diuretic therapy or severe circulatory failure. In these circumstances, stopping diuretic therapy, reducing water intake, and perhaps giving a short course of a corticosteroid may correct the electrolyte abnormality and allow diuretic therapy to be recommenced.

If the patient fails to respond, the diagnosis should always be reviewed, and complicating diseases sought. It may be difficult to distinguish widespread bronchopneumonia from pulmonary oedema. Dependent oedema in the elderly may be due to local abnormalities in the legs, and treatment for cardiac failure will be both inappropriate and ineffective. Anaemia, thyrotoxicosis, infective endocarditis, pulmonary embolism and Paget's disease of bone may precipitate or complicate cardiac failure and should be sought.

Lastly, the patient may have such extensive damage to the myocardium that despite optimum therapy the heart is incapable of sustaining a normal cardiac output or of maintaining a normal venous pressure. This will be a terminal event in many elderly people. This diagnosis should not be made until the correctable factors mentioned above have been excluded. However, when this diagnosis has been made, treatment should principally be directed towards the patient's comfort and dignity.

It is important that failure to respond should not be diagnosed too readily in older patients. Elderly people with severe heart disease may respond to treatment very slowly, and may gradually recover over a period of many weeks. Having reassured himself that the diagnosis is correct, that the prescribed treatment is appropriate and that compliance is adequate the physician should resist the temptation to make unnecessary changes in therapy. Patience, encouragement and continued rest, but not complete immobility, will frequently result in a slow but steady improvement with an eventual satisfactory result.

INFECTIVE ENDOCARDITIS

The age incidence of infective endocarditis is changing and a larger proportion of cases is now found in older people[50]. Older subjects with this disease often have atypical features and this may result in delay in diagnosis and a high mortality rate. Often the precipitating cause may not be found and in older people the source of infection may not be the mouth. Disorders of the gall bladder, colon, urinary and respiratory systems may all be sources of infection. Organisms involved include, as well as *Streptococcus viridans*, *Streptococcus faecalis* and other non-haemolytic streptococci, *Staphylococcus pyogenes* and *Escherichia coli*. Even organisms which are often thought to be contaminants, such as *Staphylococcus albus*, may cause infective endocarditis in older people. In the elderly, rheumatic valve disease is not always present and a heart damaged by ischaemia may be the site of endocarditis.

The possibility of infective endocarditis must be kept in mind when dealing with obscure pyrexia in an older patient especially in the presence of a heart murmur. However, even the fever and heart murmur may be absent. The diagnosis is made by culturing the organism from the blood. About six blood cultures should be taken in fairly rapid succession and need not coincide with the presence of pyrexia or with symptoms. In addition to bacteria, coxiella which causes Q fever, or chlamydia which causes psittacosis may also cause infective endocarditis[51]. These organisms do not grow on blood culture. In patients with bacterial infection who have already received an antibiotic the results of blood cultures may be persistently negative and drug treatment has to be based on clinical judgement.

Clinical diagnosis depends on recognizing the classical triad: signs of infection, signs of embolism and signs of a heart disorder[51]. Infective endocarditis occurs in three clinical groups[52], medical infective endocarditis, endocarditis in patients who have undergone cardiac surgery, and infective endocarditis in drug addicts. Only the first of these is likely to be relevant in the older age groups although cardiac surgery is becoming increasingly common in older patients.

Treatment
Treatment should begin as soon as the clinical diagnosis has been made and blood cultures have been taken. The choice of drugs and the duration of treatment depends on[52]:

(a)   The infecting organism;
(b)   The duration of symptoms before treatment started;
(c)   The rapidity of the patient's clinical response;
(d)   Whether the patient has had a prosthetic valve or other foreign material within the heart.

The minimum period of treatment is 3 weeks but if the patient has an artificial valve he should be treated for at least 6 weeks. The antibiotic chosen should always be bactericidal towards the isolated infecting organism and the peak plasma concentration should be at least six times the *in vitro* minimum lethal concentration. Treatment should aim at achieving high peak concentrations of the antibiotic, and parenteral treatment will usually be more effective than oral treatment. It is better to inject antibiotics as a bolus through the side arm of an intravenous needle or subclavian venous line than to add the antibiotic to the infusion bottle[52]. The exceptions are aminoglycosides which should be given intramuscularly to avoid toxicity. Indwelling cannulae in leg or arm veins should be avoided because of slow venous return and a high risk of phlebitis with secondary infection often resistant to the antibiotics given.

In most patients, treatment should begin with penicillin G 10 – 20 mega units every 24 hours combined with an aminoglycoside such as gentamicin in a dose appropriate to the patient's age and renal function. If the blood culture grows *Streptococcus viridans*, penicillin alone should be effective and the aminoglycoside can be stopped. However there is some evidence from animal experiments that a combination of penicillin and gentamycin eliminates *Streptococcus viridans* more rapidly from cardiac vegetations than penicillin alone (see Chapter 2). It may therefore be preferable to continue the combination for 3–6 weeks. If gentamycin is used the dose should be monitored by blood levels and the peaks should not exceed 14 mg/ml nor be less than 5 mg/ml. *Streptococcus faecalis* is resistant to penicillin or streptomicin alone but ampicillin or a combination of penicillin and streptomycin is effective. In staphylococcal endocarditis penicillin may be ineffective and if so cloxacillin or flucloxacillin should be used in combination with fusidic acid.

If the blood culture reports are negative, the most likely cause is recent administration of antibiotics. If this has occurred, diagnosis may have to be based solely on the clinical features. In these circumstances treatment with penicillin and an aminoglycoside is appropriate. In the absence of bacteriological proof, the diagnosis of infective endocarditis and the decision to start a prolonged course of treatment is difficult. However, once the decision has been made, it is essential that it is carried to completion and that treatment is not prematurely discontinued. *Coxiella* or *Chlamydia* infections are other causes of culture-negative endocarditis and are diagnosed by serological testing. Tetracycline is the drug of choice. Fungal endocarditis is usually caused by *Candida* but *Aspergillus* and other fungi may also occur. Fungal endocarditis most often occurs in patients with intravascular catheters who are receiving steroids, broad-spectrum antibiotics or cytotoxic agents[52]. Parenteral feeding of debilitated patients who are also receiving antibiotics carries the risk of conveying secondary fungal infection. Blood cultures are often sterile and antifungal chemotherapy with amphotericin B or flucytosine is difficult because of hepatic toxicity and because these drugs may not eradicate the infection. It is important that once the diagnosis of infected endocarditis has been made that the treatment course should be completed, and that improvement in the patients clinical condition should not result in premature cessation of antibiotic therapy.

Surgical treatment may be needed because of acute haemodynamic catastrophies particularly acute aortic regurgitation and less often acute mitral regurgitation. If a prosthesis has become infected particularly with fungi or *Coxiella*, surgery may be the only way to eliminate the infection.

Prevention
Administration of antibiotics to patients with valvular heart disease at times when bacteraemia is common prevents the development of infective endocarditis. Recently, prophylaxis of endocarditis has been reviewed by Durack[53] and the following regimes recommended. For dental manipulation, benzylpenicillin 2 000 000 units plus procaine penicillin 600 000 units plus streptomycin 1·0 g i.m. muscularly 30 min before the procedure. An alternative regime is vancomycin 1·0 g i.v. 5 min before the procedure. For urethral, gynaecological and other abdominal procedures, ampicillin 1·0 g plus gentamicin 80 mg i.m. 30 min before the procedure, both repeated 8 and 16 hours later. An alternative regime is cephazolin 1 g plus gentamicin 80 mg i.m. 30 min before the procedure, both repeated 8 and 16 hours later. Experimental evidence indicates that bacterial endocarditis can be prevented by antibiotics provided the most effective drugs are given at the appropriate time.

PULMONARY EMBOLISM AND DEEP VEIN THROMBOSIS

The clinical diagnosis of deep vein thrombosis is unreliable and special investigations using isotope scanning, doppler, or radiological techniques are necessary to obtain a correct idea of the frequency of this condition[54]. The recent development of simple techniques for detecting venous thrombosis in the leg have made possible studies on the use of anticoagulants in the prevention of this condition. A high incidence of clinically undetected venous thrombosis has been reported in all these studies. Although pulmonary embolism is not found in the absence of venous thrombosis, the risk of developing a pulmonary embolus when a deep vein thrombosis has occurred is unknown[54]. Pulmonary embolism is also not always correctly diagnosed and the symptoms and signs may be interpreted as an infective process.

There is little published information specifically dealing with pulmonary embolism and deep vein thrombosis in the older subjects. Nevertheless it would be expected that these conditions would occur with increasing frequency in the elderly as conditions which predispose to venous thrombosis in the legs themselves tend to occur more frequently with increasing age. An incidence of deep vein thrombosis as assessed by fibrinogen leg scanning of 60% in one study[55] and 45% in another[56] has been reported in stroke. Immobility from various causes, fracture, distortion of leg veins resulting from osteoarthrosis of the knees, myocardial infarction and surgery to the lower limb, particularly for reduction of fractures or for osteoarthrosis, all predispose to deep vein thrombosis.

The drugs used in both prevention and treatment of venous thromboembolism are anticoagulants. In practice only two anticoagulants need to be considered: heparin, a rapidly acting anticoagulant which has to be given by injection, and warfarin, a coumarin drug which is given orally and which acts much less rapidly than heparin.

Heparin
Heparin acts by increasing the activity of the naturally occurring alpha-2-globulin, antithrombin III heparin cofactor. Trace amounts of heparin may increase this factor 50–100-fold. Heparin and the cofactor act together to inhibit activated factor X and hence inhibit the formation of thrombin from prothrombin and thus the formation of fibrin from fibrinogen. Heparin also inhibits platelet aggregation[57].

Heparin's electronegative charge appears to have an important role in its activity and drugs such as protamine sulphate, which neutralize this charge, counteract the anticoagulant effect of heparin. As well as its anticoagulant effects, heparin has an unrelated effect of liberating lipoprotein lipase into the circulation with a resultant increase in the blood's lipolytic activity. Heparin circulates bound to plasma albumin, is inactivated in the liver and excreted in the urine as uroheparin. In conditions where albumin levels are low, binding will be diminished and hence heparin will be relatively more potent. Side-effects of heparin include excess bleeding and rarely, diarrhoea, alopecia, hypersensitivity reactions, and, with prolonged use, osteoporosis. The pharmacokinetics of heparin have not been specifically studied in the elderly. However, heparin therapy is normally controlled by the whole blood clotting time (Lee–White) rather than being given as a fixed dose, and thus any changes in sensitivity or handling of the drug resulting from age will be taken into account.

Heparin is given in two ways: in large doses intravenously for the treatment of patients who have had a pulmonary embolus or a deep vein thrombosis, or in small doses as a prophylaxis against thromboembolic disease.

High-dose heparin treatment is given by means of a constant infusion pump, or is added to an intravenous infusion of dextrose or saline: 10 000–12 500 units are given in 12 hours. Alternatively, heparin may be given as intermittent intravenous injections with an initial dose of 12 500 units followed by 10 000 units every 4 hours. The dose is adjusted to maintain the whole blood clotting time at two to three times the pretreatment value. If hypersensitivity to heparin is suspected a test dose of 1000 units may be given. Preparations of sodium heparin and calcium heparin are available and appear to have similar effects. Heparin may be used as the sole anticoagulant but the disadvantages of prolonged intravenous therapy usually mean that only a short course is given. If prolonged anticoagulation is required, heparin is given for 3 – 4 days while the anticoagulant effect of warfarin is developing.

Heparin may also be given subcutaneously in small doses as a prophylactic measure against deep vein thrombosis in patients who are predisposed to this condition[58]. A number of trials have been carried out on the use of prophylactic heparin in patients undergoing surgery. The doses of heparin used are insufficient to cause bleeding problems for the surgeon and appear to be effective in reducing the incidence of venous thrombosis and fatal pulmonary embolism[59]. The advocates of this treatment recommend that all patients undergoing surgery or other immobilization procedures should be given heparin, starting shortly before the operation and continuing for a variable period after the operation. It is not entirely clear yet as to how long the heparin has to be continued after the operation. In the majority of cases heparin is given as 5000 units 2 hours before operation and after operation 5000 units twice or thrice daily until mobilization has occurred. Low-dose heparin has also been used as a prophylaxis against deep vein thrombosis after acute stroke[60]; 5000 units of calcium heparin given 8 hourly subcutaneously for 14 days was associated with a reduction in positive leg scans from 75% to 12·5%. In the untreated group the mean time for the scans to become positive was 5·6 days. The influence of heparin on the development of pulmonary embolism or on the functional recovery from the stroke was not assessed. Apart from haematomata at injection sites, bleeding from low dose heparin regimes, even at operation, has not been a problem.

Low-dose heparin therapy has been shown to be effective in reducing deep vein thrombosis after myocardial infarction, stroke and surgery. It does not have troublesome side-effects, and appears to be well tolerated. No laboratory control is necessary. The available evidence would suggest that patients at risk of deep vein thrombosis should be given low-dose heparin until mobilization has occurred. Nevertheless a recent survey has shown that many orthopaedic surgeons did not use prophylactic measures against venous thromboembolism in patients with hip fractures[61]. There appears to be still a considerable potential for prevention of venous thromboembolism particularly in elderly patients.

Warfarin

For longer-term anticoagulation, the orally administered coumarin or inandione drugs are used. However, only the most commonly used oral anticoagulant, warfarin, will be considered in detail here.

Warfarin acts on the liver to depress vitamin K-dependent synthesis of factors II (prothrombin), III, IX and X. It is readily absorbed from the gastrointestinal tract and circulates bound to plasma albumin. It is metabolized by the liver, and the metabolites are excreted in the urine.

The most important unwanted effect of warfarin is haemorrhage, usually presenting as epistaxis or haematuria, although bleeding from any source will be worse in patients taking the drug. When haemorrhage occurs the warfarin has usually been administered in excessive amounts. The effects of warfarin may be counteracted by phytomenadione (vitamin K) which may be given orally in a dose of 2–20 mg or by slow intravenous infusion. Stimulation of hepatic prothrombin synthesis by vitamin K is not instantaneous, and if the haemorrhage is severe, blood transfusion may be required.

Two aspects of the pharmacology of warfarin are subject to variation with age – hepatic metabolism and plasma protein binding. The enzymatic degradation of warfarin in the liver may be accelerated by drugs which cause enzyme induction, including barbiturates and glutethemide. However, there is evidence that hepatic enzyme induction is less active in the elderly[19] and hence effects of other drugs on warfarin's activity are likely to be limited in older patients. The drugs which cause enzyme induction are also less likely to be prescribed to elderly patients. Recent evidence has also suggested an increase in hepatic sensitivity to warfarin in older subjects[62].

In a study on changes in warfarin binding to plasma proteins with increasing age[16] it was found that there was a very close correlation between the maximum warfarin binding sites and plasma albumin. It was also found that the maximum plasma binding of the warfarin was significantly lower in a group of older subjects than in a group of younger subjects. However, the mean plasma albumin was also significantly lower in the older subjects. It appeared that the affinity of albumin for warfarin was not changed by age and that it was the effect of age on plasma albumin levels that reduced the amount of bound warfarin. Warfarin will also be displaced from plasma albumin by occupation of the binding sites by other protein bound drugs. The effect of reduced binding would be to allow more free drug to be available at any moment for distribution to other body tissues. This would at least transiently enhance the effect of the drug whether it is active before or after metabolic transformation. As warfarin is highly bound, only 1% being in the free form at therapeutic concentrations, a reduction of only 1% in the bound fraction from 99% to 98% doubles the amount of drug available for pharmacological activity[22].

Thus there are several reasons why elderly people are more sensitive to warfarin and why lower doses should be used. However, warfarin is not prescribed in a fixed-dose regime but its activity is controlled by measurement of the prothrombin time, and hence any effect of age or plasma albumin on its activity will result in appropriate adjustment of the dose.

In adults warfarin is normally given as a loading dose of 25–30 mg, usually 10 mg/day for 3 days. However in view of the increased sensitivity of older people to warfarin smaller doses should probably be used, such as 10 mg/day for 2 days or 5 mg/day for 3 days. The prothrombin time is checked on the fourth day and the dose is then tailored to keep the prothrombin time two to two-and-a-half times the control value. Although warfarin is normally given orally, it may also be administered intramuscularly or intravenously; if parenteral anticoagulants have to be used, heparin is usually chosen.

The length of time for which patients who have had deep vein thrombosis or pulmonary embolism should remain on anticoagulants is not known. Usually an arbitrary time of about 3 months is chosen for a first episode, and 6–12 months for recurrent episodes. The anticoagulant is then gradually withdrawn to prevent the rebound hypercoagulation which may occur on sudden withdrawal of the drug.

Arterial thrombosis and embolism

While there is widespread agreement that anticoagulants have beneficial effects on venous thromboembolic disease, the effects on arterial thromboembolism are much less certain. Embolism from intracardiac thrombi in the left atrium in association with mitral stenosis and atrial fibrillation, or in the left ventricle in association with a myocardial infarction, may be prevented by anticoagulation. It has recently been suggested that the risk of embolism from a mural thrombus in the left ventricle is only significant if the myocardial infarction is large as judged by the serum creatinine phosphokinase level, and that anticoagulants should be reserved for this situation[63].

Transient cerebral ischaemic attacks are caused by microemboli composed of fibrin and platelets which originate from atheromatous plaques in the extracranial arteries. While warfarin prevents microemboli, recent attention has been focused on drugs which inhibit platelet aggregation in the hope that these drugs – which include aspirin, dipyridamole and sulphinpyrazone – will prevent emboli without causing bleeding. There is evidence that the use of aspirin in patients with transient cerebral ischaemic attacks reduces the frequency of the attacks although the effect on the incidence of stroke was less marked[64]. Sulphinpyrazone has been shown to be effective in preventing death following myocardial infarction but this aspect requires further investigation[65].

CARDIAC SURGERY IN OLDER PATIENTS

Rheumatic valvular heart disease is a condition which first becomes manifest in early life and which usually has its maximum effects in middle age. However, a proportion of patients with rheumatic heart disease will remain asymptomatic until old age when problems may develop. The condition of patients who had cardiac surgery earlier in life may deteriorate again and further surgery may be required. Calcific aortic valve disease, whose basis is a congenital bicuspid aortic valve, causes symptoms in middle age and later, when surgery may be required.

Some years ago it was stated that 'surgical treatment for valvular disease is not at present feasible for elderly patients and any treatment must therefore be medical'[66]. Since then a number of reports of open heart surgery in older patients have appeared[67–70] and in general these reports indicate a low operative mortality and considerable functional improvement. Among the factors in older patients which may adversely affect the results of cardiac surgery are coexisting coronary artery disease, chronic chest disease and cerebral vascular disease. However, these are adverse factors at any age, and it is suggested that the indications for valve surgery in the elderly should be the same as in any age group. The majority of the operations reported have been for aortic valve disease and have usually involved replacement of the aortic valve. In the earlier reports prosthetic valves were used but more recently there has been an increasing use of biological valves. These seem particularly appropriate for elderly patients as long-term anticoagulation is not needed and their durability is of less concern than in younger patients. Mitral valve replacement has been less commonly carried out but appears to have equally beneficial results. The mortality for multiple valve replacement is much higher than for single valve replacement. Closed mitral valvotomy for mitral stenosis can also be performed in older patients[71] and age does not seem to adversely effect the results of this operation.

More recently attention has been paid to surgery for coronary artery disease. This has involved grafting a saphenous vein from the aorta to the coronary artery distal to the obstruction. This operation is usually performed in patients with severe angina but may also be used for patients with severe coronary atherosclerosis as demonstrated by coronary angiography. Coronary bypass surgery has been in use for a relatively short time; the results to date indicate that anginal symptoms are relieved in a large number of patients[72]. However the effects of the operation on survival are not clear except for patients who have the prognostically very serious condition of obstruction of the left main coronary artery[73,74]. The place of this operation in elderly patients is unknown and at present it does not seem likely that there would be many indications for the operation in very old patients.

DISORDERS OF CARDIAC RHYTHM AND CONDUCTION

Cardiac arrhythmias and conduction defects are common in old age. Although some disorders of cardiac rhythm and conduction may occur in the absence of other evidence of heart disease, most of these disorders are complications of serious organic disease of the heart. In older patients this will most frequently be ischaemic heart disease but cardiomyopathy and valvular disease may also cause disorders of rhythm conduction. In the elderly the only clinical finding in thyrotoxicosis may be a disorder of cardiac rhythm, usually atrial fibrillation.

In the approach to the patient with a cardiac arrhythmia search must first be made for the underlying cause. In some cases this may be reversible and specific antiarrhythmic therapy may not be required. As far as possible, the underlying pathological process in the heart should be identified. Other disorders associated with disorders of cardiac rhythm and conduction include: electrolyte disorders, particularly of potassium; intrathoracic disease including lobar pneumonia, carcinomatous involvement of the pericardium by direct spread from a bronchogenic carcinoma or from metastatic spread, and pulmonary embolism; and change in blood volume from, for example, gastrointestinal bleeding, or in the oxygenation of the blood from respiratory disease. Drugs are a common cause of cardiac arrhythmias, and of these the most common is digoxin. Digoxin may precipitate virtually any cardiac arrhythmia but the disorders specifically associated with this drug are coupled ventricular ectopic beats (bigeminy), and atrial tachycardia with atrioventricular block.

Changes in heart rate and rhythm can have serious effects throughout the body. With a normal heart, variations in heart rate from approximately 40–160 beats/min are not associated with changes in cardiac output, but heart rates below or above these figures result in progressive decreases in output. When the heart is diseased the range of heart rates in which the cardiac output is normal is much narrower. Thus, in old age, where there are changes in cardiac function associated with the ageing process itself, and where there is an increasing likelihood of heart disease, particularly from ischaemia, changes in heart rate are likely to be less well tolerated than in younger patients. The results of changes in cardiac output will be reflected throughout the body. The brain is particularly sensitive to changes in blood supply, and confusion and syncopal attacks will be common accompaniments of respectively sustained or paroxysmal changes in heart rate. It is likely that in the elderly, changes in cardiac function are responsible for a proportion of cases of confusion and drop attacks[75,76]. The kidneys and the heart itself are other organs sensitive to changes in cardiac output.

Cardiac arrhythmias may be sustained or paroxysmal. Paroxysmal arrhythmias are difficult to diagnose as the abnormality may not be present when the patient is seen. The recent development of methods of recording the electrocardiograph (ECG) over long periods of time while the patient is carrying out his normal activities (ambulatory ECG monitoring) has revealed a high frequency of previously unsuspected cardiac arrhythmias[77]. The response to antiarrhythmic treatment can also be assessed by ambulatory ECG monitoring.

The aim of treatment of cardiac arrhythmias and conduction disorders is to control the heart rate and to return the patient's cardiac rhythm to normal. This aim is to achieve two purposes, first to improve cardiac performance, relieving the symptoms caused by the abnormal heart rate, and second, to reduce the risk of more serious or perhaps fatal arrhythmias.

The present status of treatment of cardiac arrhythmias has been recently reviewed[78]. It has been suggested that the ideal antiarrhythmic drug should demonstrate selective efficacy against a specific type of arrhythmia in a manner unassociated with general and particularly cardiovascular side-effects. It should be effective and safe following intravenous administration and when given orally should have a long therapeutic half-life. So far the ideal drug has not been developed. The effectiveness and safety of long-term antiarrhythmic therapy in the elderly has not been evaluated. Detailed discussion of the mechanism of arrhythmias and of their clinical features and diagnosis is outside the scope of this chapter.

Supraventricular arrhythmias
The commonest supraventricular arrhythmia is atrial fibrillation, but atrial flutter and supraventricular tachycardia also occur. Atrial fibrillation is usually an accompaniment of ischaemic or other heart disease but may occasionally occur without evidence of other heart disease ('lone' atrial fibrillation). The mainstay of treatment of atrial fibrillation and flutter is digoxin. This drug has been considered in detail elsewhere in this chapter and the principles of its use and its complications are no different in the treatment of rhythm disorders than in the treatment of cardiac failure. The digitalization regime for atrial fibrillation is the same as that for cardiac failure. The response to treatment is monitored by recording the heart rate at the cardiac apex so that the pulse deficit between the true cardiac rate and the radial pulse rate can be taken into account. Adequate control is achieved when the pulse deficit has disappeared and the heart rate is between 70–80 beats/min. Atrial flutter is similarly treated and is often converted to atrial fibrillation. Failure to respond to treatment may be caused by many of the factors already mentioned in the discussion of cardiac failure. In addition, atrial fibrillation resistant to digoxin may be the presenting feature of thyrotoxicosis.

An alternative to drug treatment for atrial fibrillation and other supraventricular arrhythmias is direct current conversion to sinus rhythm. This treatment is most effective when the arrhythmia is of recent onset and due to remediable heart disease, which has been adequately treated, such as mitral valve disease treated by cardiac surgery or thyrotoxicosis. If these conditions are present then the age of the patient is no contraindication to DC conversion. However, in older patients atrial fibrillation is commonly an accompaniment of chronic non-remediable heart disease and control of the heart rate with digoxin is the appropriate treatment. The risk of arterial emboli must be considered when DC conversion is to be used.

Ventricular arrhythmias

Ventricular arrhythmias consist of ventricular ectopic beats, ventricular tachycardia and ventricular fibrillation. Although ventricular ectopic beats and short episodes of ventricular tachycardia may be precipitated by emotion, smoking, coffee and other stimulants, in the elderly they are likely to be associated with serious organic heart disease. In the course of an acute myocardial infarction, ventricular ectopic beats are of serious significance as they may precipitate ventricular fibrillation. Ventricular tachycardia may also predispose to ventricular fibrillation, and has serious effects of its own as it is usually accompanied by a fall in cardiac output with deleterious effects on many organs including the heart itself. Untreated ventricular fibrillation is rapidly fatal.

Proper treatment of ventricular arrhythmias requires diagnosis of both the arrhythmia itself and the underlying heart disease[79]. Acute ventricular arrhythmias are often associated with a reversible metabolic or cardiac abnormality such as acute myocardial infarction, digoxin toxicity, electrolyte disturbances, hypoxia or cardiac failure. Chronic ventricular arrhythmias in the elderly are usually due to ischaemic heart disease.

The decision to treat ventricular arrhythmias depends on the circumstances and potential seriousness of the disorder. In acute arrhythmias treatment is usually necessary until the underlying cause can be reversed. When symptoms are present in patients with chronic ventricular arrhythmias, the aim of treatment is to abolish or reduce symptoms. In ambulatory patients with chronic asymptomatic ventricular arrhythmias, it is not known whether treatment reduces the risk of sudden death or the subsequent development of symptoms.

The pharmacokinetics of antiarrhythmic drugs have been the subject of recent comprehensive reviews[79,80]. No specific studies on the pharmacokinetics of these drugs appear to have been performed in the elderly. However, it is possible to predict how the elderly will handle these drugs. None of the commonly used antiarrhythmic drugs is excreted predominantly by the kidney but most are metabolized by the liver. Thus when hepatic function is impaired or hepatic blood flow reduced by cardiac failure elimination of drugs such as lignocaine and propranolol will be impaired. Drugs, such as phenytoin, which are highly protein bound will be affected by changes in plasma protein levels common in ill elderly patients.

All drugs used in the management of ventricular arrhythmias are cardiac depressants. All have significant side-effects, particularly with chronic use. Thus quinidine causes hypotension, tinnitus and vertigo, procainamide causes a syndrome similar to systemic lupus erythematosis (SLE) and phenytoin has effects on the central nervous system. Of the newer drugs, mexiletine is structurally similar to lignocaine and has similar side-effects. Disopyramide is a recently introduced antiarrhythmic drug which is well tolerated and effective. However, it should not be used in the presence of heart block and its negative inotropic properties may cause problems with cardiac failure. In the elderly its anticholinergic properties may cause unwanted effects on the eye or the bladder, precipitating glaucoma or urinary retention respectively. Lignocaine is also effective and well tolerated but can only be administered parenterally, usually intravenously, and thus its use is limited to acute short-term treatment. Beta-adrenoreceptor blocking drugs may also be used in the treatment of arrhythmias[81].

With the information available at present it is difficult to make firm recommendations on the drug treatment of ventricular arrhythmias in the elderly. For rapid suppression of acute ventricular arrhythmias, particularly in the presence of an acute myocardial infarction, lignocaine is the drug of choice. It should be given intravenously as a 100 mg loading dose followed by a 2–4 mg/min constant infusion aimed at achieving blood levels of 1·4–6·0 μg/ml[79]. In patients with cardiac failure or hepatic disease the dose should be reduced. For long-term prophylaxis or suppression, disopyramide 300–800 mg/day may be the drug of choice, but procainamide, 3–6 g/day, phenytoin 300–400 mg/day or quinidine, 1·0–2·4 g/day may also be used.

If ventricular tachycardia does not rapidly respond to drug treatment, DC conversion should be used – this is the only effective treatment for ventricular fibrillation.

Disorders of conduction
Heart block is classically divided into first degree block, in which there is prolongation of conduction through the AV node but all

beats are conducted, second degree block, subdivided into Mobitz type 1 (Wenckebach) where the PR interval progressively lengthens until a ventricular beat does not occur and Mobitz type 2 where the PR interval is constant but there are periodic dropped beats, and complete or third degree block where there is no conduction between the atria and the ventricles and each is controlled by its own pacemaker. First degree heart block and Mobitz type 1 block are benign disorders which cause no symptoms, are often transient, and require no treatment except in presence of acute myocardial infarction. Mobitz type 2 heart block is of more serious prognostic significance, as it may be a precursor to complete heart block.

The most serious consequences of heart block are Stokes–Adams attacks in which there is a sudden cessation of the circulation with loss of consciousness. The circulatory failure is caused by ventricular asystole or fibrillation. Apart from the obvious hazards of unpredictable episodes of syncope Stokes–Adams attacks may themselves be fatal, and they frequently occur when the block is changing from second to third degree. They may also occur in patients in whom complete heart block is always recorded. Sometimes the heart block is transitory so that unless the patient is seen during an attack the ECG is recorded as normal.

The other main consequence of complete heart block is a reduction in cardiac output. This usually precipitates congestive cardiac failure but in elderly patients especially it may be associated with a decline in cerebral perfusion and consequent impairment of mental function.

The treatment of heart block depends on the circumstances in which it occurs, its duration and its consequences. Heart block is of most serious prognostic significance when it occurs in the course of an acute myocardial infarction. Although it is often transient, while it is present there is risk of ventricular asystole or fibrillation. In these circumstances a transvenous pacing catheter is inserted. Heart block is sometimes diagnosed incidentally in patients who have had no symptoms which could be related to it. It may not be possible to estimate its duration, and in these circumstances treatment is not required. If complete heart block is present and the patient has exercise intolerance, but not Stokes – Adams attacks, increasing the heart rate by the use of a long-acting preparation of isoprenaline hydrochloride in a dose which controls the heart rate without producing side-effects may be beneficial.

When Stokes–Adams attacks are occurring, or are suspected, in a patient with Mobitz type 2 or complete heart block, insertion of a permanent pacemaker is essential. Age is of no relevance in the decision to insert a pacemaker in a patient with an appropriate disorder and symptoms. If the patient has Mobitz type 2 or complete heart block and is in cardiac failure, the use of digoxin is hazardous as it may convert second degree to third degree heart block or slow the heart further. In these circumstances a pacemaker should be inserted. The increase in heart rate and cardiac output may itself correct the cardiac failure. If not it can then be treated in the usual way.

In a patient who is confused and has complete heart block, the confusion may be the result of a reduction in cerebral blood flow resulting from the slow heart rate. On the other hand older patients may have heart block and dementia from unrelated causes. The appropriate procedure is to undertake a trial of pacing in which a temporary transvenous pacemaker is inserted and changes in the patient's mental state are assessed. When such a trial is carried out it is important that it should be of adequate duration. Improvement of mental state, particularly if the heart block and confusion have been of any duration, is not likely to occur very rapidly. Thus the pacemaker should be functioning for at least 1 week before a true assessment of its value in treatment of the patient's mental impairment can be made. If the mental state improves, a permanent pacemaker should be inserted.

Stokes–Adams attacks may terminate spontaneously but emergency treatment may have to be instituted to resuscitate the patient before the pacemaker can be inserted. Regular thumping of the patient's chest with the closed fist may stimulate effective cardiac contractions but if this is not effective closed chest cardiac massage may be necessary. Ventricular fibrillation will require electrical conversion.

ISCHAEMIC HEART DISEASE

Angina pectoris
Angina is not a common symptom in older patients. This may be due to the diminished activity which occurs with increasing age, or may be related to the frequent absence of pain with myocardial infarction in the elderly[23].

Glyceryl trinitrate remains the best drug for angina. It is a vasodilator, but probably relieves the pain of angina by reducing the blood pressure and cardiac work rather than by dilating the coronary arteries. For maximum effect the patient has to be carefully instructed in its use. The tablet (0·5 mg) should be chewed or allowed to dissolve in the mouth as it is absorbed by the buccal mucosa. Glyceryl trinitrate is most effective when it is taken as soon as possible after the onset of the pain, or even better, taken prophylactically before an expected attack of angina occurs. Reassurance that neither addiction nor tolerance is a risk of regular use of glyceryl trinitrate may be necessary as patients are sometimes reluctant to take enough tablets. The headache and facial flushing which occurs on first use of glyceryl trinitrate usually becomes less marked with regular use. However, being a vasodilator, glyceryl trinitrate may cause hypotension and hence lightheadedness, unsteadiness or falling in elderly patients. Patients should be warned that if the pain persists despite the use of glyceryl trinitrate, they should not take more of the drug but should seek medical help as a myocardial infarction may have occurred. Long-acting and slow-release preparations of nitrites and nitrates are available but appear to offer no advantages over glyceryl trinitrate.

If glyceryl trinitrate does not give adequate relief of pain in angina, beta-adrenoreceptor blocking drugs may be used. These drugs probably reduce pain by interrupting the sympathetic drive on the heart and hence reducing the oxygen consumption of the myocardium. A number of beta-blocking drugs is available, but none appear to have significant advantages over propranolol. Propranolol is prescribed in an initial dose of 15 mg four times daily, gradually increasing to 80–120 mg four times daily or until symptoms are relieved. The hazards of precipitating cardiac failure or bronchospasm in patients predisposed to these conditions are of particular importance in older patients. Propranolol should not be stopped suddenly as rebound angina or myocardial infarction may occur.

Surgical management of angina pectoris has already been discussed.

Atherosclerosis
Atherosclerosis is the pathological condition which causes the greatest burden of disease and disability in old age. It is a chronic slowly progressive disorder which probably starts in childhood. Although the pathogenesis of atherosclerosis is not completely understood, a number of factors which predispose to its premature development have been identified[82]. Efforts at treating or preventing atherosclerosis have been directed to modifying these risk factors in the hope that the progression of the vascular disease will be reduced. The results have been disappointing[83,84]. Most attention has been paid to reducing serum lipid levels by diet or drugs. Although some studies have produced encouraging results, these have not been

repeated by other investigations. In addition, previously unsuspected side-effects have emerged from these studies, in some cases resulting in the mortality in the treated group being as high as that in the control group despite a reduction in the frequency of non-fatal ischaemic heart disease[85].

Because of the disappointing results of the best designed trials, and because in most older people atherosclerosis will have reached a relatively advanced stage of its development, the use of diets or drugs to lower serum lipids cannot be recommended. Once coronary, cerebral or peripheral vascular disease has become clinically manifest, there is little evidence that the underlying pathological process can be altered.

References

1 Caird, F. I. and Kennedy, R. D. (1976). Epidemiology of heart disease in old age. In F. I. Caird, J. L. C. Dall and R. D. Kennedy (eds). *Cardiology in Old Age*, pp. 1–10. (New York, Plenum Press)

2 Goodwin, J. F. (1970). Congestive and hypertrophic cardiomyopathies. *Lancet*, i, 731

3 Krasnow, N. and Stein, R. A. (1978). Hypertrophic cardiomyopathy in the aged. *Am. Heart J.*, **96**, 326

4 Hodkinson, H. M. and Pomerance, A. (1977). The clinical significance of senile cardiac amyloidosis: a prospective clinico-pathological study. *Q. J. Med.*, **46**, 381

5 Caird, F. I., Dall, J. L. C. and Kennedy, R. D. (1976). *Cardiology in Old Age*. (New York, Plenum Press)

6 Caird, F. I. and Dall, J. L. C. (1978). The cardiovascular system. In J. C. Brocklehurst (ed). *Textbook of Geriatric Medicine and Gerontology*, 2nd ed., pp. 125–157. (Edinburgh: Churchill Livingstone)

7 Burch, G. E. (1975). Interesting aspects of geriatric cardiology. *Am. Heart J.*, **89**, 99

8 Urthaler, F., Walker, A. A. and James, T. N. (1978). The effect of aging on ventricular contractile performance. *Am. Heart J.*, **96**, 481

9 Wade, O. L. (1972). Drug therapy in the elderly. *Age Ageing*, **1**, 65

10 Crooks, J., Shepherd, A. M. M. and Stevenson, I. H. (1975). Drugs and the elderly. The nature of the problem. *Health Bull.*, **33**, 222

11 Ritschel, W. A. (1976). Pharmacokinetic approach to drug dosing in the aged. *J. Am. Geriatr. Soc.*, **24**, 344

12 Caird, F. I. (1977). Prescribing for the elderly. *Brit. J. Hosp. Med.*, **17**, 610

13 Judge, T. G. and Caird, F. I. (1978). *Drug Treatment of the Elderly Patient*. (London: Pitman)

14 Taylor, B. B., Kennedy, R. D. and Caird, F. I. (1974). Digoxin studies in the elderly. *Age Ageing*, **3**, 79

15 Vestal, R. E., McGuire, E. A., Tobin, J. D., Andres, R., Norris, A. H. and Mezey, E. (1977). Ageing and ethanol metabolism. *Clin. Pharmacol. Ther.*, **31**, 343

16 Hayes, M. J., Langman, M. J. S. and Short, A. H. (1975). Changes in drug metabolism with increasing age: 1: Warfarin binding and plasma proteins. *Br. J. Clin. Pharmacol.*, **2**, 69

17 Hayes, M. J., Langman, M. J. S. and Short, A. H. (1975). Changes in drug metabolism with increasing age: 2: Phenytoin clearance and protein binding. *Br. J. Clin. Pharmacol.*, **2**, 73

18 Farah, F., Taylor, W., Rawlins, M. D. and James, O. (1977). Hepatic drug acetylation and oxidation: effects of aging in man. *Br. Med. J.*, **2**, 155

19 Salem, S. A. M., Rajjayabun, P., Shepherd, A. M. M. and Stevenson, I. H. (1978). Reduced induction of drug metabolism in the elderly. *Age Ageing*, **7**, 1

20 Baylis, E. M., Hall, M. S., Lewis, G. and Marks, V. (1972). Effects of renal function on plasma digoxin levels in ambulant patients in domiciliary practice. *Br. Med. J.*, **1**, 338

21 Castleden, C. M., George, C. F., Marcer, D. and Hallett, C. (1977). Increased sensitivity to nitrazepam in old age. *Br. Med. J.*, **1**, 10

22 Hepner, G. W., Vesell, E. S. and Tantum, K. R. (1978). Reduced drug elimination in congestive heart failure. *Am. J. Med.*, **65**, 271

23 Pathy, M. S. (1967). Clinical presentation of myocardial infarction in the elderly. *Br. Heart J.*, **29**, 190

24 Smith, T. W. and Haber, E. (1973). Digitalis. *N. Engl. J. Med.*, **289**, 945; 1010; 1063; 1125

25 Greenblatt, D. J. and Koch-Weser, J. (1976). Intramuscular injection of drugs. *N. Engl. J. Med.*, **295**, 542

26 Caird, F. I. (1972). Metabolism of digoxin in relation to therapy in the elderly. *Gerontol. Clin.*, **16**, 68

27 Hurwitz, N. (1969). Predisposing factors in adverse reactions to drugs. *Br. Med. J.*, **1**, 536

28 Ewy, G. A., Kapadia, G. G., Yao, L., Lullin, M. and Marcus, F. I. (1969). Digoxin metabolism in the elderly. *Circulation*, **39**, 449

29 Aronson, J. K., Grahame-Smith, D. G. and Wigley, F. M. (1978). Monitoring digoxin therapy – the use of plasma digoxin concentration measurements in the diagnosis of digoxin toxicity. *Q. J. Med.*, **47**, 111

30 Brown, D. D. and Juhl, R. P. (1976). Decreased bioavailability of digoxin due to antacids and kaolin-pectin. *N. Engl. J. Med.*, **295**, 1034

31 Brown, D. D., Juhl, R. P. and Warner, S. L. (1978). Decreased bioavailability of digoxin due to hypocholesterolemic interventions. *Circulation*, **58**, 164

32 Manninen, V., Apajalahti, A., Melin, J. and Karesoja, M. (1973). Altered absorption of digoxin in patients given propantheline and metoclopramide. *Lancet*, i, 398

33 Caird, F. I. and Kennedy, R. D. (1977). Digitalisation and digitalis detoxication in the elderly. *Age Ageing*, **6**, 21

34 Editorial. (1976). Foxglove saga (continued): *Lancet*, ii, 405

35 Dall, J. L. C. (1970). Maintainance digoxin in elderly patients. *Br. Med. J.*, **2**, 705

36 Johnston, G. D. and McDevitt, D. G. (1979). Is maintenance digoxin necessary in patients with sinus rhythm. *Lancet*, i, 567

37 Wade, A. (ed). (1977). Martindale. *The Extra Pharmacopoeia*, 27th edn. (London: Pharmaceutical Press)

38 Goodman, L. S. and Gilman, A. (eds). (1975). *The Pharmacological Basis of Therapeutics*, 5th edn. (New York: Macmillan)

39 Binnion, P. F. (1975). Hypokalaemia and digoxin-induced arrhythmias. *Lancet*, i, 343

40 Dargie, H. J., Roddy, K., Kennedy, A. C., King, P. C., Read, P. R. and Ward, D. M. (1974). Total body potassium in long-term frusemide therapy: is potassium supplementation necessary? *Br. Med. J.*, **4**, 316

41 Ibrahim, I. K., Ritch, A. E. S., MacLennan, W. J. and May, T. (1978). Are potassium supplements for the elderly necessary? *Age Ageing*, **7**, 165

42 Davidson, C., McLachlan, M. S. F., Burkinshaw, L. and Morgan, D. B. (1976). Effect of long-term diuretic treatment on body-potassium in heart-disease. *Lancet*, **ii**, 1044

43 Lawson, D. H., Boddy, K., Gray, J. M. B., Mahaffey, M. and Mills, E. (1976). Potassium supplements in patients receiving long-term diuretics for oedema. *Q. J. Med.*, **45**, 469

44 MacLennan, W. J., Lye, M. D. W. and May, T. (1977). The effect of potassium supplements on total -body-potassium levels in the elderly. *Age Ageing*, **6**, 46

45 Lawson, D. H. (1974). Adverse reactions to potassium chloride. *Q. J. Med.*, **43**, 433

46 Editorial. (1975). Picking a diuretic. *Br. Med. J.*, **1**, 521

47 Burr, M. L., King, S., Davies, H. E. F. and Pathy, M. S. (1977). The effects of discontinuing long-term diuretic therapy in the elderly. *Age Ageing*, **6**, 38

48 McDevitt, D. G. and Johnston, G. D. (1979). Digoxin-compliance as a factor in drug utilisation. In Duchene-Marullaz, P. (ed.) *Advances in Pharmacology and Therapeutics, Vol. 6, Clinical Pharmacology*, p. 143. (Oxford and New York: Pergamon Press)

49 Wandless, I. and Davie, J. W. (1977). Can drug compliance in the elderly be improved? *Br Med. J.*, **1**, 359

50 Wedgewood, J. (1976). Remediable heart disease. In F. I. Caird, J. L. C. Dall and R. D. Kennedy (eds). *Cardiology in Old Age*, pp. 249–265. (New York: Plenum Press)

51 Oakley, C. M. (1974). Infective endocarditis. *Br. J. Hosp. Med.*, **11**, 101

52 Oakley, C. (1978). Use of antibiotics – endocarditis. *Br. Med. J.*, **2**, 489

53 Durack, D. T. (1975). Current practice in prevention of bacterial endocarditis. *Br. Heart J.*, **37**, 478

54 LeQuesne, L. P. (1974). Relation between deep vein thrombosis and pulmonary embolism in surgical patients. *N. Engl. J. Med.*, **291**, 1291

55 Warlow, C., Ogston, D. and Douglas, A. S. (1972). Venous thrombosis following strokes. *Lancet*, **i**, 1305

56 Denham, M. J., Farran, H. and James, G. (1973). The value of ^{125}I fibrinogen in the diagnosis of deep venous thrombosis in hemiplegia. *Age Ageing*, **2**, 207

57 McNicol, G. P. (1974). Low-dosage heparin. In J. G. G. Ledingham (ed). *Advanced Medicine 10*, pp. 281–287. (London: Pitman)

58 Mitchell, J. R. A. (1978). The prevention of thrombosis. In D. J. Weatherall (ed). *Advanced Medicine 14*, pp. 228–235. (London: Pitman)

59 International Multicentre Trial. (1975). Prevention of fatal postoperative pulmonary embolism by low doses of heparin. *Lancet*, **ii**, 45

60 McCarthy, S. T., Robertson, D., Turner, J. J., Hawkey. C. J. and Macey, D. J. (1977). Low-dose heparin as a prophylaxis against deep-vein thrombosis after acute stroke. *Lancet*, **ii**, 800

61 Morris, G. K. and Mitchell, J. R. A. (1976). Prevention and diagnosis of venous thrombosis in patients with hip fractures. *Lancet*, **ii** 867

62 James, O. F. W. (1978). Drug metabolism in the elderly. *Age Ageing*, **7**, 81

63 Thompson, P. L. and Robinson, J. S. (1978). Stroke after acute myocardial infarction: relation to infarct size. *Br. Med. J.*, **2**, 457

64 Canadian Cooperative Study Group. (1978). A randomized trial of aspirin and sulfinpyrazone in threatened stroke. *N. Engl. J. Med.*, **299**, 53

65 Anturane Reinfarction Trial Research Group (1978). Sulfinpyrazone in the prevention of cardiac death after myocardial infarction. *N. Engl. J. Med.*, **298**, 289

66 Editorial. (1968). Systolic murmurs in the elderly. *Br. Med. J.*, **4**, 530
67 Ahmad, A. and Starr, A. (1969). Valve replacement in geriatric patients. *Br. Heart J.*, **31**, 322
68 Austen, W. G., DeSanctis, R. W., Buckley, M. J., Mundth, E. D. and Scannel, J. G. (1970). Surgical management of aortic valve disease in the elderly. *J. Am. Med. Assoc.*, **211**, 624
69 Oh, W., Hickman, R., Emanual, R., McDonald, L., Somerville, J., Ross, D., Ross, K. and Gonzalez-Lavin, L. (1973). Heart valve surgery in 114 patients over the age of 60. *Br. Heart J.*, **35**, 174
70 De Bono, A. H. B., English, T. A. H. and Milstein, B. B. (1978). Heart valve replacement in the elderly. *Br. Med. J.*, **2**, 917
71 Ellis, L. B., Benson, H. and Harken, D. E. (1968). The effect of age and other factors on the early and late results following closed mitral valvuloplasty. *Am. Heart J.*, **75**, 743
72 Seides, S. F., Borer, J. S., Kent, K. M., Rosing, D. R., McIntosh, C. L. and Epstein, S. E. (1978). Long-term anatomic fate of coronary-artery bypass grafts and functional status of patients five years after operation. *N. Engl. J. Med.*, **298**, 1213
73 Murphy, M. L., Hultgren, H. N., Detre, K., Thomsen, J., Takaro, T. and participants of the Veterans Administration Cooperative Study. (1977). Treatment of chronic stable angina. *N. Engl. J. Med.*, **297**, 621
74 Detre, K., Murphy, M. L. and Hultgren, H. (1977). Effect of coronary bypass surgery on longevity in high and low risk patients. *Lancet*, **ii**, 1243
75 Goldberg, A. D., Raftery, E. B. and Cashman, P. M. M. (1975). Ambulatory electrocardiographic records in patients with transient cerebral attacks or palpitation. *Br. Med. J.*, **2**, 569
76 Walter, P. F., Reid, S. D. and Wenger, N. K. (1970). Transient cerebral ischaemia due to arrhythmia. *Ann. Intern. Med.*, **72**, 471
77 Harrison, D. C., Fitzgerald, J. W. and Winkle, R. A. (1976). Ambulatory electrocardiography for diagnosis and treatment of cardiac arrhythmias. *N. Engl. J. Med.*, **294**, 373
78 Jewitt, D. E. (1977). Limitations of present drug therapy of cardiac arrhythmias – a review. *Postgrad. Med. J.*, **53**, 12
79 Winkle, R. A., Glantz, S. A. and Harrison, D. C. (1975). Pharmacologic therapy of ventricular arrhythmias. *Am. J. Cardiol.*, **36**, 629
80 Harrison, D. C., Meffin, P. J. and Winkle, R. A. (1977). Clinical pharmacokinetics of antiarrhythmic drugs. *Prog. Cardiovasc. Dis.*, **20**, 217
81 Singh, B. N. and Jewitt, D. E. (1977). β-Adrenoreceptor blocking drugs in cardiac arrhythmias. In: *Cardiovascular Drugs*, **2**, (Sydney: ADIS Press) 119
82 National Heart and Lung Institute Task Force on Arteriosclerosis. (1971). Arteriosclerosis. (Washington: National Institutes of Health)
83 Ahrens, E. H. (1976). The management of hyperlipidemia: whether, rather than how. *Ann. Intern. Med.*, **85**, 87
84 Mann, G. V. (1977). Current concepts: diet–heart: end of an era. *N. Engl. J. Med.*, **297**, 644
85 Committee of Principal Investigators. (1978). A co-operative trial in the primary prevention of ischaemic heart disease using clofibrate. *Br. Heart J.*, **40**, 1069

Review articles

Detailed accounts of the pharmacology, use and side effects of drugs are given in two classical reference books:

Wade, A. (ed). (1977). Martindale. *The Extra Pharmacopoeia.* 27th Edn. (London: Pharmaceutical Press)

Goodman, L. S. and Gilman, A. (eds). (1975). *The Pharmacological Basis of Therapeutics.* 5th Edn. (New York: MacMillan)

Other reviews on the topics of this chapter include:

Burch, G. E. (1975). Interesting aspects of geriatric cardiology. *Am. Heart J.*, **89,** 99

Caird, F. I. (1972). Metabolism of digoxin on relation to therapy in the elderly. *Geront. Clin.*, **16,** 68

Caird, F. I. (1977). Prescribing for the elderly. *Br. J. Hosp. Med.*, **17,** 610

Caird, F. I. and Dall, J. L. C. (1978). The cardiovascular system. In J. C. Brocklehurst (ed.). *Textbook of Geriatric Medicine and Gerontology*, 2nd En., pp. 125 – 157. (Edinburgh: Churchill Livingstone)

Caird, F. I., Dall, J. L. C. and Kennedy, R. D. (1976). *Cardiology in Old Age.* (New York: Plenum Press)

Editorial. (1976). Focglove saga (continued). *Lancet*, **ii,** 405

Editorial. (1978). Digoxin – more problems than solutions. *Lancet*, **ii,** 1288

Goodwin, J. F. (1970). Congestive and hypertrophic cardiomyopathies. *Lancet*, **i,** 731

Lawson, D. H. (1974). Adverse reactions to potassium chloride. *Q. J. Med.*, **43,** 433

LeQuesne, L. P. (1974). Relation between deep vein thrombosis and pulmonary embolism in surgical patients. *N. Engl. J. Med.*, **291,** 1291

McDevitt, D. G. and Johnstone, G. D. (1978). Digoxin – compliance as a factor in drug utilisation. In Duchene-Marullaz, P. (ed.) *Advances in Pharmacology and Therapeutics, Vol. 6, Clinical Pharmacology*, p. 143. (Oxford and New York: Pergamon Press)

McNicol, G. P. (1974). Low-dosage heparin. In J. G. G. Ledingham (ed). *Advanced Medicine 10.* pp. 281 – 287 (London: Pitman)

Mitchell, J. R. A. (1978). The prevention of thrombosis. In D. J. Weatherall

4

The management of hypertension in the elderly

B. Moore-Smith

INTRODUCTION

If the aetiology of essential hypertension in the middle aged is an enigma, its ill-effects are, epidemiologically, all too apparent. In the elderly the uncertainty about causation extends also to the sequelae. Hypertension in those of advanced years is widely regarded as benign and devoid of serious consequences especially in women.

Much of the published work on the consequences of hypertension concerns only the middle-aged, but such work as has been carried out on the elderly does not always lead to the conclusion that high blood pressure in the older age range is innocuous, does not require treatment, and that in any case its treatment is hazardous and likely only to make the patient worse.

The most immediate problem is that of definitions. For the sake of convenience the term 'elderly' will be taken to imply a chronological age exceeding 65 years, unless otherwise stated, if only because there is such a paucity of information about hypertension in those aged over 75, and even less over 85.

Hypertension as a state is incapable of definition solely in terms of a sphygmomanometer reading; it is a continuously distributed variable [1-3] which is associated with an increasing risk of cardiovascular catastrophe the higher is the pressure[1,4], and so far as is known there is no lower limit below which no such sequelae are ever seen.

From the practical point of view the problem in the elderly, as in younger age groups, is to establish what levels of blood pressure are

117

associated with an unacceptable risk of serious complications, whether treatment reduces this risk and, if so, what forms of treatment are available and devoid of a tendency to worsen the lot of the patient.

PREVALENCE OF HYPERTENSION WITH AGE

All societies
Is a tendency to a rising blood pressure an inevitable concomitant of age? The balance of the evidence suggests that this is not the case.

MacCulloch[5] reported contrasting rates of change of blood pressure with age between many areas of the world. In general blood pressure was lower where the culture was stable, traditional forms were honoured, and group members were secure in their roles and adapted to them by early experience. This association of continuing low blood pressure with advancing age was seen most strongly in so-called 'primitive' societies. In contrast the prevalence of raised blood pressure in an urban population could be related to the rate of growth of a city; the rapidly expanding urban environment seemed to be stressful.

There have been various attempts based on anthropological studies, to link the simple, stable and primitive lifestyle with a low sodium intake. A low salt intake in 'primitive' societies in many parts of the world, and a low prevalence of hypertension, was contrasted with a high salt intake and high prevalence in 'civilized' societies[6,7]. Application of such differences between 'primitive' and 'civilized' societies to subgroups of 'westernized' cultures failed to yield convincing evidence of such an important role for sodium. The ability remains, however, for some societies almost entirely to escape a rise in blood pressure with increasing age.

In a longitudinal survey in South Wales Miall and Lovell[8], employing multiple regression analysis, examined the relative contribution of age and pressure in predicting change of pressure, and drew the conclusion that changes in pressure are highly significantly related to mean pressure but only indirectly related to age. Age seemed to play a part solely because blood pressure changes on average were positive, increased with higher pressures, and the higher the pressure the greater the rate of increase. A further conclusion was that there might be a level, only above which this self-perpetuating mechanism operated, and this might offer another explanation of the low pressures found throughout life in some primitive communities.

Also in a developed society Harlan et al.[9] in a 30 year study of blood pressure in a white male cohort of 1000 aviators, found that an increase in blood pressure was not related to age *per se*. Approximately half of the cohort experienced a rise of 3 mmHg or less over the 30-year period, although their age at the latest examination was only 54. They agreed with Miall and Lovell[8] that those with the highest initial pressures suffered the greatest increases. Other than the level of the blood pressure itself, weight gain stood out as the most important factor related to pressure increase.

It seems therefore that mankind is not conditioned to a rise in blood pressure by advancing years alone. In 'developed' societies however there is evidence to suggest that, perhaps because of environmental and other influences, there is an important tendency to rising blood pressure with age and its attendant risks, although some of the evidence is apparently contradictory.

Developed societies
Hamilton et al.[10] found in 2031 patients attending outpatient clinics at St Mary's Hospital, London that systolic pressures increased throughout the age range (10 to 85), although the increase of diastolic pressures was less pronounced. Pressures were greater in women than in men, except for systolic pressures in men under the age of 30 (Figure 1). Their results accorded with those of other investigators and where there were divergencies these were explicable by the methods used for selection of the samples. All these studies were cross-sectional.

Heller and Rose[11] employing a criterion of systolic pressure equal to or greater than 160 mmHg, or diastolic pressure equal to or greater than 100 mmHg, or both, found a prevalence of hypertension in unselected hospital practice, rising from 3% at age 15–39 to 41% at age 60 or more. Kitchin, Lowther and Milne[12] in a group aged 62–90 found prevalence rates of systolic hypertension (blood pressure more than 160) of 38% in males, 57% in females. Diastolic hypertension (blood pressure more than 100 mmHg), occurred in 11% of males and 19% of females. Over the age span studied the prevalence of systolic hypertension in women rose from 46% to 68% at the top of the age range, while in males it fell from 41% to 33%.

Russek and Zolman[13] studied 3691 white men between the ages of 50 and 95. Using a cut-off level of 150/95 mmHg to divide normotension from hypertension they found that there was a steady and progressive rise in the proportion of hypertensives so defined

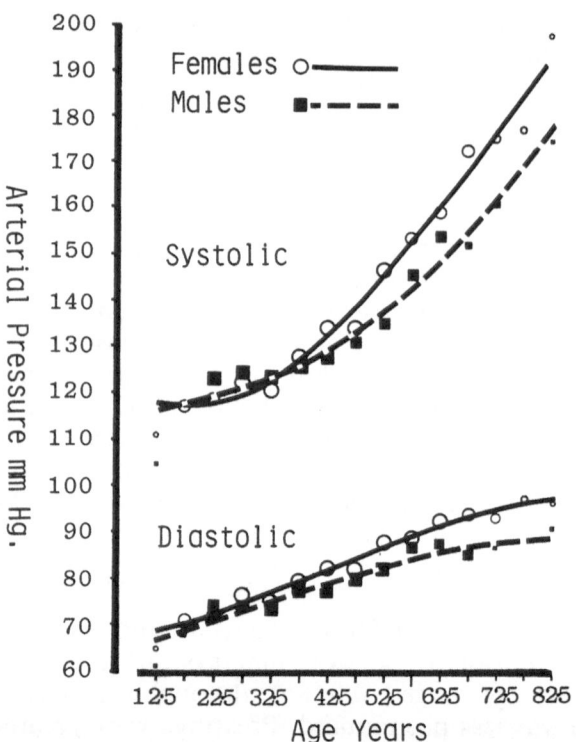

Figure 1 Systolic and diastolic pressures for females (open circles) and males (black squares) for each 5 year age group of the population sample, together with the fitted curves. The area of each circle or square is proportional to the number of subjects in that age group

from 25·2% (age 50–54) to 72·2% (age 85–95). In the group as a whole average systolic pressure rose from 138·9 mmHg (age 50–54) to 164 mmHg (age 85–95). Average pulse pressure rose progressively with age but there was no significant elevation of diastolic pressure with advancing years. Even in the 'normotensives' average systolic pressures rose from 129·6 mmHg (age 50–59) to 134·1 (age 80–95). In these normotensive subjects however average diastolic pressures fell with age from 80·1 mmHg (age 50–59) to 74·5 (age 80–95).

Droller *et al.*[14] found in Sheffield pensioners a trend towards slightly higher mean systolic blood pressure with advancing age but their results in a small sample did not reach the level of significance.

Master, Lasser and Jaffe[15] examined the blood pressure in 5757 white people aged 65–106, considered to be basically healthy and specifically without cardiovascular disease. They found that the systolic pressure did not rise after age 75, or the diastolic pressure after age 70. Mean systolic pressure reached a maximum of 150 mmHg in women aged 70–74 falling therafter, reaching 149 mmHg at age 95. In men mean systolic pressure reached 145 mmHg at age 70–74 remaining constant thereafter. In both sexes diastolic pressure was practically constant after age 65 at mean values of 85 mmHg in women and 83 mmHg in men. The mean pressure of all these apparently normal subjects was 145/82 in men and 156/84 in women, and the modal blood pressure was 140/80 in both sexes. It was not possible to establish a sharp demarcation between normal and abnormal. They considered that subjects in the middle 80% range of pressure (115/70 to 175/95 in men and 120/65 to 192/102 in women) did not require treatment if there were no other factors requiring consideration.

Anderson and Cowan[16] in a survey of 546 healthy people aged 60–89 attending the Rutherglen Health Centre found higher pressures than Master and colleagues. The middle 95% range of pressure distribution was 111/70 to 216/109 in men and 120/70 to 236/113 in women, which however compares with a middle 95% range of 100/62 to 190/102 for men and 100/55 to 212/112 for women in Master and colleagues[15].

Allowing for the multiphysician involvement in the American series, populations examined in two different continents, and the preselection of the American population to be free of cardiovascular disease, these two series are more nearly comparable than appears at first sight. In a later paper Anderson and Cowan[17] confirmed the increase in systolic pressure and the small variation of diastolic pressure with age in another apparently healthy group of 631 people aged 60–89. Again pressures were higher in women.

Babu *et al.*[18] examined the blood pressure in 199 people aged from 50 to over 100 in a hospital for the elderly and those with chonic diseases. They were selected not to be hypertensive (in contrast to Anderson and Cowan's study) and to be in all respects otherwise healthy. In this preselected group the systolic blood pressure rose slightly with age from an average of 120/75 aged 50–59 to an average of 130/75 aged 90–99. There was no appreciable change in diastolic pressure with age.

There is general agreement that systolic pressure in both sexes in the groups studied rises as age advances and that diastolic pressure is relatively stable. There are differences chiefly relating to whether the systolic rise is continuous or levels off in the 70s[15] and what levels of blood pressure can be accepted as occurring normally in a population. The main differences can be attributed to the methods used to select the samples, particularly the exclusion of those with cardiovascular disease[15], or those with hypertension[18]. None of these studies assesses the risk associated with the levels found.

CHARACTERISTICS OF THE ARTERIAL PRESSURE WAVE CAUSING SYSTOLIC ACCENTUATION

The reason for the predominant rise in systolic pressure was examined by O'Rourke[19] who noted that increased peripheral resistance led to an increase in mean pressure and if arterial distensibility was unaltered both systolic and diastolic pressures rose. When, however, arterial distensibility was reduced, for instance by atherosclerosis, the increase in mean pressure was reflected in a much greater rise in systolic than diastolic pressure and the latter might not rise at all or might indeed fall. It was the increase in impedance (determined by the inertial properties of the blood and by the elasticity, viscosity and geometry of arteries as well as by the viscous properties of blood in small vessels) of the systemic circulation, caused in large part by the loss of arterial distensibility, which produced an increase in the amplitude of the aortic pressure wave and alteration in its shape, giving rise to a systolic peak while the diastolic part of the wave fell almost exponentially. Such changes were seen in the proximal aorta of patients with hypertensive arterial degenerative disease and aortic coarctation.

THE RISKS ASSOCIATED WITH SYSTOLIC HYPERTENSION

These characteristics of the circulation have given rise to distinctions between 'classical' and 'systolic' hypertension. Dyer *et al.*[20] defined systolic hypertension as a systolic pressure equal to or exceeding 160 mmHg with a diastolic of less than 95 mmHg. So defined the prevalence rose steeply from age 45–79, reaching 27% in white males and 43% in black females at the upper age limit. They quoted the Chicago People's Gas Company study on employed males as confirming increased risk with systolic elevation of blood pressure, and the Chicago Heart Association Detection Project in Industry as finding higher rates of ECG abnormality in subjects age 65–74 with systolic hypertension.

Colandrea *et al.*[21], defining systolic hypertension as a systolic pressure of 160 mmHg or greater and diastolic less than 90, investigated prospectively 3246 subjects in a retirement community at

Seal Beach, California (mean age 69·7 for men, 68·3 for women). They found that the 'hypertensive' subjects had an average systolic pressure of 172·2 mmHg while that of the controls was 127·3 mmHg and agreed with Gubner[22] that systolic hypertension was a significant risk factor for the development of cardiovascular disease and mortality. This study[21] was remarkable for the marked lability of the systolic pressure, the prevalence of hypertension, as defined, falling from 14% on the initial screening to 2·7% on the third clinic visit.

Consideration of mortality experience in insured males (aged at the time of policy issue 15–69) in the Build and Blood Pressure Study of the Society of Actuaries, (Chicago 1959) led Gubner[22] to the conclusion that moderate elevation of systolic pressure alone had a decidedly adverse significance, mortality increasing progressively with successive increments of systolic pressure, and a greater significance than diastolic pressure elevation over the levels studied (the maximum systolic pressure was 167 mmHg and the maximum diastolic pressure 102 mmHg). The relative increase in mortality was as great in women as in men.

The Chicago stroke study[23], on an admittedly atypical low income urban population age 65–74, found no association between systolic pressure and total mortality, for those with a diastolic pressure of less than 95, until systolic pressures reached 180 mmHg or above, when there was a large jump in mortality rates.

In another investigation at Seal Beach, California Cutler[24] undertook a survey of premonitory signs and symptoms of stroke and found a higher incidence of mean blood pressure, cervical bruits and abnormal ECGs in the stroke victims. While both systolic and diastolic pressures were higher in the stroke group the differences were statistically significant only for systolic blood pressure.

Friedman *et al.*[25], again at Seal Beach, matched patients at the time of their stroke with two controls; the matching included age, sex, systolic blood pressure and the interval between initial examination and the date of the stroke or selection as a control. With blood pressure thus excluded as a factor at the time of the stroke they found a significant difference in previous systolic hypertension between strokes and controls in men but not in women, and a significant association of stroke with atrial fibrillation and with other forms of cardiac disease and non-cerebral atherosclerosis.

Miall and Chinn[2] continuing a longitudinal survey in South Wales noted in the 65–74 age range the important prognostic significance of systolic pressures of 180 mmHg or more and of diastolic pressures of 110 mmHg or more.

Fry[26] in a South London general practice adopted a policy of non-treatment of hypertension between 1949 and 1969. He discovered 704 hypertensives, defined as having a diastolic blood pressure of 100 mmHg or more on at least three occasions, 35 of whom received treatment for various reasons and were excluded from review, leaving 669 whose blood pressure presumably followed a natural course. No control group was constructed for comparison of morbidity and mortality and the observed mortality rate of the group was therefore compared with the expected mortality for the population at large from the figures of the Office of Population Censuses and Surveys.

The observed/expected death rate ratio of these hypertensive patients was inversely related to age, being highest in those aged 30–39, only a little greater than one for the decade 60–69 and actually less than one in the over-70s. The mortality rate was higher in males at all ages. The inference drawn was that the risk to life of hypertension varied with the age at which the hypertension was first observed and that over the age of 60 there was no extra risk. The mortality rate rose with the initial level of diastolic pressure and young males were the most severely affected. In the over-60s there was no relationship between diastolic pressure and observed mortality rate. As other observers had found there was no noticeable rise of diastolic pressure with age.

It must be noted that the diagnosis was based on diastolic pressures and in the elderly it is systolic pressures which are both commonly raised and associated with cardiovascular sequelae. It is perhaps here that the lack of a control group is most keenly felt and there was also an 18% removal rate in the series, these patients being lost to follow-up. The probable inapplicability of national life tables to a middle-class suburb of high mobility, and the misleading effect of mortality ratios as an index of excess mortality risk are commented on elsewhere[27]. Half of the hypertensives were diagnosed when they were aged 60 or more suggesting an age relationship but the conclusion of Miall and Lovell[8] that pressure changes are related to pre-existing pressure rather than to age is apposite. It is also to be noted that in this untreated series the chief causes of morbidity and mortality were cardiac and cerebrovascular.

Kannel *et al.*[28] investigated prospectively the risk factors in the blood pressure in 5127 people in the Framingham study. Normotension was defined as a blood pressure below 140/90 and hypertension as a blood pressure equal to or exceeding 160 and a diastolic in excess of 95. All other values were regarded as being borderline.

The risk of coronary heart disease was related to antecedent blood pressure in both sexes and there was no evidence that hypertension was innocuous in older people. Blood pressure was a potent independent contributor to coronary heart disease. There was nothing to suggest the incidence increased abruptly at some critical level of pressure. It was the actual level which mattered[1] and the proportion of fatal attacks rose with the level of blood pressure. Discriminate analysis showed that the association of coronary heart disease with blood pressure was stronger for the systolic component, and even mean arterial pressure (diastolic pressure plus one-third of the pulse pressure) was a less good discriminator, though better than diastolic pressure. Only for men aged less than 45 was diastolic pressure a better discriminator, between 45 and 59 the two pressures were of equal value, while above 60 years systolic pressure was an increasingly better predictor of coronary heart disease. They pointed out that the systolic pressure associated with the same risk as a diastolic pressure of 95 mmHg shifted with age from 144 mmHg age 40 to 158 mmHg at age 68, because of the factors described by O'Rourke[19], but considered that the risk of coronary heart disease was simply proportional to the level of blood pressure. Likewise there was no doubt that hypertension was a precursor and predisposing factor contributing powerfully to the occurrence of strokes[29], assuming grave significance when attended by left ventricular hypertrophy on ECG, cardiac enlargement or congestive cardiac failure. Pointing out that prudent reduction of elevated blood pressure, even in persons with completed strokes, can actually improve cerebral blood flow by decreasing cerebrovascular resistance, Kannel and colleagues[31] considered that fear of futility and danger in reducing blood pressure in people with cerebroatherosclerosis was unjustified, as moderate to severe hypertension may actually reduce cerebral flow by invoking excessive cerebral autoregulation[30].

The Framingham study[29] showed a similar sex incidence of stroke due to atherothrombotic brain infarction, with women being more vulnerable in the older age groups as distinct from the situation with coronary heart disease. Again there was no safe level of blood pressure, systolic pressure was the best single prognostic discriminator, there was no indication that the impact of diastolic pressure was greater than systolic or that the effect of systolic pressure decreased with age. The same general conclusions were drawn in respect of congestive cardiac failure[31]. They urged re-evaluation of the beliefs that systolic pressure was unimportant, that women tolerated hypertension well, that an elevated pressure was a normal concomitant of ageing and that labile hypertension was of little consequence.

In summary, the Framingham study[4] showed a rising risk of death from cardiovascular disease with both age and level of blood pressure in both sexes, patients being aged 30–62 at entry to the study (Table 1). No critical value of blood pressure dividing normotension from hypertension was found. The WHO criterion of essential hypertension as a blood pressure of 160/90 or more merely identified a high risk group, though among hypertensives so defined risk was strikingly related to the degree of blood pressure elevation. Furthermore the contention that risk was related to diastolic rather than systolic pressure could not be supported (Table 2).

In the context of the elderly in particular, the Framingham data gave no indication of a lessening impact of blood pressure, whether systolic or diastolic, with advancing age (Figure 2). Nor was there any support for the thesis that increasing blood pressure was a normal accompaniment of ageing.

Table 1   Risk of death from cardiovascular disease (coronary disease, brain infarction, congestive heart failure) according to hypertensive status. Men and women aged 45–74 (Framingham study: 18-year follow up)

	Average annual incidence (rate per 10 000) at age			
	45–54	55–64	65–74	45–74
Men				
Normotensive.	29	78	108	58*
Borderline	40	106	226	97*
Hypertensive	95	216	260	160*
Totals	44	118	118	91†
Women				
Normotensive	9	24	25	22*
Borderline	10	45	107	40*
Hypertensive	38	55	199	72*
Totals	14	40	123	40†

* Age-adjusted rates
† Actual rate

The often quoted concept of the relative immunity of women to the malign effects of hypertension received no support when regression coefficients of cardiovascular morbidity and mortality on systolic blood pressure according to age were calculated (Table 3).

Statistical techniques (despite their hazards[32,33]) showed that neither age nor their femininity protected hypertensive women, premenopausally or postmenopausally, from the effects of their

Table 2 Risk of death from cardiovascular disease according to level of systolic and diastolic blood pressure at biennial examination. Men and women aged 45–74 (Framingham study: 18-year follow-up)

Blood pressure (mmHg)		Average annual incidence per 10 000			
		Men		Women	
Systolic	Diastolic	Systolic	Diastolic	Systolic	Diastolic
74–109	20–69	52	64	20	27
110–119	70–74	60	70	23	30
120–129	75–79	70	77	27	33
130–139	80–84	82	85	32	37
140–149	85–89	96	93	38	41
150–159	90–94	111	103	44	45
160–169	95–99	130	113	52	50
170–179	100–104	151	124	61	55
180–189	105–109	176	136	72	61
190–300	110–160	204	150	84	67
Total population		91	91	40	40

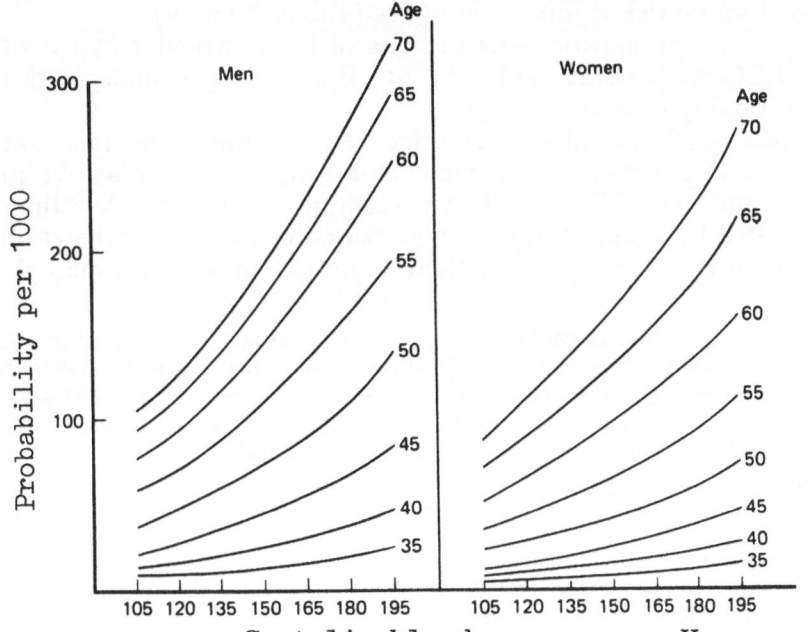

Figure 2 Probability of cardiovascular disease in an 8 year period according to systolic blood pressure at specified ages in each sex. Low-risk subjects: serum cholesterol < 185 mg/100 ml, nonsmokers, no glucose intolerance, no ECG evidence of left ventricular hypertrophy (Framingham heart study: 18-year follow up)

Table 3 Regression of cardiovascular morbidity and mortality on systolic blood pressure according to age. Men and women aged 45–74 (Framingham study: 18-year follow-up)

Age	Men	Women	Men	Women
	Age-specific regression coefficients			
	Cardiovascular disease		*Cardiovascular mortality*	
45–54	0·021	0·019	0·020	0·018
55–64	0·020	0·019	0·020	0·011
65–74	0·012	0·016	0·007	0·023
	Overall mortality		*Coronary mortality*	
45–54	0·017	0·008	0·022	−0.001
55–64	0·013	0·006	0·021	0·015
65–74	0·009	0·015	0·019	0·021

hypertension as compared with normotensive females. The differences in the two groups were as striking in women as in men even if the absolute risk is greater in males (Tables 3 and 4).

The dire prognostic effect of signs of left ventricular hypertrophy on ECG were noted (Table 5). At all ages 38% of males with this abnormality died within 8 years.

Anderson[32] recently re-examined the Framingham data statistically and concluded that 'the relationship between diastolic pressure and morbidity is almost certainly more complex than is indicated by a simple logistic regression line and it may therefore be premature to conclude that there is no threshold of normality'. He

Table 4 Regression of cardiovascular morbidity on systolic and diastolic blood pressure. Men and women aged 45–74 (Framingham study: 18-year follow-up)

Blood pressure	Brain infarction		Congestive failure		Coronary disease		Intermittent claudication	
	Men	Women	Men	Women	Men	Women	Men	Women
Multivariate regression coefficients								
Systolic	0·027	0·019	0·016	0·016	0·012	0·016	0·007	0·013
Diastolic	0·044	0·042	0·018	0·022	0·021	0·023	−0·005	0·018
Standardized regression coefficients								
Systolic	0·694	0·688	0·606	0·596	0·352	0·478	0·250	0·536
Diastolic	0·643	0·703	0·423	0·451	0·300	0·364	−0·021	0·388

Table 5 Five-year mortality according to ECG evidence of left ventricular hypertrophy. Men and women aged 45–74 (Framingham study: 18-year follow-up; from *Monograph No. 30*)

ECG signs of left ventricular hypertrophy	Cardiovascular mortality		Coronary mortality		Sudden death		Overall mortality	
	Men	Women	Men	Women	Men	Women	Men	Women
None	3·58	1·62	1·44	0·52	0·80	0·19	6·70	3·62
Possible*	11·06	5·24	3·73	0·97	2·11	0·36	16·39	8·58
Definite†	31·85	16·43	9·50	1·80	5·53	0·68	37·57	19·71

* Possible = voltage criteria
† Definite = voltage criteria plus ST and T abnormalities

also pointed out that the apparently superior prognostic indications of systolic pressure might be in part due to the mathematical methods employed.

These considerations may well be a source of potential confusion in relation to mild hypertension, but do not invalidate the overall importance of raised blood pressure in cardiovascular, and especially cerebrovascular, morbidity and mortality in both sexes. It must be noted however that the Framingham study deals mostly with the middle-aged and the report in 1970[29], for instance, assessing the epidemiological role of blood pressure in stroke, had only accumulated 16 cases of stroke aged over 65. Whether the data for the middle-aged can safely be extrapolated to those aged, say, over 75 remains uncertain but it would seem unlikely that so powerful a risk factor would entirely disappear at more advanced ages.

As concluded earlier the consensus is that as age increases systolic blood pressure rises, but that diastolic pressure is relatively unaffected. While selection of elderly subjects not to be hypertensive seems to yield an elite group whose blood pressure does not rise with age[15,18,34], perhaps for the reasons advanced by Miall and Lovell[8], there is general agreement that there is an increased risk of untoward cardiovascular events with increased systolic pressure in middle-aged and elderly subjects[1,2,4,20–25,28,29,31].

THE EFFECTS OF TREATMENT OF RAISED BLOOD PRESSURE

In predominantly younger age groups the Veterans' Administration Cooperative Study Group reporting in 1967[35] on experience in 143 males, average age 51, with diastolic pressures of 115–129 mmHg found two morbid events and no deaths in the treated group compared with 27 morbid events and four deaths in the controls.

In 380 males, average age 51, with lower diastolic pressures of 90–14 mmHg they found[36] the risk of morbid events was 18% in the treated group against 55% in the untreated. While the incidence of congestive cardiac failure, stroke and progressive renal damage was reduced by treatment that of myocardial infarction and sudden death was unaffected[37].

With regard to the elderly, approximately one-fifth of both groups in this latter study[37], was aged between 60 and 75. Systolic blood pressure was apparently related to age rising to an average of 178 mmHg in the 70–75 age group. Diastolic pressures were unaffected by age.

In the untreated group 62·8 % of patients of 60 or over developed morbid events compared with 28·9 % in the treated group, treatment being 54% effective at this age. Cardiovascular and renal abnormalities were noted in 78% of the over-60s at entry to the trial and their presence greatly increased the risk of developing morbid events. The risk factors contributing to the development of morbid events were: (a) age over 50, (b) cardiovascular/renal abnormalities, (c) diastolic blood pressure 105–114 mmHg. The risk increased progressively with the numbers of risk factors present, while the effectiveness of treatment likewise increased with the number of factors, from nil when no factor was present, to 66% when all three were. The overall conclusion drawn was that all patients with any sign of cardiovascular disease, or diastolic blood pressure averaging in excess of 104 mmHg should be found and treated irrespective of age. Toxic reactions with drugs used (hydrochlorothiazide, reserpine and hydrallazine), all given concurrently, were relatively high but such a choice of treatment regimen would be unusual now.

Beevers *et al.*[38,39] in a group of hypertensives of average age 55 found that the incidence of stroke was closely related to the adequacy of the control of the blood pressure and was independent of the presenting diastolic pressure. The incidence of cardiac infarction and angina was not affected. Like Pickering[1] they pointed out that the protective role of hypertensive treatment lies in the prevention of cerebral haemorrhage from Charcot–Bouchard aneurysms first described in 1868[40], rediscovered by Russell in 1963[41] and further considered in 1967 by Cole and Yates[42], the importance of which frequently seemed to be overlooked, especially in the context of systolic hypertension.

Marshall[43] found a significant improvement in prognosis for cerebrovascular disease with long term hypotensive therapy and without unfortunate sequelae atrributable to treatment. However, the oldest patient was only 68 and the average age of the treated group was 41·2 years (control group 59·7).

Hamilton, Thompson and Wisniewski[44] found, again in the under-60s with diastolic pressures of at least 110, a significant improvement in the prognosis of essential symptomless hypertension with effective treatment.

Priddle *et al.*[45] carried out a controlled trial of treatment on 183 elderly patients (90% aged over 70, 86% female) in residential homes in Toronto, who had a systolic pressure of 180 mmHg or a diastolic of 100 on at least two occasions. The mortality rate of the treated group was about half of that of the controls. The drugs used were thiazides producing an average reduction of 20 mmHg systolic and 10 mmHg diastolic. Although this was not a random study and only mortality rates were studied, moderate falls in blood pressure were achieved without noticeable side-effects with a significant fall in the death rate.

It seems therefore that treatment of hypertension at all ages carries an improved prognosis and that in particular the protective effect is most important in the prevention of intracerebral haemorrhage from Charcot – Bouchard aneurysms. The Toronto trial[45] on elderly patients is especially encouraging as the protective effect was considerable with only a modest pressure drop.

Antihypertensive treatment after a stroke
The Hypertension–Stroke Cooperative Study Group[46] found no evidence that treatment of blood pressure averaging 167/100 (range 140/90 to 220/115), after a stroke, had any effect on the recurrence rate. The only positive effect was on the incidence of congestive cardiac failure. In this study the mean age was 59, 9 % being over 70 and 75 % aged 50–70; 80 % were black and 60 % were male.

Carter[47], also looking at the effects of hypotensive therapy after stroke, found better results in untreated patients aged over 65 with systolic hypertension (blood pressure more than 160 systolic and less than 110 diastolic). In this he agreed with Adams[48] who, recording the prognosis for hypertensive hemiplegics, felt that hypertension might almost be a positive factor for survival, 72 % of female survivors having systolic pressures of more than 185 mmHg, and 52 % diastolics of more than 110 mmHg. Adams felt that there were more important factors than the blood pressure alone in considering treatment after a stroke. He also noted the tendency for the untreated blood pressure to fall to lower levels over a 2–3 month period in hospital, rising again 1 month after discharge to levels still below those at onset. Merrett and Adams[49] comparing mortality rates after stroke found a higher mortality for the first 2 months after a stroke in normotensives than hypertensives (blood pressure more than 180/110), but after this time there was no difference. Treatment of diastolic hypertension (more than 110 mmHg) in the over-65s in Carter's series produced better results in the treated group but the numbers were small.

In strokes not treated for hypertension the recurrence rates were about 50 % over a follow-up period of 4 years[50–53] but Beevers et al.[38], aiming at diastolic pressures of less than 110 or preferably less than 100, obtained recurrence rates over 4 years with treatment of 29 % overall and 16 % in the well controlled. The average age however was only 56 and there was a marked contrast with Adams[48] and Merrett and Adams[49] whose subjects presumably were older, and with Carter's older subjects[47].

Treatment of hypertension after a stroke is therefore found to be variable in its results: the Hypertension–Stroke Cooperative Study Group[46] found no effect on recurrence rate in the middle-aged; Carter[47] in systolic hypertension found better results without treatment in the over-65s; while Adams[48] and Merrett and Adams[49] considered hypertension post-stroke in the elderly to be at worst innocuous and at best a positive factor for survival.

Conversely Beevers *et al.*[38] in younger subjects obtained much better results with treatment.

The conclusion seems to be that, after a stroke, treatment of hypertension is valuable in preventing recurrence in younger subjects but that the benefits of treatment wane with age and over 65 may be positively harmful[47–49].

CEREBRAL AUTOREGULATION

One of the closest associations with a raised blood pressure is the occurrence of stroke[24,25,29,38,39,43]. Consideration of the mechanism by which cerebral blood flow is maintained at a constant level, and the disorders to which it is prone in the elderly is therefore important in relation to the treatment of hypertension.

The maintenance of a constant cerebral blood flow in the face of varying systemic blood pressure (the Bayliss effect), has been demonstrated both in animals and in man[54]. As blood pressure increases, cerebral vessels constrict and as it is reduced they dilate; this phenomenon is termed autoregulation.

Lassen and Skinhøj[55] pointed out that the average whole brain blood flow in man was practically constant at 50 ml/100 g per min at a constant arterial partial pressure of carbon dioxide ($aPCO_2$). Within this overall value there were local increases in areas of increased function, that is regional cerebral blood flow (rCBF) was variable as the increased metabolism was matched by an increase in local flow. In brain infarction there was a decrease of function, metabolism and flow, in both the ipsilateral and contralateral hemispheres – 'transhemispheric depression'.

These two authors[55] and Obrist[56] examined the control of rCBF finding that $aPCO_2$ exerted a profound effect from maximal vasodilatation in hypercapnia, to vasoconstriction to hypoxic levels in hypocapnia. CO_2 reactivity was mediated by cerebrospinal fluid (CSF) periarteriolar pH changes which in turn were dependent on local

CSF bicarbonate concentration. This formed a homeostatic mechanism guarding brain pH against the effects of respiratory acidosis and alkalosis. Chronic $aPCO_2$ changes were so completely compensated that CSF pH was normal. It was therefore unwise rapidly to reduce a chronically raised $aPCO_2$ as the patient would probably develop signs of hypocapnia.

In contrast to the effects of $aPCO_2$ in which an alteration of pressure of 1 mmHg produced a 5% alteration in rCBF, arterial partial pressure of oxygen (aPO_2) produced little effect on rCBF until a threshold level of aPO_2 of 50 mmHg. At this level of aPO_2 progressive brain tissue lactacidosis occurred suggesting that in hypoxia rCBF was once more regulated by periarteriolar pH. There was a rich autonomic nerve supply to the intracranial extracerebral vessels. Obrist[56] quoted work which indicated increasing evidence of the role of autonomic activity in autoregulation, and it is probable that both metabolic and autonomic mechanisms act in series to maintain a constant cerebrovascular resistance.

Lassen and Skinhøj[55] found that brain lactacidosis resulted from even very short periods of underperfusion of brain tissue and it was obvious after resuscitation from cardiac arrest, in focal brain ischaemia, injury, tumour, haematoma, meningitis and subarachnoid haemorrhage. The lactacidosis might lead to local cerebral vasomotor paralysis with a danger of 'intracranial steal' following the exhibition of vasodilators, or 'inverse steal' after vasoconstrictors. Such lactacidosis could lead to a local or general 'luxury perfusion' when flow was in excess of metabolic demands, to local or general loss of autoregulation and to cerebral oedema. Adequate oxygenation was the most rational therapeutic approach; hyperventilation to reduce $aPCO_2$ was usually apparent as part of the body's homeostatic effort. It was equally important to avoid vasodilator drugs because of their adverse effect on intracranial pressure and so on rCBF, while the use of vasoconstrictor drugs might be considered in order to produce an 'inverse steal' situation.

Cerebral autoregulation in hypertension
In normotensives there was both a lower and an upper limit of autoregulation, that is below and above these levels cerebral blood flow passively followed the perfusion pressure. In hypertension cerebrovascular resistance was increased in proportion to the increased blood pressure so maintaining normal cerebral blood flow. Normally the lower limit of autoregulation was 60–70 mmHg but in hypertension this might rise to 110 or 130 mmHg. At the higher end the limit was raised[57] but when this was exceeded there was a

sudden increase in cerebral blood flow suggesting that the symptoms of hypertensive encephalopathy might be due to overdistension of vessels and oedema[55], and not due to vascular spasm[58], although no direct confirmation of this was obtained.

In ten patients with blood pressure levels of 160/110 to 250/145 Stranguaard *et al.*[59] also found the lower level to be reset at 120 mmHg. This rise also occurred in cerebral hypoxic states. They postulated that the upward shift of autoregulatory levels might be caused by arteriolar hypertrophy and might explain why patients cannot tolerate too rapid a lowering of blood pressure although a gradual lowering might reset the autoregulatory level. They also suggested that at the higher end a failure of autoregulation could give rise to sudden overperfusion, exudation, focal oedema, capillary compression and acute encephalopathy.

These observations are not specifically related to elderly subjects but establish the existence of cerebral autoregulation which maintains a normal cerebral blood flow in hypertension, brought about by an increase in cerebrovascular resistance, and define the means by which this resistance is controlled. The important practical implications include the dangers of vasodilator drugs and equally the dangers of too rapid a reduction of blood pressure in hypertension. This may lead to a sudden failure of adequate cerebral perfusion as systemic blood pressure falls below the raised lower limit of autoregulation.

For example, Graham[60] described two hypertensive patients in whom a precipitous fall of blood pressure in one instance to unrecordable levels and the other to 120/80 produced boundary infarction in the cerebral cortex. In the latter case in a normotensive patient no harm should have resulted but with the upward resetting of autoregulatory levels in hypertension, symptoms and signs of ischaemia developed with a sudden fall in blood pressure.

Jackson *et al.*[61] quoted six elderly patients (aged 64–84) who were admitted to hospital after episodes of unconsciousness within 1 week of starting vigorous hypotensive therapy for asymptomatic hypertension. All had presented symptoms of postural hypotension and had become housebound. Sheehy[62] described five patients with similar effects from overenthusiastic treatment.

Cerebral autoregulation in elderly hypertensives

Fazekas *et al.*[63] investigated cerebral blood flow, oxygen delivery and cerebral vascular resistance in both normotensive and hypertensive patients aged over 50 (mean age 74 for normotensives, 67 for hypertensives), before and after the inhalation of 5% CO_2, during hyperventilation and after the administration of intravenous aminophylline. They found the changes elicited were similar to, but less marked, than those seen in younger subjects without cerebrovascular disease. They concluded that the cerebrovasculature in the presence of arteriosclerosis can still respond to appropriate stimuli. There was a marked reduction of cerebral blood flow, metabolic rate and oxygen delivery and a marked increase in cerebrovascular resistance as compared with younger normal groups. The only significant difference between their normotensive and hypertensive groups was the greater cerebrovascular resistance in the latter, which was also seen in younger hypertensives. The greater cerebrovascular resistance in hypertensives of all ages, together with a lower cerebral blood flow implied a reduced calibre of the cerebral vessels in arteriosclerosis.

Meyer et al.[30], knowing that the cerebral vasodilator response to carbon dioxide was maintained, even if to a diminished degree, in subjects with cerebrovascular disease and hypertension[63], wondered if moderate to severe hypertension might reduce cerebral blood flow by excessive autoregulation, and if the cautious reduction of blood pressure in such subjects might increase the cerebral blood flow.

They investigated two groups of patients with stable cerebrovascular pathology, one group hypertensive (mean arterial pressure over 110 – average age 60·8 years), and one group normotensive (mean arterial pressure below 110 – average age 61·2 years). In both groups cerebral blood flow and oxygen and glucose consumption were decreased as compared with normal values. Cerebrovascular resistance was however significantly greater in the hypertensive than in the normotensive group.

In a further group of 13 hypertensive patients (average age 61·9 years) with stable or recovered cerebrovascular disease they measured cerebral blood flow and metabolism before and after reduction of blood pressure with α-methyldopa. A statistically significant decrease in blood pressure was achieved and the cerebrovascular resistance fell significantly in every case. In the group as a whole there was an increase in cerebral blood flow to a significant degree.

These changes suggested that autoregulation was maintained even to a diminished degree in these subjects, and that reduction of the hypertension reduced excessive vasoconstriction. They concluded that the occurrence of severe hypertension may cause such a degree of vasoconstriction that cerebral blood flow may be reduced, leading to local tissue acidosis, oedema and spasm, as is seen in hypertensive encephalopathy, in contrast to the mechanism suggested by Stranguaard *et al.*[59] and Lassen and Skinhøj[55].

Also in the elderly Sokoloff[64] found that healthy old people have similar cerebral blood flow to young controls, while Obrist[56] found that elderly subjects with mild symptomatic cerebrovascular disease, organic dementia and senile and presenile dementia without focal neurological signs, all had reduced cerebral blood flow.

Wollner[65] reported a failure of autoregulation in some elderly patients with symptomatic postural hypotension. In others with postural hypotension but no symptoms no such loss could be demonstrated.

Kendell and Marshall[66] using hexamethonium to paralyse the sympathetic ganglia, and a tilting table, failed to reproduce symptoms of previously experienced transient ischaemic attacks before generalized symptoms of hypotension developed, presumably because of the maintenance of cerebral autoregulation and perhaps provided further evidence for the relative safety of hypotensive therapy in cerebrovascular disease.

In summary, autoregulation of cerebral blood flow can be demonstrated to be normal in healthy elderly subjects[64], to be maintained even if to a diminished degree in elderly hypertensives[63] and to be inappropriate in degree and effects in some instances[30,65]. An increased cerebrovascular resistance in the face of a rise in the systemic blood pressure is a common, and indeed expected, finding in all age groups.

Importantly, the restrictive effects on cerebral blood flow can be reduced by appropriate hypotensive therapy[30] without producing the fell effects so graphically described by Graham[60], Jackson[61], and Sheehy[62], who demonstrate that too sudden reduction of systemic blood pressure may precipitate disaster.

Local variations in autoregulation within the brain may result in intracerebral 'steal' of blood supply from areas already threatened, especially with vasodilator drugs[55]; in others loss of autoregulation may produce symptoms of postural hypotension in patients who would be unaware of the drop in systemic blood pressure if autoregulation was maintained[65].

THE ASSESSMENT OF HYPERTENSION IN THE ELDERLY

The successful management of the elderly hypertensive depends primarily on correct assessment. It is not sufficient merely to record the blood pressure on one occasion and institute treatment, such a course is only too likely to produce the hypotensive disasters referred to earlier. The elderly hypertensive whose lower level of cerebral autoregulation may be elevated[57,59] and whose homeostatic mechanisms are failing is especially prone to a harmful fall in cerebral blood flow if systemic blood pressure is suddenly reduced. Contrariwise there is general agreement that there is an increased risk of untoward cardiovascular events with increased systolic blood pressure in elderly subjects. The problem facing the doctor, dealing with an elderly patient, is how to proceed safely to avoid the risks associated with a raised blood pressure on the one hand and the risks of the treatment itself on the other.

Simpson[67], discussing the treatment of high blood pressure in the over-60s advised asking four questions: (1) How high is the blood pressure really? (2) Is there a treatable cause? (3) How much organ damage is there? (4) Are there any associated conditions influencing treatment or prognosis?

The height of the blood pressure

The first of these, how high is the blood pressure really, is extremely pertinent. In younger age groups there is wide acceptance of the prognostic importance of casual blood pressure readings, even though they may mask very wide swings in pressure in both normotensives and hypertensives[1], and there is also a marked circadian rhythm[68]. In the elderly casual blood pressure readings may not be so reliable either prognostically or as an indication for treatment. Personal experience shows that high levels of blood pressure found by chance, for example at a domiciliary visit, may disappear on admission to hospital or at day hospital attendance. Adams[48] noted the tendency for blood pressure to fall spontaneously over a period after a stroke. Coleandrea *et al.*[21] reported the marked lability of the blood pressure in elderly subjects (average age almost 70); the prevalence of systolic hypertension, as defined, fell from 14% at initial screening to 2·7% on the third clinic visit. Pickering[1], referring to the same phenomenon in some younger subjects, considered that it was a manifestation of a defence reflex, followed by its gradual extinction with repeated visits and blood pressure measurements; this may well be equally applicable to the elderly.

Blood pressure readings in the elderly should be repeated, until on at least three occasions the figures obtained are consistent and indicate that a relatively stable state has been reached. The readings should be obtained over a period of time, and while a sustained diastolic pressure, in excess of 120 mmHg for example, for some days indicates a need for appropriate treatment, more prolonged observation extending to several weeks or even a month or two is advisable when diastolic or systolic pressures are less severely elevated or their trend is still uncertain. Having established the stable level of blood pressure, consideration then needs to be given to the other questions raised by Simpson[67].

Treatable causes
The likelihood of a treatable cause in the elderly is small (as indeed is almost as true in younger age groups and certainly in the middle-aged), and unless there is a clinical suspicion of endocrine disturbance or evidence of a renal lesion of recent onset, particularly pyelonephritis, little is likely to be gained by extensive investigation.

Organ damage
The question of organ damage as an indication for treatment is a vexed one. If it has occurred it ought to be regarded as a failure of treatment (in the widest sense), or certainly of prevention, rather than forming an indication to institute treatment in the hope of preventing a recurrence. In the case of stroke for instance, the evidence suggests that treatment, as a preventive factor against recurrence, is of value in younger subjects but may be positively harmful in the elderly[47]. The consequences of a stroke to the individual and to the community are severe. There is increased risk, notably of stroke, with increasing blood pressure. The inference must be that reduction of risk before the damage occurs by appropriate control of blood pressure is required. These considerations should apply as much to the elderly as to the middle-aged, as the former and their spouses are even less able to cope with the effects of a stroke than those who are younger. There can be no doubt, at any age, that prevention of a stroke is preferable to living with the results as a stroke survivor. Similar considerations apply to hypertensive cardiac and renal disease.

Associated factors
The fourth question of Simpson related to associated factors influencing treatment or prognosis. He quoted smoking, alcohol, hyperlipidaemia, diabetes, anaemia, asthma and depression, but, oddly, omitted consideration of weight.

Obesity and blood pressure

Kannel *et al.*[69], like Harlan *et al.*[9], remarked that obesity was a significant contributor to a raised blood pressure and that obesity went hand in hand with rising blood pressure and advancing age. This was true throughout the range of blood pressure and weight. They noted that there was an increase in blood pressure with weight gain and a fall with weight loss, and that this was true in the non-obese as well as in the obese, and was more striking in men than in women.

Reisen *et al.*[70], noting the Framingham evidence and other studies that equated blood pressure reduction by weight loss with reduction in dietary sodium, carried out a study on 107 middle-aged hypertensives (140/90 mmHg or more), all of whom were at least 10% overweight, using salt-unrestricted reducing diets. In a group on no drug therapy the blood pressure reduced to normal in 75% after a mean weight loss of 8·8 kg. In a group initially poorly controlled by hypotensive drugs a mean weight loss of 9·8 kg resulted in 61% of the blood pressures returning to normal levels. No such reduction was obtained in a poorly controlled group who did not lose weight.

They achieved blood pressure reductions ranging from 28/19 mmHg/6·7 kg weight loss in the moderately obese to 48/24 mmHg/10·3 kg weight loss in the very obese. They concluded that weight reduction by dietary restriction was both highly cost-effective in reducing blood pressure and independent of sodium levels in the diet.

Ramsay *et al.*[71], in patients on average 15·7% overweight (no age range stated) using 800 kcal diets achieved an average weight loss of 6 kg and a reduction in blood pressure of 20/15 mmHg/10 kg weight loss, which is of the same order as Reisin and colleagues obtained. The difference in blood pressure reduction between this group and a group who lost less than 3 kg was statistically highly significant, although blood pressures in the latter group also fell slightly.

Ballantyne, Devine and Fife[72] from Glasgow, on the other hand, found a relationship between obesity and blood pressure only in male non-smokers. They also found that their data from Scotland suggested that weight reduction was unlikely to reduce blood pressure significantly in hypertensives. This study, however, was on relatively small numbers aged in the middle to late 40s.

The Framingham study showed a relationship between blood pressure and weight and Reisin and colleagues[70] and Ramsay and colleagues[71] confirmed that blood pressure reduction was obtainable by weight loss. All these studies, including the less favourable results of Ballantyne and colleagues[72] were performed on the middle-aged but as with the risk factors from hypertension there is no reason to suppose that the effects of weight reduction would be entirely extinguished in the elderly.

The difficulty of achieving weight loss is no less in the elderly, and indeed may be greater after a lifetime of unsuitable eating habits, but the evidence suggests that this approach to blood pressure re-duction should be fundamental as without weight reduction it may be difficult to achieve any lowering of blood pressure at all[70].

The good effects of weight reduction are of course not confined to the blood pressure; the patients' joints and general mobility, their tendency to hiatal herniation and pelvic prolapse, their respiratory effort and glucose tolerance, no less than their cardiovascular system, are all likely to benefit. It seems that dietitians are more successful than doctors in achieving weight loss[70,71] and their help is especially important in trying to influence the feeding habits of a lifetime. A nihilistic approach to weight loss in hypertension is not justified, and intervention of any kind has some effect[71].

Associated prognostic factors

The adverse prognostic effects of factors associated with hyperten-sion have also been commented on in respect of atrial fibrillation and other forms of cardiac disease and non-cerebral atherosclerosis[25], and cervical bruits and abnormal ECGs[24]. Ander-son and Cowan[17] noted the relation of peripheral arterial disease to blood pressure. They recorded: (1) the presence of abnormality on ophalmological examination and (2) on radial artery palpation, and (3) the absence of pulsation in one or more of the dorsalis pedis and posterior tibial arteries. When all three criteria were abnormal the upper limits of systolic blood pressure were appreciably higher in both sexes (Table 6). In men diastolic pressure was not influenced significantly by the number of abnormalities; in women it increased by 2 mmHg for each vascular attribute which was abnormal.

The finding of such cardiac and extracardiac-associated factors should lead to careful consideration of the indication for treatment in doubtful cases.

Age itself, illogically it would seem, is often quoted prognostically as an indication for or against treatment, usually against, in the elderly. Thus Hamilton[73], while awaiting the results of current trials, described his and others' reluctance to impose a therapeutic regimen on the elderly remarking that it was an emotional rather than a logical attitude. Simpson[67] quoted age over 70 as a factor against

Table 6 The relation of abnormalities of the peripheral circulation to systolic blood pressure in apparently healthy men and women – see text (from Anderson and Cowan[17])

| | Systolic blood pressure (mmHg) | | |
| | No abnormal criteria | Three abnormal criteria | |
Age	Males and females	Males	Females
60 years	185	204	211
85 years	200	218	225

treatment in borderline cases. Isaacs[74], having divided the elderly population into those likely and unlikely to comply with treatment, recommended treatment of the compliant asymptomatic only if the blood pressure was rising and the age less than 75. He would treat those with symptoms, aged less than 75, and would consider treatment of symptomatic and compliant patients over 75. The evidence[2,4,20-25] of increased risk of morbidity and mortality with rising systolic pressure suggests however that age *per se* should not be the overriding factor.

Clinical assessment

The assessment of an elderly patient with a raised blood pressure, whether symptomatic or not, requires a full history including enquiry about angina, claudication, dyspnoea, oedema and earlier cardiac disease; examination of the peripheral vascular system for bruits and absence of peripheral pulses, and of the retina for signs of hypertensive retinopathy. The heart should be examined for signs of cardiac disorder including coronary and rheumatic heart disease, cardiac enlargement or heart failure and particularly atrial fibrillation[25]. ECG abnormalities should be sought, especially left ventricular hypertrophy. General examination should look for evidence of obesity, nephropathy, neurological involvement, hyperlipidaemia, smoking, diabetes and gout, and include appropriate investigations. It should also establish the presence or absence of major abnormalities affecting other systems of the body. Unless there is an excessive and sustainedly high pressure requiring early treatment, such as a diastolic blood pressure of 120 mmHg, or the presence of hypertensive cardiac failure, which is a major indication for treatment, the blood pressure should be measured and observed until stable values are obtained.

Blood pressure levels requiring treatment in the elderly
Having achieved a stable blood pressure and having fully assessed
the patient what levels of blood pressure should be treated even in
the asymptomatic?

Diastolic blood pressure
In younger age groups the evidence is that reduction of diastolic
pressures of less than 105 mmHg does not result in significant lowering of morbidity risks[36]. Simpson considered treatment to be
advisable in a diastolic range of 105–115 mmHg in the over-60s
and to be mandatory above this level. Chrysant, Frohlich and
Papper[75] recommended treatment of diastolic pressure over
95 mmHg at any age. They seem not to have recognized that the
excess risks which are statistically related to diastolic elevations over
this level are not significantly reduced by treatment below diastolic
pressures of 105 mmHg. The adverse prognostic effect of diastolic
pressures of 110 mmHg or more was noted by Miall and Chinn[2]. In
fact, largely for the reasons advanced by O'Rourke[19] diastolic pressures of more than 110 mmHg are not commonly found in the
elderly as compared with systolic elevations, the former occurring in
about 3% of whites and about 10% of blacks over the age of 65[76].
    For sustained diastolic pressures exceeding 105 mmHg, unrespon-
sive to weight loss, treatment should be instituted cautiously to
reduce the pressure to less than 105 mmHg. This is indicated at any
age in the elderly population, even in the asymptomatic, as there is
no evidence of declining risk with advancing years[4,20].

Systolic blood pressure
In contrast to diastolic pressure systolic elevations of 160 mmHg or
more vary in prevalence from 26·9% in males aged 75–79 in
America[77] to 68% in women aged 90 in Scotland[12]. There is much
evidence of increasing morbidity and mortality with increasing
systolic pressures but there is no evidence available yet as to the
protective effects of treatment of elevated systolic pressures in the
elderly, or if effective whether there are levels below which the gain
from treatment becomes insignificant.
    A priori it would seem that any reduction in pressure would be
advantageous in a patient who for instance has Charcot – Bouchard
aneurysms and Priddle's experience in Toronto[45] treating systolic
pressures in excess of 180 mmHg, in which the mortality rate was
halved, is promising. Apart from this study there is some evidence
that a systolic pressure of 180 mmHg or more is associated with a
sharply increased risk. The Chicago Stroke Study[20], and Miall and

Chinn in Wales[2] both noted the sudden jump in mortality rates above the 180 mmHg level. In Jamaica, in 1065 men and women aged 35–64, Ashcroft and Desai[78] found significantly increased mortality only at pressures over 180 systolic and 110 diastolic but warned against comparisons between dissimilar populations. Gubner's[22] examination of insurance statistics found too few instances of higher levels of systolic pressure for reliable conclusions to be drawn, though as he reported steadily increasing mortality at lower systolic levels; it would seem unlikely that this tendency would disappear or be reversed as pressures continued to rise. Indeed the very absence of subjects with higher pressures suggests that insurance companies regard them as uninsurable because of the risk of mortality.

The conclusion at present, on epidemiological grounds, is that elderly subjects who are found to have a consistently elevated blood pressure should be appropriately treated in order to maintain the pressure at levels below 180 mmHg systolic, or 105 mmHg diastolic, either singly or together. The results of clinical examination and assessment referred to above may modify the action to be taken in the individual patient. Thus the finding of a condition of severely limited prognosis, such as carcinoma of the lung or stomach, would probably preclude treatment of hypertension of any grade. Carcinoma of the prostate, for instance, often carrying quite a long prognosis, would have a much slighter impact on the decision whether to treat. The possible prevention of a stroke in a patient already disabled by rheumatoid arthritis might form a positive indication.

Contraindications to treatment

The most important contraindication to treatment is the production of hypotensive ill-effects of any degree. Close supervision of the blood pressure when treatment is begun or altered is mandatory.

A major contraindication is the presence of hypertensive brain failure which has a bad prognosis and is frequently made worse by pressure reduction[34,79][82]. Lesser degrees of intellectual impairment likewise warrant caution not least because of possible problems of compliance with treatment[81]. Treatment after a stroke has already been referred to and is best avoided in the elderly[47]. Due note should be taken of evidence of failing renal function in elderly patients as a drug-induced fall in renal blood flow may precipitate uraemia and the renal excretion of drugs may be affected.

A possible contraindication to treatment is often thought to arise from the reassessment of the needs of elderly patients who have grown old with their raised blood pressure and its therapy. The criterion should not be some arbitrary age alone but assessment should include the whole patient and his wellbeing.

If treatment is withdrawn it should be done gradually and the effects on the control of the blood pressure closely followed. The problems which may arise from psychological dependence on long standing drug therapy should be borne in mind.

There are clear benefits to be gained from the reduction of treatment in an age group, one of whose major problems is frequently polypharmacy, and a policy of regular review of the indications for continuing treatment in individual patients is to be commended.

TREATMENT

The approach to the treatment of raised blood pressure in the elderly was epitomized in a *Lancet* leading article[27]: 'blood pressure reduction (in the elderly) should be planned as gentle seduction rather than an acute battle'.

With increasing blood pressure (especially systolic in the elderly), there is increasing risk of coronary artery disease, cardiac failure, and stroke. It is in the prevention of the last of these in particular, that the cautious approach to pressure reduction is so important, because of the twin dangers of a raised lower level of cerebral autoregulation on the one hand, or markedly diminished cerebral autoregulatory function on the other. In both instances abrupt reductions of systemic blood pressure may rob the brain of its blood flow with catastrophic results.

It is thus reassuring that several studies have failed to show hypotensive ill-effects with carefully regulated treatment[30,39,43,45,47,63] or even under quite severe experimental conditions[66]. Equally there is universal condemnation of the use of the powerful sympatholytic agents in the elderly[35,62,75,79,81-87] and their use should not be considered unless in the most exceptional circumstances. These drugs therefore will not be discussed, but should their use be necessary the dose must be titrated most carefully against the response and a careful watch kept for any signs of postural or exertional hypotension.

When, after full assessment, it is decided to treat an elevated blood pressure of 180/105 or more in an elderly patient, the first step is to undertake weight reduction, especially if the patient is obese. If successful, there is evidence in the middle-aged[70,71] that this alone will significantly reduce blood pressure, and if omitted the presence of obesity will make drug therapy less effective[70]. Again such effects are unlikely to be totally abolished by advancing years.

If weight reduction is unlikely to be achieved, or while awaiting its effects, drug therapy may be begun, the blood pressure being closely monitored, and treatment can be adjusted later in the light of progress made. Those who advise against the use of sympatholytic agents in the elderly are equally consistent, with occasional reservations, in agreeing that thiazide diuretics are the drugs of first choice – step 1 agents.

Step 1 treatment

Thiazide diuretics

The benzothiadiazines, acting on the cortical diluting segment of the renal tubule, are intermediate in diuretic potency between the 'loop' diuretics (frusemide and ethacrynic acid) and those acting on the distal tubule and collecting duct (spironolactone, triamterene and amiloride). The antihypertensive mechanisms of all these orally administered diuretics are uncertain but initially they produce negative sodium and water balance, resulting in a fall in body weight, extracellular fluid and plasma volumes, and in cardiac output. Renal blood flow and glomerular filtration rate fall slightly and plasma renin activity increases[86].

These effects occur in both normotensive and hypertensive subjects, but only in the latter is there an accompanying fall in blood pressure. The same effects may be produced by dietary salt restriction.

After about a month of treatment both cardiac output and the fluid compartment volumes return to normal. The sustained antihypertensive effect appears to be due to the development of a diminished peripheral resistance from a reduction in vascular reactivity to pressor amines, together with a persistent reduction of total body sodium content and of plasma volume.

Appropriate doses of this group of drugs in the elderly include bendrofluazide 5–10 mg/day; hydrochlorothiazide 50–100 mg/day; and cyclopenthiazide 0.25–0.5 mg/day, to produce an equivalent hypotensive effect.

The 'loop' diuretics are of equivalent hypotensive potency but their greater diuretic effects increase the risk of dehydration, hypokalaemia and metabolic alkalosis. They should be reserved for the early treatment of hypertensive cardiac failure or for patients with marked renal insufficiency and are not suitable for prolonged treatment of hypertension.

The hypotensive effects of the distal diuretics are the subject of varying opinion[87], and they are not commonly used as drugs of first choice.

Side effects of the thiazide diuretics Of the oral diuretics the benzothiadiazines are the most suitable for the long-term treatment of hypertension. Apart from the initial dangers of water and sodium depletion in the first month of treatment they share three main unwanted side effects:

(i) Hypokalaemia In the elderly dietary potassium intake is often reduced and its renal conservation impaired. The concurrent administration of potassium supplements is therefore strongly advised especially in patients on digitalis, or when using chlorthalidone which has the same site of action as the thiazides and is particularly prone to give rise to hypokalaemia. Suitable preparations of potassium include slow-release tablets of potassium chloride 600 mg 2–6 tablets/day yielding 16–48 mmol of potassium, or effervescent tablets containing potassium bicarbonate and potassium chloride yielding 12 mmol of potassium per tablet, 1–4 tablets/day. A number of thiazide diuretics are marketed in combination with slow-release potassium tablets, with the advantage of ease of dosage, but they share the problem of a fixed and probably insufficient dose of potassium to counteract the kaliuretic effects of the diuretic combined with it. An alternative approach is to administer a potassium-retaining diuretic at the same time, such as spironolactone 50–100 mg/day, or triamterene 100–200 mg/day, to counteract the hypokalaemic effect of 100 mg/day of hydrochlorothiazide or its equivalent. Amiloride 5 mg is combined in the same tablet as hydrochlorothiazide 50 mg, as Moduretic and has much to commend it for the simplicity of dosage, an important point in the elderly.

(ii) Hyperglycaemia Since diabetics and suspected prediabetics are common in the elderly this side-effect should be looked for by regular blood sugar estimations while on treatment.

(iii) Hyperuricaemia and gout The former is said to occur in 65 to 70% of patients treated with thiazides[88] but overt gout is probably only seen in one-tenth of these. Less common side-effects include hypercalcaemia and skin rashes.

The exhibition of oral diuretics during or after weight loss will probably suffice to reduce the blood pressure of many elderly patients to acceptable levels.

Reported experience with diuretics as hypertensive agents in the elderly

Reported trials of diuretic therapy for hypertension in the elderly are few but Priddle *et al.*[45] achieved a reduction in mortality of 50% in a treated group of elderly patients against controls by pressure reductions of 20 mmHg systolic and 10 mmHg diastolic using chloro-thiazide, 250 mg/day in the majority of patients. Pressures treated were those in excess of 180 mmHg systolic or 100 mmHg diastolic. Amery *et al.*[83] reported the pilot trial of the European Working Party on High Blood Pressure in the Elderly. The drugs used were hydrochlorothiazide 25 mg, and triamterene 50 mg, combined in one capsule, with methyldopa added if the blood pressure failed to respond after 1 month on diuretics only, and after the initial dose of diuretic had been doubled. After 1 year 55% of the treatment group were still on diuretics alone. A significant decrease in systolic and diastolic blood pressure was found in both treated and placebo groups in the first 3 months, but there was a significant difference in favour of the treated group thereafter, although placebo group pressures also continued to fall.

Electrolyte disturbances were not significant, and there was no difference in glucose tolerance between the treatment and control groups and though serum uric acid levels were significantly raised after 1 year in the treatment group no attack of gout was reported.

The ability of the two diuretics, alone or in combination with methyldopa, to produce a significant hypotensive action in the elderly, confirmed the earlier work of Corman and Sversky[89].

Step 2 treatment
In those cases where a satisfactory fall of blood pressure is not obtained with diuretics alone, the addition of further drugs in step-wise fashion should be considered. It needs to be emphasized that these further drugs should be given in addition to, and not instead of, the baseline diuretic drugs of first choice, in order to obtain a potentiating effect. In Great Britain the choice of step 2 drugs lies between α-methyldopa and the β-adrenergic blockers, as the rauwolfia compounds are generally considered to carry an unaccept-able risk of depression, extrapyramidal disturbance and fluid reten-tion in the elderly[75,81,82,87,88,90,91]

α-Methyldopa
This drug interferes with chemical neurotransmission at postgang-lionic nerve endings by producing a false and less potent neuro-transmitter, which blocks the adrenergic receptors, resulting in a decrease in peripheral arteriolar resistance. It also has a sedating effect on the central nervous system reducing the outflow of sym-pathetic activity[91].

It is effective in reducing blood pressure in both standing and supine positions, with little exertional hypotension, and in small doses postural hypotension is unusual.

Appropriate doses in the elderly should not exceed 125 mg twice daily to start with and may be increased by 125 mg/day, every 4 or 5 days, titrating the dose against the level of blood pressure obtained. It should rarely be necessary to exceed a total dose of more than 1·5 g/day in elderly patients already taking a diuretic, which is in any case advisable to counteract the tendency of methyldopa to cause sodium and fluid retention.

Side-effects of α-methyldopa
(i) Somnolence, decreased mental acuity, depression   These effects are dose related and daytime sedation may occur in two-fifths or more of patients. They may subside after a few weeks but in the elderly the results can be very troublesome, the daytime sedation leading to forgetfulness and problems of behaviour, and compliance with this and other drug therapy. The necessity to start with small doses and increase slowly is obvious.
(ii) Sodium and fluid retention   The incidence is high and may occur in as many as two-thirds of subjects. The necessity for baseline diuretic therapy before embarking on methyldopa is self-evident.
(iii) Dry mouth   This is very common and may be troublesome and again may result in non-compliance with treatment.
(iv) Sexual dysfunction   Widely varying incidence of this problem is reported and it should not be overlooked in the fit elderly.
(v) Less common side-effects   These include liver damage and hepatitis, which may be severe though fortunately are rare. A positive direct Coombs test is said to occur in 20% of patients, though only 0·1 to 0·2% of those with a positive Coombs test ever develop haemolytic anaemia[88].

In the elderly who are prone to the effects of polypharmacy, the tendency of methyldopa to interact with phenothiazines, tricyclic antidepressants and lithium should not be forgotten.

Methyldopa is widely accepted as a hypotensive agent for use in the elderly[62,75,79,81-84,90,92] and the guidelines are: (1) always add it to pre-existing diuretic therapy; (2) start with a small dose and only increase slowly, titrating the dose to the blood pressure.

β-adrenergic blockers
The mode of action of this group of drugs, the major alternative to methyldopa, in the second step control of hypertension in the elderly, is still a matter for debate. Their actions include a reduction

in cardiac output, primarily through a reduction in heart rate, a reduction in plasma renin activity, and a central nervous system effect[93,94], although Barritt and Marshall[95] remark that there is little evidence that these are the true reasons for their hypotensive action.

β-blockers show little difference in their hypotensive activity whether they have intrinsic sympathomimetic activity (ISA) or whether they lack it, or indeed whether they are cardioselective or not. However those with ISA (acebutolol, oxprenolol, pindolol) are perhaps less likely to cause extreme bradycardia while cardioselective β-blockers (acebutolol, metroprolol) are less likely to cause bronchospasm. Propranolol, though lacking either of these attributes, has a long history of safe use when used with due care and the avoidance of situations in which it is likely to be harmful, such as patients in heart failure, with atrioventricular conduction defects, or with a history of bronchospasm. Despite the claims made for the later drugs of this class none is immune from precipitating danger in these circumstances.

As with methyldopa the addition of a β-blocker to a diuretic should be made gradually, again titrating the dose against the blood pressure response. Treatment should always begin with small doses, for example, propranolol 40 mg/day in divided doses and increments should be limited to 10–20 mg/day at not less than weekly intervals. Illustrative final doses which should be approached gradually over a period of time include propranolol 120–240 mg/day, oxyprenolol 160–320 mg/day, pindolol 10–45 mg/day, and acebutolol 200–600 mg/day given in a single dose.

Side-effects of β-adrenergic blockers To a varying degree these drugs share the same side effects:

(i) Aggravation or precipitation of heart failure In no circumstances should elderly patients in cardiac failure and not on diuretic or digitalis treatment be given beta-blockers, and their use should be avoided after control of heart failure unless essential.

(ii) Aggravation or precipitation of bronchoconstriction This is said to occur in 2 to 10% of patients even without a previous history of asthma[88]. In the elderly in particular a minor chest infection can precipitate bronchospasm even when beta-blockers have been previously well tolerated[96].

(iii) Interference with diabetic control β-Blockers may prolong hypoglycaemia in insulin-dependent diabetics, and hypoglycaemia has been reported even in non-diabetics[88]. Confusingly they can also block the insulin response to hyperglycaemia. These drugs should be avoided in insulin-dependent diabetics and the blood sugar of elderly patients checked before use.

(iv) Bradyarrthythmias   As with heart failure these constitute a contraindication to use, and as they are not uncommon in the elderly they should be excluded before treatment is begun.

(v) Central nervous system (CNS) disturbances   A wide variety of symptoms may occur including insomnia, vivid dreams, confusion and hallucinations. Many of these are common in the elderly and enquiry about their presence should always be made before starting treatment lest they should be worsened.

(iv) Less severe side-effects   These include cold extremities and Raynaud's phenomenon. The former can be troublesome. Skin rashes, gastrointestinal disturbances and sodium and fluid retention also occur and the serious complications experienced with practolol demand vigilance during the use of all drugs of this class.

Reported experience of β-adrenergic blockers as hypotensive agents in the elderly

Eisalo, Heino and Munter[97] reported the use of a β-blocker in elderly hypertensives in a Finnish home for the elderly. In an uncontrolled series, 38 patients (average age 72) were treated with alprenolol 400 mg/day. Average systolic pressures fell from 204 mmHg to 184 mmHg over the 3 month period of treatment, and average diastolic pressures from 114 mmHg to 103 mmHg. Three out of the 38 (8%) developed cardiac failure in the first week of treatment and had to be withdrawn.

The fall in pressure in this elderly group is similar to that observed by Barritt and Marshall[95] who, in younger subjects, reported that the average blood pressure drop was 20 mmHg with a range of up to 40 mmHg. They found that the effective dose range was narrow and the full effect in any given patient was known in a fortnight. They noted that of the side-effects complaints of cold hands and feet occurred in a quarter of patients. No large-scale trial of β-blockers as hypotensives has been reported in the elderly.

Step 3 treatment

In the uncommon event of the blood pressure of an elderly patient failing to respond to a diuretic (step 1), plus methyldopa or a β-blocker (step 2), consideration should be given to the addition of vasodilators such as hydrallazine or prazosin. These and other drugs of this class given by mouth act on arteriolar smooth muscle causing vasodilatation and a fall in peripheral resistance. Hitherto the vasodilators have not been widely used because of their associated effects of reflex tachycardia, increased cardiac output, loss of hypotensive effect, exacerbation of angina or heart failure and sodium and fluid retention. Apart from their reflex effects on pulse rate and cardiac output the sole use of vasodilators should also be avoided because of their likely adverse effect on the cerebral circulation in causing intracerebral 'steal'.

Since the advent of the β-blockers and of 'stepped' therapy however, the position has changed and a vasodilator given concurrently with a β-blocker combine in their hypotensive effect, thus enabling the use of lower doses of each, while each compensates for the effects on the pulse rate of the other.

Suitable doses of hydrallazine for the elderly are 25–50 mg twice or thrice daily, once agian starting with small doses and increasing slowly over a period of time. As such patients would already be on diuretics sodium and fluid retention should not be a problem.

The well known SLE syndrome is unusual with doses of hydrallazine of less than 200 mg/day. The newer introduction prazosin has been associated with sudden collapse and unconsciousness in about 1% of patients after the first dose; it should therefore only be started while the patient is under continuous supervision. A suitable starting dose of the latter would be 0·25 mg three times daily.

CONCLUSIONS

Far from being innocuous raised blood pressure in the elderly carries an increased risk of cardiovascular morbidity and mortality, and this is true in both sexes. However, largely because of the effects on the blood pressure wave of a stiffening arterial tree, it is the level of systolic blood pressure which is predominantly associated with untoward events, and which tends to increase with increasing age (though the two may not be directly related). For the same reasons diastolic pressures are uncommonly severely elevated in the elderly.

At present the levels of blood pressure which are known to be associated with a significantly increased risk in elderly subjects, are over 180 mmHg systolic, and over 110 mmHg diastolic. Reduction of the diastolic blood pressure below 105 mmHg does not achieve any further lessening of risk. It is uncertain whether reduction of systolic blood pressure below 180 mmHg in the elderly is advantageous in terms of risk or not.

The recommendation at present is therefore cautiously to treat elderly patients whose blood pressure is consistently in excess of

180/105 mmHg in order to reduce it to, or if judged safe, to below this level, provided there are no contraindications or modifying factors, after full assessment of the whole patient.

Treatment should begin with weight loss if at all possible, and where drugs are used a 'stepped' approach to therapy should be employed, at all times titrating the dose of the agents used to the effect on the blood pressure. Rapid reduction of the systemic blood pressure must at all costs be avoided in the elderly hypertensive because of the probable malign effects on the cerebral circulation whose autoregulatory functions may be compromised.

References

1 Pickering, Sir G. (1972). Hypertension – definitions, natural histories and consequences. *Am. J. Med.*, **52**, 570

2 Miall, W. E. and Chinn, C. (1974). Screening for hypertension, some epidemiological observations. *Br. Med. J.*, **3**, 595

3 Miall, W. E. and Oldham, P. D. (1963). The hereditary factor in arterial blood pressure. *Br. Med. J.*, **1**, 75

4 Kannel, W. B. (1974). Assessment of hypertension as a predictor of cerebrovascular disease: the Framingham Study. In: D. M. Burley, G. F. B. Birdwood, J. H. Fryer, S. H. Taylor (eds.). *Hypertension – its Nature and Treatment*, pp. 69–86. (Horsham: Ciba Laboratories)

5 MacCulloch, M. J. (1972). Psychosomatic aspects of hypertension. *Practitioner*, **208**, 704

6 Leading article (1978). Hypertension – salt poisoning? *Lancet*, **i**, 1136

7 Tudge, C. (1978). The biggest risk factor of them all? *World Med.*, **13, (12)**, 21

8 Miall, W. E. and Lovell, H. G. (1967). Relation between change of blood pressure and age. *Br. Med. J.*, **2**, 660

9 Harlan, W. R., Oberman, A., Mitchell, R. E. and Graybiel, A. (1973). A thirty year study of blood pressure in a white male cohort. In: G. Onesti, K. E. Kim, J. H. Moyer (eds). *Hypertension: Mechanisms and Management*, p. 85. (New York: Grune and Stratton)

10 Hamilton, M., Pickering, G. W., Fraser Roberts, J. A. and Sowry, G. S. C. (1954). The arterial pressure in the general population. *Clin. Sci. Molec. Med.*, **13**, 11

11 Heller, R. F. and Rose, G. (1977). Current management of hypertension in hospital. *Br. Med. J.*, **1**, 1441

12 Kitchin, A. H., Lowther, C. P. and Milne, J. S. (1973). Problems of clinical and electrocardiographic evidence of ischaemic heart diseases in the older population. *Br. Heart J.*, **35**, 946

13 Russek, H. I. and Zohman, B. L. (1946). Normal blood pressure in senescence. *Geriatrics*, **1**, 113

14 Droller, H., Pemberton, J., Roseman, C. and Grout, J. L. A. (1952). High blood pressure in the elderly. *Br. Med. J.*, **2**, 968

15 Master, A. M., Lasser, R. P. and Jaffe, H. L. (1958). Blood pressure in white people over 65 years of age. *Ann. Intern. Med.*, **48**, 284

16 Anderson, W. F. and Cowan, N. R. (1959). Arterial pressure in healthy older people. *Clin. Sci.*, **18**, 103

17 Anderson, W. F. and Cowan, N. R. (1972). Arterial blood pressure in healthy older people. *Gerontol. Clin.*, **14**, 129

18 Babu, T. N., Nazir, F., Rao, D. B. and Luisada, A. A. (1977). What is 'normal' blood pressure in the aged. *Geriatrics*, **32 (1)**, 73

19 O'Rourke, M. F. (1970). Arterial haemodynamics in hypertension. *Circ. Res.*, **26 and 27** (Suppl. 2), 123

20 Dyer, A. R., Stamler, J., Shekelle, R. B., Schoenberger, J. A. and Farinaro, E. (1977). Hypertension in the elderly. *Med. Clin. N. Am.*, **61 (3)**, 513

21 Colandrea, M. A., Friedman, G. D., Nichaman, M. Z. and Lynd, C. N. (1970). Systolic hypertension in the elderly. *Circulation*, **41**, 239

22 Gubner, R. S. (1962). Systolic hypertension: a pathogenetic entity. *Am. J. Cardiol.*, **9**, 773

23 Shekelle, R., Ostfield, A. and Klawans, H. (1974). Hypertension and risk of stroke in an elderly population. *Stroke*, **5**, 71

24 Cutler, J. L. (1967). Cerebrovascular disease in an elderly population. *Circulation*, **36**, 394

25 Friedman, G. D., in Hyg, S. M., Loveland, D. B. and Ehrlich, S. P. Jr. (1968), Relationship of stroke to other cardiovascular disease. *Circulation*, **38**, 533

26 Fry, J. (1974). Natural history of hypertension – a case for selective non-treatment. *Lancet*, **ii**, 431

27 Leading article. (1977). Hypertension in the elderly. *Lancet*, **i**, 684

28 Kell, W. B., Gordon, T. and Schwartz, M. J. (1971). Systolic versus diastolic blood pressure and risk of coronary heart disease – the Framingham Study. *Am. J. Cardiol.*, **27**, 335

29 Kannel, W. B., Philip, A. W., Verter, J. and McNamara, P. M. (1970). Epidemiologic assessment of the role of blood pressure in stroke – the Framingham Study. *J. Am. Med. Assoc.*, **214**, 301

30 Meyer, J. S., Sawada, T., Kitamura, A. and Toyoda, M. (1968). Cerebral blood flow after control of hypertension in stroke. *Neurology*, **18**, 772

31 Kannel, W. B., Castelli, W. P., McNamara, P. M., McKee, P. A. and Feinleib, M. (1972). The role of blood pressure in the development of congestive cardiac failure. *N. Engl. J. Med.*, **287**, 781

32 Anderson, T. W. (1978). Re-examination of some of the Framingham blood pressure data. *Lancet*, **ii**, 1139

33 Leading article, (1978). The anomaly that wouldn't go away. *Lancet*, **ii**, 978

34 Kennedy, R. D. (1974). Hypertension. *Mod. Geriatr.*, **4**, 360

35 Veterans' Administration Cooperative Study Group on antihypertensive agents. (1967). Effects of treatment on morbidity in hypertension. I. Results in patients with diastolic blood pressure averaging 115 to 129 mmHg. *J. Am. Med. Assoc.* **202**, 1028

36 Veterans' Administration Cooperative Study Group on antihypertensive agents. (1970). Effects of treatment on morbidity in hypertension. II. Results in patients with diastolic blood pressure averaging 90 to 114 mmHg. *J. Am. Med. Assoc.*, **213**, 1143

37 Veterans' Administration Cooperative Study Group on antihypertensive agents. (1972). Effects of treatment on morbidity in hypertension. III. Influence of age, diastolic pressure, and prior cardiovascular disease. Further analysis of side-effects. *Circulation*, **45**, 991

38 Beevers, D. G., Fairman, M. J., Hamilton, M. and Harpur, J. E. (1973). The influence of antihypertensive treatment over the incidence of cerebral vascular disease. *Postgrad. Med. J.*, **49**, 905

39 Beevers, D. G., Fairman, M. J., Hamilton, M. and Harpur, J. E. (1973). Antihypertensive treatment and the course of established cerebral vascular disease. *Lancet*, **i**, 1407

40 Charcot, J. M. and Bouchard, C. (1868). Nouvelles recherches sur la pathogenie de l'haemorrhagie cerebrale. *Arch. Physiol. Normale Patholog.*, **1**, 110, 643, 725

41 Russell, R. W. R. (1963). Observations on intracerebral aneurysms. *Brain*, **86**, 425

42 Cole, F. M., Yates, P. O. (1967). The occurrence and significance of intracerebral microaneurysms. *J. Pathol. Bacteriol.*, **93**, 393

43 Marshall, J. (1964). A trial of long-term hypotensive therapy in cerebrovascular disease. *Lancet*, **i**, 10

44 Hamilton, M., Thompson, E. N. and Wisniewski, T. K. M. (1964). The role of blood pressure control in preventing complications of hypertension. *Lancet*, **i**, 735

45 Priddle, W. W., Liu, S. F., Breithaupt, D. J. and Grant, P. G. (1968). Amelioration of high blood pressure in the elderly. *J. Am. Geriatr. Soc.*, **16**, 887

46 Hypertension – Stroke Cooperative Study Group. (1974). Effect of antihypertensive treatment on stroke recurrence. *J. Am. Med. Assoc.*, **229**, 409

47 Carter, A. B. (1970). Hypotensive therapy in stroke survivors. *Lancet*, **i**, 485

48 Adams, G. F. (1965). Prospects for patients with strokes with special reference to the hypertensive hemiplegic. *Br. Med. J.*, **2**, 253

49 Merrett, J. D., Adams, G. F. (1965). Comparison of mortality rates in elderly hypertensive and normotensive hemiplegic patients. *Br. Med. J.*, **2**, 802

50 Acheson, J., Hutchinson, E. C., (1971). The natural history of focal cerebral vascular disease. *Q. J. Med.*, **40**, 15

51 Robinson, R. W., Cohen, W. D., Higano, N., Mayer, R., Lukowsky, G. H., McLaughlin, R. B. and MacGilpin, H. H. (1959). Lifetable analysis of survival after cerebral thrombosis; ten year experience. *J. Am. Med. Assoc.*, **169**, 1149

52 Pierson, E. C. and Hoobler, S. W. (1957). Significance of transient encephalopathy in cases of benign hypertension. *Univ. Michigan Med. Bull.*, **23**, 446

53 Carter, A. B. (1971). Strokes and hypertension. *Am. Heart J.*, **82**, 1

54 Lassen, N. A. (1959). Cerebral blood flow and oxygen consumption in man. *Physiol. Rev.*, **39**, 183

55 Lassen, N. A. and Skinhøj, E. (1975). Regional cerebral circulation in man and its regulation. *Mod. Trends Neurol.*, **6**, 59

56 Obrist, W. D. (1975). Cerebral blood flow and its regulation. *Clin. Neurosurg.*, **22**, 106

57 Skinhøj, E. (1973). Haemodynamic studies within the brain during migraine. *Arch. Neurol.*, **29**, 95

58 Byrom, F. B. (1969). *The Hypertensive Vascular Crisis* (London: Heinemann).

59 Stranguaard, S., Olesen, J., Skinhøj, E., Lassen, N. A. (1973). Autoregulation of brain circulation in severe arterial hypertension. *Br. Med. J.*, **1**, 507

60 Graham, D. I. (1975). Ischaemic brain damage of cerebral perfusion failure after treatment of severe hypertension. *Br. Med. J.*, **4**, 739

61 Jackson, G., Pierscianowski, T. A., Mahon, W. and Condon, J. (1976). Inappropriate antihypertensive therapy in the elderly. *Lancet*, **ii**, 1317

62 Sheehy, T. W. (1977). To treat or not to treat hypertension in the aged. *J. Med. Assoc. State of Alabama*, **46 (12)**, 27

63 Fazekas, J. F., Bessman, A. N., Cotsonas, N. J. Jr. and Alman, R. W. (1953). Cerebral haemodynamics in cerebral arteriosclerosis. *J. Gerontol.*, **8**, 137

64 Sokoloff, L. (1966). Cerebral circulatory and metabolic changes associated with ageing. *Res. Publ. Assoc. Res. Nerv. Ment. Dis.*, **41**, 237

65 Wollner, L. (1978). Managing postural hypotension: four effective lines of treatment. *Mod. Geriatr.*, **8(4)**, 16

66 Kendell, R. E., Marshall, J. (1963). Role of hypotension in the genesis of transient focal cerebral ischaemic attacks. *Br. Med. J.*, **2**, 344

67 Simpson, F. O. (1978) Hypertension. *Br. Med. J.*, **2**, 882
68 Millar-Craig, M. W., Bishop, C. N. and Raftery, E. B. (1978). Circadian variation of blood pressure. *Lancet*, **i**, 795
69 Kannel, W. B., Codbrand, N., Skinner, J. J. Jnr., Dawber, T. R. and McNamara, P. M. (1967). The relation of adiposity to blood pressure and development of hypertension – the Framingham study. *Ann. Intern. Med.*, **67**, 48
70 Reisin, E., Abel, R., Modan, M., Silverberg, D. S., Eliahou, H. E. and Modan, B. (1978). Effect of weight loss without salt restriction on the reduction of blood pressure in overweight hypertensive patients. *N. Engl. J. Med.*, **298**, 1
71 Ramsay, L. E., Ramsay, M. H., Hettiarachchi, J., Davies, D. L., Winchester, J. (1978). Weight reduction in a blood pressure clinic. *Br. Med. J.*, **2**, 244
72 Ballantyne, D., Devine, B. L. and Fife, R. (1978) Interrelation of age, obesity, cigarette smoking, and blood pressure in hypertensive patients. *Br. Med. J.*, **1**, 880
73 Hamilton, M. (1976). When to treat hypertension. *Br. J. Hosp. Med.*, **16**, 516
74 Isaacs, B. (1978). Results of treating hypertension in the elderly. Presented at a *Symposium on Hypertension in the Elderly* 20 October, Leicester Royal Infirmary
75 Chrysant, S. G., Frohlich, E. D. and Papper, S. (1976). Why hypertension is so prevalent in the elderly – and how to treat it. *Geriatrics*, **108**, 101
76 Stamler, J., Stamler, R., Riedlinger, W. F., Algera, G. and Roberts, R. H. (1976). Hypertension screening of one million Americans – community hypertension evaluation clinic (CHEC) programme, 1973–1975. *J. Am. Med. Assoc.*, **235**, 2299
77 Blood pressure of adults by race and area. United States 1960–1962 (1964). *Natl. Health Survey*, Series 11, No. 5
78 Ashcroft, M. T. and Desai, P. (1978). Blood pressure and mortality in a rural Jamaican community. *Lancet*, **i**, 1167
79 Coope, J. (1976). Blood pressure in the elderly. *Journal of J. R. Coll. Gen. Practit.*, **26**, 745
80 Hughes, W., Dodgson, M. C. H. and MacClellan, D. C. (1954) Chronic cerebral hypertensive disease. *Lancet*, **ii**, 770
81 Caird, F. I. (1977). Treatment of hypertension in the elderly. *Prescribers J.*, **17**,
82 Kennedy, R. D. (1975). Drug therapy for cardiovascular disease in the aged. *J. Am. Geriatr. Soc.*, **23**, 113
83 Amery, A., Berthaux, P., Birkenhager, W., Bulpitt, C., Clement, D., De Schaepdryver, A., Dollery, C., Ernould, H., Fagard, R., Forette, F., Hellemans, J., Kho, T., Lund-Johansen, P., Meurice, J. A. and Pierquin, L. (1977). Antihypertensive therapy in elderly patients: pilot trial of the European working party on high blood pressure in the elderly. *Gerontology*, **23**, 426
84 Dall, J. L. C. (1978). In the elderly, a gradual reduction in B. P. is the answer. *Mod. Med. Hypertension Suppl.*, **April**
85 Livesley, B. (1975). Hypertension in the elderly. *Update*, **11**, 1343
86 Page, L. B., Yager, H. M. and Sidd, J. J. (1976). Drugs in the management of hypertension, part I. *Am. Heart J.*, **91**, 810
87 Holloway, D. A. (1974). Drug problems in the geriatric patient. *Drug Intelligence and Clin. Pharm.*, **8**, 632
88 Riddiough, M. A. (1977). Preventing, detecting and managing adverse reactions of antihypertensive agents in the ambulant patient with essential hypertension. *Am. J. Hosp. Pharm.*, **34**, 465
89 Corman, L. A. and Sversky, N. J. (1973). Methyldopa-hydrochlorothiazide therapy in hypertensive geriatric patients. *J. Am. Geriatr. Soc.*, **21**, 36
90 Luxton, D. E. A. (1977). The arterial blood pressure in old age. *Update*, **14**, 83

91 Page, L. B., Yager, H. M. and Sidd, J. J. (1976). Drugs in the management of hypertension, part II. *Am. Heart J.*, **92**, 114
92 Goldberg, L. I. (1975). Current therapy of hypertension. *Am. J. Med.*, **58**, 489
93 Kelly, K. L. (1976). Beta blockers in hypertension: a review. *Am. J. Hosp. Pharm.*, **33**, 1284
94 Page, L. B., Yager, H. M. and Sidd, J. J. (1976). Drugs in the management of hypertension, part III. *Am. Heart J.*, **92**, 252
95 Barritt, D. W. and Marshall, A. J. (1977). Treating hypertension, the place of beta blockade. *Br. Heart J.*, **39**, 821
96 James, I. (1978). When angina is the problem. *Mod. Geriatr.*, **8 (No. 4)**, 60
97 Eisalo, A., Heino, A. and Munter, J. (1974). The effect of alprenolol in elderly patients with raised blood pressure. *Acta Med. Scand.*, **195**, 23

Review articles on hypertension in the elderly

Chrysant, S. G., Frohlich, E. D. and Papper, S. (1976). Why hypertension is so prevalent in the elderly – and how to treat it. *Geriatrics*, **108**, 101
Coope, J. (1976). Blood pressure in the elderly. *J. R. Coll. Gen. Pract.*, **26**, 745
Dall, J. L. C. (1978). In the elderly, a gradual reduction in B. P. is the answer. *Mod. Med. Hypertension Supplement*, April, 1978
Dyer, A. R., Stamler, J., Shekelle, R. B., Schounberger, J. A. and Farinaro, E. (1977). Hypertension in the elderly. *Med. Clin. N. Am.*, **61**, 513
Kannel, W. B., Codbrand, N., Skinner, J. J. Jr., Dawber, T. R. and McNamara, P. M. (1967). The relation of adiposity to blood pressure and development of hypertension – the Framingham study. *Ann. Intern. Med.*, **67**, 48
Kennedy, R. D. (1974). Hypertension. *Mod. Geriatr.*, **4**, 360
Kennedy, R. D. (1976). Longterm consequences of asymptomatic hypertension in the elderly. *Update*, **12**, 25
Lassen, N. A., Skinhøj, E. (1975). Regional cerebral circulation in man and its regulation. *Mod. Trends Neurol.*, **6**, 59
Leading article. (1977) Hypertension in the elderly. *Lancet*, **i**, 684
Livesley, B. (1975). Hypertension in the elderly, *Update*, **11**, 1343
Luxton, D. E. A. (1977). The arterial blood pressure in old age. *Update*, **14**, 83
Obrist, W. D. (1975). Cerebral blood flow and its regulation. *Clin. Neurosurg.*, **22**, 106
Sheehy, T. W., (1977). To treat or not to treat hypertension in the aged. *J. Med. Assoc. State Ala.*, **46**, 27

Review articles on the treatment of hypertension in the elderly

Barritt, D. W. and Marshall, A. J. (1977). Treating hypertension, the place of beta blockade. *Br. Heart J.*, **39**, 821
Caird, F. I. (1977). Treatment of hypertension in the elderly. *Prescribers J.*, **17**, 52
Goldberg, L. I. (1975). Current therapy of hypertension. *Am. J. Med.*, **58**, 489
Kelly, K. L. (1976). Beta blockers in hypertension: a review. *Am. J. Hosp. Pharm.*, **33**, 1284
Kennedy, R. D. (1975). Drug therapy for cardiovascular disease in the aged. *J. Am. Geriatr. Soc.*, **23**, 113
Page, L. B., Yager, H. M. and Sidd, J. J. (1976). Drugs in the management of hypertension, part I. *Am. Heart J.*, **91**, 810
Page, L. B., Yager, H. M. and Sidd, J. J. (1976). Drugs in the management of hypertension, part II. *Am. Heart J.*, **92**, 114

Page, L. B., Yager, H. M. and Sidd, J. J. (1976). Drugs in the management of hypertension, part III. *Am. Heart J.* **92**, 252

Riddiough, M. A. (1977). Preventing, detecting and managing adverse reactions of antihypertensive agents in the ambulant patient with essential hypertension. *Am. J. Hosp. Pharm.*, **34**, 465

Simpson, F. O. (1978). Hypertension. *Br. Med. J.* **2**, 882

Turner, P. (1975). Drug treatment of hypertension. *J. Clin. Pathol.*, **9** (Suppl.), 36.

5

Treatment of the elderly diabetic

R. A. Jackson

INTRODUCTION

The complexities in management of diabetes in the elderly present a
2-fold challenge; firstly the condition itself lacks precise definition,
and secondly the total care required involves considerations which
extend far beyond pure metabolic control. Thus while the same
general principles of treatment apply to diabetics of all ages, in the
elderly the approach and priorities are somewhat changed. The
main aim of therapy is the relief of symptoms of hyperglycaemia and
the maintenance of a sense of wellbeing. The goal should be to
achieve a degree of diabetic control that is acceptable to both patient and physician through an approach built around the patient's
established pattern of living. Emphasis should be placed more on
the overall welfare of the person and less on the metabolic disorder.
Whether or not complications are preventable 15 years hence by
excellent control is of secondary importance in a person who
develops diabetes at the age of 65.

Since diabetes is a lifelong disease, continuing medical supervision
at regular intervals is essential in order to render patients symptom-
free and to allow them to lead as normal a life as possible within the
constraints set by their disease. As in all other areas of geriatric care,
treatment of the elderly diabetic is essentially a team responsibility,
shared on the one hand by the doctor and staff in the hospital and
in the community, on the other hand, by the general practitioner,
the social workers and most importantly, the patient's family.
Clearly, the provision of adequate care to large numbers of patients
who frequently suffer from multiple pathology, requires a well-
organized multidisciplinary approach.

159

Management of elderly diabetics depends, as in younger patients, on dietary restriction, oral therapy and insulin. The clinical types of diabetes in the elderly include those patients *with* symptoms either previously diagnosed or presenting for the first time in old age and those patients, a large and important though ill-defined group, *without* symptoms but who demonstrate impaired glucose tolerance. In the majority of elderly diabetics, the metabolic disturbance is mild and many patients remain asymptomatic in apparently good health with elevated blood glucose levels which would be unacceptable in younger patients. Indeed one may question whether in many such patients treatment is really necessary at all. Obesity is less common in the elderly and this is fortunate since as a rule older patients cannot comply with stringent therapeutic recommendations whether with regard to dietary regulation or drug administration, however desirable their application may be. Strict dietary control is almost impossible to enforce and acceptance of this and other constraints in elderly patients will avoid unrealistic demands being made on the patient and promote the development of a good doctor – patient relationship.

In any event, it is generally agreed that a less rigid approach should be adopted to blood glucose regulation in the elderly in order to take due account of all aspects of the patient's physical and mental condition and social circumstances. As already indicated the principal aim of therapy is to maintain wellbeing at the expense, if necessary, of achieving absolute normoglycaemia while nevertheless taking adequate precautions to prevent the more serious complications of clinical hypoglycaemia and ketoacidosis.

While the care of patients over 80 years of age is clearly the responsibility of the geriatrician, it is a matter for consideration whether the supervision of diabetic control of the 'young' elderly diabetic should be the responsibility of the geriatrician or the diabetologist. There are no strict rules in this regard and in such patients the precise division of responsibility will depend on local preferences, the general condition and social circumstances of the patient and the severity of the diabetes. Where social problems arise, there is no doubt that the geriatrician should take charge of the case but in many patients who are otherwise well, diabetic control could be supervised either by the geriatrician interested in diabetes, the physician with an interest in geriatrics or the interested general practitioner. Overall, however, management may be best undertaken by the geriatrician who may choose to consult with the physician in the diabetic clinic from time to time during periods of marked deterioration in metabolic control.

Conventional classification of primary diabetes is based predominantly on age of onset, recognizing two main groups – 'juvenile-onset' where patients are characteristically insulin-requiring and 'maturity-onset' where patients are typically not insulin-dependent. These terms are unsatisfactory, however, since some patients in the seventh and eighth decades may develop insulin-dependent diabetes while the presentation of a 'maturity-onset' variety in the young has been described[1]. Furthermore, recent evidence[2] suggests that *irrespective* of age of onset, insulin-requiring diabetics have the *same* HLA-determined susceptibility to insulin deficiency and emphasizes environmental factors (such as viruses) and autoimmunity in pathogenesis. In contrast, maturity-onset diabetes is not associated with any particular HLA haplotype but has a strong familial inheritance. Thus Cudworth[2] has proposed the term 'Type I' diabetes to include all insulin-dependent patients regardless of age and 'Type II' diabetes to include those insulin-independent patients previously classified as 'maturity-onset' and which includes the vast majority of elderly diabetics.

GLUCOSE TOLERANCE AND AGE

The decline in glucose tolerance with increasing age in apparently normal persons is well established[3-5] (Figure 1 and Table 1). The rise in fasting and postprandial blood glucose levels is of questionable significance since it amounts to no more than 0·1 mmol/l (2 mg/100 ml) and 0·2 mmol/l (4 mg/100 ml) per decade respectively through the adult years[7]. Glucose levels occurring 1 or 2 hours after a 50 g oral glucose load, however, rise by about 0·06 mmol/l (1 mg/100 ml) with each year of age, that is about 0·3–0·7 mmol/l (6–13 mg/100 ml) per decade, and levels tend to be about 0·6 mmol/l (10 mg/100 ml) higher for women than men at all ages.

It is generally agreed that the incidence of diabetes mellitus appears to be rising steadily partly because of increasing obesity, partly because of increasing longevity, and probably also because of more efforts to detect diabetes. Diagnosis relies principally on three tests – the detection of glycosuria, estimates of fasting or random blood sugar levels and the glucose tolerance test. Unfortunately, glycosuria is not a useful screening test for diabetes in the elderly since as a result of the frequent elevation in renal threshold for glucose in old age it is absent in 50% of patients with significant hyperglycaemia[8]. Table 2 shows the frequency of glycosuria after 50 g glucose but the random (midmorning) blood sugar may be a

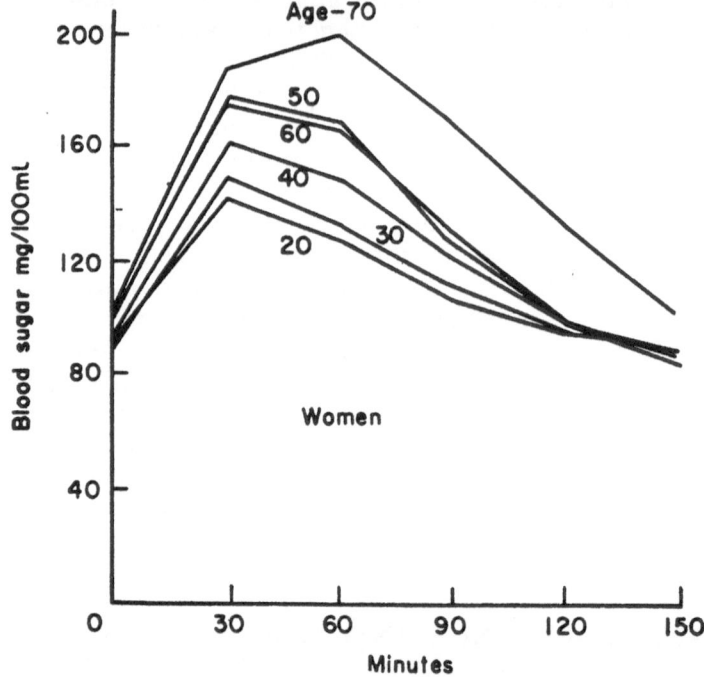

Figure 1   Glucose tolerance by age in 281 normal women[4] (reproduced by permission of the publishers)

Table 1   Per cent of all cases diagnosed at various ages[6]

Age group	Per cent of total
0–20	5
20–40	10
40–60	40
60 +	45
Total	100

(Reproduced by permission of the publishers)

Table 2 Number of adults (per cent) showing glycosuria to testape after 50 g glucose by mouth[3]

Age	Both sexes	Men	Women
18–79	14·3	17·9	10·8
18–24	8·7	11·4	6·3
25–34	11·1	13·8	8·7
35–44	15·3	20·0	10·9
45–54	16·2	20·4	12·0
54–64	14·8	17·3	12·4
65–74	19·3	26·4	13·4
75–79	23·1	21·8	23·4

(Reproduced by permission of the publishers)

more effective screening test suggesting in one study[8] an estimate of total prevalence of 11%.

The finding of declining glucose tolerance with age and uncertainty about its significance has resulted in controversy over the criteria which should be used to diagnose mellitus in older people – that is, at which levels and at which ages plasma glucose concentrations should be considered 'abnormal' and diagnostic of diabetes. One approach has been to use the same standards that have been applied to younger populations but even here standards quoted by different authors differ somewhat. Normal upper limits for the glucose in capillary blood after 50 g or 100 g glucose load have been set as follows: fasting – 5·6 mmol/l (100 mg/100 ml); 1 hour – 8·9 mmol/l (160 mg/100 ml) and 2 hours – 6·7 mmol/l (120 mg/100 ml); wider limits have also been quoted, in other words that diabetes is present if the blood glucose levels fasting and 1 and 2 hours after the oral glucose exceed 6.7 mmol/l (120 mg/100 ml), 10 mmol/l (180 mg/100 ml) and 6·7 mmol/l (120 mg/100 ml) respectively, and impaired tolerance is said to be present if values exceed the limits at only 1 hour and 2 hours[9]. Because in the elderly these values are so frequently exceeded, some upward revision of standards of normality with age has been recommended particularly of the 2 hour figure to 7·5 mmol/l (135 mg/100 ml)[10], or of standard normal limits by 0·56 mmol/l (10 mg/100 ml) for each decade over 40 years[11].

Thus, since the condition has not been precisely defined, it is hardly surprising that estimates of the prevalence of diabetes in the elderly on the basis of glucose tolerance remain somewhat uncertain and, indeed, fraught with error[12]. The evidence summarized by Andres and Tobin[13] has suggested that over half the population at age of 70 would have abnormal 1 or 2 hour plasma glucose values if the standards developed for younger people are used. Several authors[4,14-17] are in agreement indicating that after age of 60 well over 50% of a normal population will have 'abnormal' glucose tolerance with a prevalence ranging from 50–100%. These figures suggest that diabetes is seriously overdiagnosed in the aged and clearly the criteria for normal glucose tolerance in the younger age group cannot be used to define a statistically abnormal response in the elderly.

With this in mind Siperstein[12] has suggested that only persons with an elevated fasting plasma glucose level should be diagnosed as diabetic. He points out the variability of the oral glucose tolerance test including the changes with age and bases his rationale for ignoring it as a diagnostic standard on the fact that, if common statistical approaches to defining normality and abnormality are used (that is, defining 95% of a tested population as normal), then 1 and 2 hour plasma glucose levels as high as 13·3 mmol/l (240 mg/100 ml) or higher would fall in the 'normal' range. Indeed, the wide variability of plasma glucose levels after a standard glucose level may be very misleading and this seems to be particularly true of the elderly[18]. There are thus ample data[12] to conclude that glucose tolerance in the elderly may become statistically abnormal only when blood glucose levels exceed 14·4 mmol/l (260 mg/100 ml) at 1 hour and 11·1–12·2 mmol/l (200–220 mg/100 ml) at 2 hours. Williams[19] has also emphasized use of fasting plasma glucose concentrations and recommended that the diagnosis of diabetes mellitus in older people should not be made unless fasting hyperglycaemia, that is, a plasma glucose level of more than 7·8 mmol/l (140 mg/100 ml) is found on at least two occasions.

Normal fasting blood glucose concentrations do not exclude impaired glucose tolerance, though the defect clearly will not be severe. When fasting levels are not elevated, a glucose tolerance test may be indicated in older persons who have borderline values in non-fasting screening procedures, symptoms of diabetes, glycosuria, strong family histories of diabetes, obesity or evidence of cerebral, coronary or peripheral vascular disease. There is no precise information available, however, regarding the degree to which the decline in glucose tolerance will progress to unequivocal diabetes mellitus, and such information will only come from adequate longitudinal studies. Limited published evidence to date suggests that a significant number of such persons will eventually be clearly diabetic including the development of characteristic diabetic complications. Thus, the results of a 10 year follow-up confirm that while the vast majority of patients with an abnormal glucose tolerance test remain unchanged and some even become normal, a notable percentage of patients convert to florid diabetes within this period[20]; prediction of the outcome, in any one individual, however, is impossible. Whenever diabetes is first discovered in older people, however, it is important to consider the possibility that it may be secondary to a pancreatic neoplasm or less common conditions which may predispose to diabetes and which may be seen at any age.

It is not clear whether the effect of age on glucose tolerance is a characteristic of normal ageing or may in fact represent a high prevalence of genetic predisposition to diabetes with appearance of the chemical manifestations of the disease as age advances, or both. However, the possibility that the deterioration in glucose tolerance is due solely to the increased prevalence of diabetes requires the assumption of an absurdly high incidence of diabetes of approximately 70–100%[16,17] – for which there is no support whatsoever. Studies of the mechanism of the impairment in glucose tolerance have given conflicting results and its basis remains obscure. The most definitive studies have been those by Andres and Tobin, and Tobin *et al.*[13,21] which did not suggest a change in tissue sensitivity to insulin with age or a decreased insulin release with a glucose challenge. Other workers[22] have confirmed a prompt and normal insulin response to an oral glucose load in elderly patients showing a hyperglycaemic tendency; while this response is impaired in the elderly clinical diabetic, it is not more so than in younger patients, so that factors other than impaired insulin release must be involved. The decay in glucose tolerance with age is also seen on cortisone-glucose tolerance testing[23] as well as in the intravenous glucose tolerance test, and it is therefore not due to differences in absorption[24]. Thus the mechanism for the decay in glucose tolerance with age remains uncertain at the present time.

ORGANIZATION OF DIABETIC CARE –
GENERAL CONSIDERATIONS

Broadly, diabetics are treated in one or more of the following environments: (a) as a hospital inpatient where initial stabilization or restabilization in the course of treatment is achieved or where control is maintained during admission for unrelated factors; (b) as a hospital outpatient attending the geriatric clinic and/or diabetic clinic; (c) as an outpatient attending the interested general practitioner (GP); and (d) being seen at home as an outpatient who is housebound.

Hospital care

Although the emphasis on particular aspects of care will vary from time to time according to the patient's general health and metabolic control, the care of the elderly diabetic must remain the dual responsibility of those physicians with an interest in diabetes and those with special experience in geriatric care. Precisely how the division of responsibility is ultimately determined will depend, as already indicated, on the particular preferences and interests of the individual geriatrician and diabetologist involved. It may be that where the patient's general condition remains good and the major management problem is confined to diabetes, the patient will remain predominantly under the care of the diabetologists. However, in mild diabetics, whose general condition is poor or who deteriorates for one reason or another, such as due to a superimposed cerebrovascular disease, the geriatrician will assume overall care of the patient. Inevitably there will be a third group of patients more difficult to define but whose optimum care will require the combined attention of the diabetologist and geriatrician. If an attending physician has an interest both in diabetes and geriatrics so much the better. In any event this collaboration in the care of elderly diabetics should continue whether the patients are hospitalized as an inpatient or attending the clinics on an outpatient basis, and this can be reassuring to patients and doctors alike.

The hospital diabetic clinic

Traditionally patients with diabetes have been managed almost exclusively in the diabetic clinic of a hospital and this is particularly so in the elderly, where the majority of patients are mild diabetics not requiring insulin. The facilities of the hospital diabetic clinic have not increased at a rate commensurate with the expanding diabetic population. In a growing population with an age structure biased towards the elderly the number of known diabetics is rising rapidly. Undoubtedly many diabetic clinics are now overcrowded and many are becoming unmanageable with the result that many patients are kept waiting unduly long and are often seen by a different doctor each visit. The relief of some of the pressure on time is of fundamental importance in dealing with elderly patients where the need for repetition of instructions and explanations, the gaining of confidence and provision of reassurance is basic to successful management. The importance of not hurrying a consultation or showing a sense of urgency in seeing the next patient cannot be overestimated. Old people take longer to enter and leave the consulting room and to dress and undress, and adequate time and assistance must be available for this. Nevertheless, the diabetic clinic provides a centre for clinical assessment of new patients, follow-up of old patients, regulation of therapy and the opportunity for discussions with the general practitioner and relatives as well as the opportunity to see other members of staff with special interests in aspects of diabetic care.

In addition to the physician and junior doctors, other staff should include:

(1) A *dietitian* to give advice to new patients and reassess others in whom weight control is unsatisfactory and who should be accessible to patients and general practitioners without the necessity for prior reference to the doctors in the clinic.

(2) *Technicians* – a technician should be available to measure blood glucose at the clinic so that the results are available when the patient is seen by the doctor.

(3) A trained *chiropodist* – who is needed particularly in the elderly neuropathic patient requiring instruction as to the care of the feet. Danger signs can be detected early and medical colleagues will be available for immediate consultation.

(4) *Health visitors* – whose attendance at the clinic can provide a valuable service in meeting patients and arranging for home visits where this is advisable.

(5) An *ophthalmologist* – the attendance, where possible, of an eye surgeon is invaluable for the proper inspection of eyes at regular intervals. Alternatively arrangements must be made available for referral to the eye clinic without further notice.

(6) Other *specialists* – similar special arrangements should be possible with the *dental department* for the care of the teeth, an *orthopaedic surgeon*, a *general surgeon* interested in care of the feet and vascular disease, a *neurologist* for appropriate consultation, etc.

(7) *Specialist nurses* – may work as part of the diabetic clinic[25].

(8) The social services department – *social workers* should be available to help patients adjust to their disabilities and to arrange social support where necessary.

Specific aspects of follow-up care are considered elsewhere in this chapter (page 194). In general, however, at follow-up appointments the patient should be asked about their symptoms and particularly about hypoglycaemic attacks. When appropriate patients must be specifically asked to produce their weight and urine charts. Most important of all, the patients should be asked to bring their bottles of tablets or insulin to the clinic so that it can be ensured that the prescribed treatment is being taken. One of the major difficulties in treating some elderly patients is the frequent confusion about their medication, despite adequate explanation, and the resultant taking of incorrect doses; errors are even more likely to occur when more than one doctor prescribes for the patient.

Frequency of attendance is clearly related to the severity of the condition and response to treatment, but it is vital that all missed appointments be investigated immediately and a further appointment arranged unless events more serious than forgetfulness or transport difficulties have taken place.

Education of the patient
The education of the patient has clearly been the stepchild of the diabetes world for too long. In order to teach the patient it is first necessary to emphasize diabetes to the physician, especially the non-diabetologist. Indeed the Report of the National Commission on Diabetes to the Congress of the United States (10 December 1975)[26] contained the unqualified statement that 'the cornerstone of good medical treatment practice is the acceptance by the health professionals, patients and their families that, for diabetes, *patient education is treatment*'. The italics are those of the Commission.

Since diabetes remains a lifelong problem, it is clearly of fundamental importance that patients be taught to become as expert as possible in the day-to-day management of their own disease. Ideally, education of the patient must be the shared responsibility of the hospital and/or diabetic clinic on the one hand and the general practitioner or district nurse on the other, and should begin, at least, at the first encounter or clinic visit. Furthermore, other members of the family or close friends always should be similarly involved and informed at an early stage and sufficient time must be allowed for the necessary explanations to take place. Repeated instruction and ongoing education will be needed with some forgetful patients and should always be undertaken with the same patience and understanding for the patient's feelings as must accompany the initial consultation; here, not only the general practitioner and district nurse, but a close relative or friend of the patient should be encouraged to accept some responsibility for care and become a member of the care 'team'. This approach alone will tend to allay any fears of being able to cope with a new disease and the need, in the more severe cases, to adopt a new way of life. Reassuring the patient that they will be supported in living with their disease is of crucial importance at this stage.

The diabetic clinic therefore, apart from offering supervision of the diabetic state and general health, should provide educational facilities for the patient dealing with all aspects of their disease. Often a half-hour discussion using illustrative slides with ten or twelve patients in a group can be more constructive than a 5 minute talk to each individually. However, with some elderly patients it will be necessary to spend some time on an individual basis in order to ensure than some appreciation of the problem is obtained. Where appropriate the patient must be taught in detail the technique of insulin administration and the method of urine testing and recording results and verbal instruction must be supplemented with practical demonstration. Patients should be taught how different situations, for example intercurrent infections and steroid therapy, may alter diabetic control and increase insulin requirements. The patient must be aware of the warning signs of hypoglycaemia and how to deal with it and that loss of appetite may lead to hypoglycaemia if insulin dosage remains unchanged. The patient and family should have some basic understanding regarding drug action and where appropriate the use of hypoglycaemic agents. Most important of all, drug interactions and their associated hazards must be explained clearly.

Diet is another problem which may affect the whole family and should be discussed with the patient's spouse who may be responsible for preparing meals. The district nurse has no formal training in diabetes but can reinforce advice given by the hospital dietitian and, because she is in the home, can offer really practical help. Five minutes spent going through the food cupboard can have more impact on the patient than an hour of theoretical dietary advice. Where the patient receives meals-on-wheels obvious allowance must be made regarding dietary adherence. Indeed, the home visit is an ideal time for reinforcing information previously imparted and for again renewing contact with the family.

Care of the feet is an area of particular concern in the elderly and this is discussed in detail below (page 203). In long-term care, treatment is often taken over entirely by the nursing staff, but even here many patients are capable of some degree of self-management and wish to retain as much a sense of independence as possible. In such patients self-management should be encouraged as if the patient were in their own homes.

In the UK an educational programme is available as a slide/tape package from the British Diabetic Association and an active local branch of the Association can also contribute fully to the education of diabetic patients. Detailed booklets of all the implications of being a diabetic are available and should be supplied to every patient.

Care in the community

A major development in the management of diabetes has been the shift of emphasis from hospital to community care of patients. The reasons for this are several: many diabetic clinics, as noted above, have become 'overloaded' with patients such that the clinician is frequently dissatisfied with the quality of patient care and many patients feel that they are paid insufficient attention. In many centres insufficient hospital beds are available to allow admission for initiation of insulin therapy when not indicated as an emergency. The developments to accommodate this need have included the general practitioner based miniclinic (see below, page 171), community care schemes and the use of specially trained diabetic health visitors and district nurses liaising between the hospital clinic, the general practitioner, the patient and the various community services (social, medical, dietetic, chiropodial, etc.)[25,27].

The passage of time will establish the merits of these various schemes but such developments are of particular importance in relation to the elderly. Waiting for hours in the diabetic clinic is exhausting for older patients particularly after a journey, possibly in an ambulance, to the hospital itself. This, added to the feeling which some patients have that they are being dealt with abruptly, makes the hospital visit an unpleasant experience. With relief of some of the pressure on the hospital diabetic clinic, more time can be given to those patients who do need to attend while those seeing their general practitioner will be spared the journey to the hospital and have their contact with their doctor reinforced.

The full potential for diabetic care in the community depends on good communication and an efficiently functioning team. The telephone therefore must be exploited to allow diabetics easy access to advice from the general practitioner and district nurse or the hospital doctor or diabetic clinic nurse. Patients must be encouraged to seek advice when concerned as many will refrain from asking for help.

The interested practitioner or specialist nurse can also measure blood glucose levels on the spot and can make recommendations regarding the dose of oral agents or adjust the dose of insulin to re-establish control without requiring the patient to reattend the hospital. An Ames reflectance meter or equivalent piece of apparatus is thus an essential item of equipment. Through the capacity of the nurse or doctor to intervene when insulin requirements are changing rapidly, as may occur with intercurrent infections, a critical situation may be avoided. Alternatively a domiciliary visit by the hospital doctor may be required to give advice when difficulties arise in housebound patients or patients who become ill and cannot easily visit the hospital.

Patients who are debilitated by eye or diabetic complications usually find each trip to the diabetic clinic an irksome experience often requiring transport by ambulance. Yet it is just these diabetics who require close contact with the diabetic team. This contact can be provided in the home by the district nurse who can check diabetic control and perform such vital tasks as inspecting the feet. In insulin-requiring subjects preset 'blocked' syringes may be required to assist management and eliminate the burden of drawing up the correct dose for people with poor or deteriorating vision. Not only that, but as mentioned above, premixed solutions of soluble and isophane insulin may be provided in more severe cases where twice daily injections are required.

Role of the general practitioner
A family doctor who is interested in diabetes and who is familiar with the emotional and personal background of his patient is best placed to provide continuity of care and undertake supervision of his diabetic patients once the initial clinical and biochemical assessment is completed[28]. The doctor may fulfil this duty in his own surgery or the patient's home or in the diabetic clinic itself by attending as a clinical assistant. In order to undertake this responsibility in the community the doctor must have adequate facilities for arranging blood sugar estimations, etc., and in some practices a specific time can be set aside for the purpose in the form of a diabetic miniclinic. These miniclinics[27] are less inhibiting to most patients than hospital clinics and reduce travelling time and expense so important to the elderly. With regard to the care of patients in their own homes, the doctor can assist follow-up by communicating with health visitors and practice-linked or district nurses. Certainly most maturity-onset diabetics can be supervised in this way, perhaps with an occasional visit to the hospital when a particular problem arises requiring a second opinion or further investigation.

Domiciliary visits
Domiciliary visits may be required from time to time by a doctor
from the geriatric team and such a visit usually takes place at the
request either of the general practitioner or district nurse. Such visits
are likely to take place primarily in regard to the patient's general
health (which clearly may secondarily influence diabetic control)
rather than in respect of a deterioration in diabetic control as such.
In the latter instance, the patient may well need to attend the hospital diabetic clinic despite any home consultation, unless other local
facilities are available.

Emotional impact of illness on the patient
The diagnosis of an illness, however mild, can be a threatening and
frightening experience at any age but particularly so in the elderly in
whom the awareness of age and the possibility of death is that much
greater and intensified in many cases by the presence of multiple
pathology. The emotional reaction of the patient to his or her
illness, therefore, is central to the management of the elderly diabetic
and may take several forms. The patient may not respond with
undue anxiety and regardless of the severity of the disorder, decide
to make the best of the situation in the assurance and knowledge
that help and support, when needed, will be forthcoming from the
doctor and nurses as well as close relatives and friends. The illness is
seen as a challenge to be met and the necessary adjustments will be
made without undue disruption of daily life. For some patients,
however, the discovery of illness is a devastating blow and, however
mild, may represent a misfortune which is too great to be coped
with. The patient may either deny the existence of the disorder
altogether or regress to a more helpless form of behaviour. Undue
depression, introversion and withdrawal from the reality of the situation may follow. On the other hand, the illness may be exploited
and used as a means of attracting attention in a manipulative way
where purely medical indications are not correspondingly pressing.
    The difficulty of distinguishing truly organic factors from psycho-
somatic aspects of the case cannot be overestimated, yet a judgement has to be made and is an essential prerequisite to optimal care.
The doctors, nurses and social workers will need all their skill and
experience in managing difficult situations related to the individual
personality of each patient – and in supporting and advising the
patient as well as family and friends in a balanced approach to the
illness. Of the various complications to which the diabetic is susceptible, perhaps blindness and amputation carry the most serious
social implications. Both situations produce feelings of inadequacy,

overdependence and anxiety not only about coping with the specific disability but also with general activity and life itself. Thus, where poor vision or blindness is present or where amputation is indicated and major physical disability and rehabilitation are added challenges to be met, management will be even more complex, and from time to time the help of an experienced psychotherapist or psychiatrist may become essential.

TREATMENT – SPECIFIC CONSIDERATIONS

Diet

Diet is the key element in treatment of the elderly diabetic. The initial step entails taking a careful dietary history based on which the appropriate persons, that is physician, dietitian, specialist nurse, can work with the patient. Dietary advice should always be based on the patient's habitual food patterns and a modification in eating patterns is prescribed in order to achieve (a) weight reduction to ideal body weight as far as possible, (b) avoidance of refined sugar, (c) adequate intake of vitamins, minerals and protein and (d) reasonable regular distribution of meals.

Exchange lists for meal planning prepared by the American and British Diabetic Associations are a valuable guide to patients for alternative food choices and emphasize the potential for individualization of meal planning under the guidance of experienced workers, rather than a fixed diet schedule. Individual recommendations should be written out for the guidance of the patient and those who help prepare the food. The recommendations should be reviewed regularly and continuing efforts made to arrive at meal plans which are acceptable to patients and will achieve therapeutic goals.

Obesity requires treatment by weight reduction as much in the elderly as in other age groups though for reasons mentioned below, adequate dietary restriction is unlikely to be achieved. Some physicians believe the elderly will never adhere indefinitely to dietary controls and this fact influences them in advising the use of drugs or insulin. Nevertheless many elderly patients are taking an unreasonably large proportion of carbohydrate in their diets when first seen and in any mild or moderately severe case simple dietetic control should be tried first. Suitable regimes bearing in mild the circumstances and the usual degree of activity of old people, are either 1400 kcal/day with 140 g carbohydrate, or 1200 kcal/day with 120 g carbohydrate or, for the obese, 1000 kcal/day with 80 g carbohydrate (or even less). In non-obese patients or those who have

achieved weight reduction by more vigorous dieting, a daily carbohydrate intake of up to 180 g can be allowed on a long-term
basis. The appointing of this total between the various meals of the
day depends on whether insulin or other drugs are also to be used.
Depending on the severity of the carbohydrate restriction, a total
ban should be imposed on sugar, sweets, chocolates, jam, sweet
biscuits, cakes, puddings and pastry, and advice given as to a
quantified restriction of bread, potatoes, rice, spaghetti and other
farinaceous foods.

A new element in dietary composition has been added by increasing knowledge of the role of fibre. Dietary fibre consists of plant cell
walls and being non-absorbable and fluid-retaining adds bulk to the
bowel contents. Adequate dietary roughage reduces intraluminal
pressure in the bowel and where the diet contains an adequate fibre
content, the rate of absorption of saccharides is decreased[29]. Clearly
recommendations regarding diet should take account of the quality
and type of food as well as the quantity. Roughage and fibre content
must be considered with wholemeal bread rather than white bread,
wholegrain cereals, coarse vegetables either lightly cooked or eaten
raw, fresh fruit and perhaps the addition of bran itself.

The protein content of the diet is important only in so far as an
adequate intake must be ensured; protein food is expensive and is
likely to be deficient in the diet of the elderly.

Dietary fat provides the most concentrated form of food energy
and when carbohydrate is restricted the fat intake will also fall
considerably, for example, with decreased intake of butter on bread
and cooking fat used in cakes, puddings, etc. Knowledge of the
relationship of dietary to blood lipids and atherosclerosis has
altered the approach not only to the amount of fat to be taken but
also the quality. The Royal College of Physicians Working Party's
recommendations[30] for the community in general are that dietary
fat should not form more than 35% of total calories and that this
reduction should apply particularly to saturated fats from animal
sources or hydrogenated fats of vegetable or maize origin. In practice this will mean mainly the substitution of butter by margarine
composed predominantly of polyunsaturated fats of vegetable origin
or the use of corn oil or sunflower oil in cooking or salad dressing.
Milk should be skimmed and lean meat grilled; eggs should be
restricted to three per week and cottage cheese should replace ordinary cheese. These recommendations are particularly applicable to
maturity-onset diabetics, but the degree to which they should be
encouraged will vary with the particular patient involved; in
general, therapy aimed at preventing or retarding atherogenesis does

not apply to the same extent to the elderly diabetic as it does in younger patients.

In summary, the first step in the elderly diabetic is to recommend dietary carbohydrate restriction, the severity depending on the degree of obesity, while giving consideration also to the fibre, protein and fat content of the food.

Although diet is important, older patients can be allowed a little more latitude than younger diabetics because the variety of diabetes found in the elderly is usually mild and stable. As noted above, this is fortunate, since the restrictions similar to those advised in younger diabetics cannot be applied as rigidly in the elderly and even in middle-aged subjects the effectiveness of dietary therapy falls far short of expectations. In the elderly there is often a lack of motivation and not infrequently this is due in part to the lack of enthusiasm on the part of the doctor prescribing treatment. Emotional problems are frequent in the elderly and loneliness, depression, lack of interest after death of the spouse may be dominant features. Cost may be a factor in non-compliance and in addition the diets prescribed may be frequently unrealistic and inflexible. Patients often have domestic difficulties, and keeping up a rigorous regime which requires the weighing of foodstuffs is usually beyond their competence or inclination. The patient may have practical problems such as difficulty in obtaining the correct food, as in the case of those having meals-on-wheels and while residential care may solve some problems it may also create others related to incorrect feeding. In any event, the indices of success will be a reduction in weight and the return of blood sugar towards the normal range.

Patients who remain hyperglycaemic do so either because they are unable to adhere to the diet or because their supply of endogenous insulin is inadequate to meet the requirements of even a meagre diet. The lack of success with dietary treatment has been well documented in the literature. In one study, less than a third of even those diabetics who agreed to participate ate within 10% of the prescribed diet[31], and in another investigation long-term weight reduction was achieved by only a fraction of those patients who were advised to slim[32].

Exercise

Sustained, regular physical activity is of major importance in the management of diabetes and assurance of general good health in older people. An increased amount of exercise of even a modest degree, if maintained, will facilitate both weight reduction and metabolic control by increasing glucose utilization. Part of the plan for every older diabetic, where possible, should be a programme of physical activity.

Oral hypoglycaemic agents

General approach

Oral hypoglycaemic agents (OHA) now have an established place in treatment and are used by 30–50% of all diabetics and a higher proportion of elderly diabetics. In general these drugs have an excellent record of safety with a minimum of side-effects or toxicity. OHA should only be prescribed when simple dietary restriction has failed to restore normoglycaemia or, at least, an acceptable fasting blood glucose concentration. The great value of OHA is that in many diabetics they obviate the need for insulin injections and all that this implies.

Thus maturity-onset diabetics can be treated satisfactorily with OHA and diet when they fail to respond to dietary restrictions alone. Failure of dietary treatment has been defined as a persistence of glycosuria with repeated postprandial blood glucose levels of more than 8·3 mmol/l (150 mg/100 ml), although these stringent criteria may be relaxed a little in some elderly patients. Thus, in addition to little or no glycosuria, reasonable goals are fasting plasma glucose values under 140 mg/100 ml and 2 to 3 hour postprandial levels of less than 160–180 mg/100 ml.

In practice most patients who respond to simple dietary restriction do so within a few weeks and unless OHA are contraindicated it is preferable to spend a number of weeks if necessary in attempting to achieve satisfactory control through diet alone (and exercise, if possible) before introducing OHA. If, however, an adequate reduction in blood and urinary glucose is not obtained, the need for further therapy will soon become apparent. The presence of symptoms and weight loss in particular indicates a more pressing need for prescribing OHA, but absence of symptoms does not necessarily indicate optimal wellbeing of the patients.

OHA are absolutely contraindicated in: (a) the presence of or liability to ketoacidosis – a single episode of ketosis or even coma in the past, however, is not necessarily a contraindication and occasionally such patients may subsequently remain well controlled on drugs and diet alone; (b) uncontrolled diabetes in emergencies; (c) acute onset of diabetes with severe hyperglycaemic symptoms and weight loss; and (d) after total pancreatectomy.

There are no absolute rules regarding the type of drug to be used and this depends entirely on the preferences of the physicians concerned. Two types of OHA are in common use, the biguanides and the sulphonylureas. In many clinics the choice of agent in the initial treatment of maturity-onset diabetes is determined to a large extent by the body weight of the patient. The sulphonylureas, part of whose action is to stimulate insulin production, tend to increase body weight, clearly undesirable in the obese, whereas the biguanides, by causing anorexia and delaying intestinal absorption, tend to cause weight loss. Thus the sulphonylureas should be used as primary treatment in non-obese patients, reserving the biguanides for those who are overweight. If primary failure occurs, that is after 3 to 6 weeks control remains poor despite satisfactory dietary adherence and the administration in maximum doses of either a sulphonylurea or biguanide alone, the second type of drug should be added in combination and dosage increased as required to maximum levels.

The use of combined therapy has greatly widened the scope of oral treatment in maturity-onset diabetics and since the biguanides and sulphonylureas have different modes of action (see pages 181 and 187) their hypoglycaemic effects are additive. In newly diagnosed patients who fail to respond adequately to dietary restriction and maximum doses of a sulphonylurea, the addition of a biguanide will often restore satisfactory control. Thus, if for example 15 mg/day glibenclamide does not restore control, the addition of metformin 1–2 g/day may prove effective.

A proportion of maturity-onset diabetics adequately controlled initially by a sulphonylurea show gradual relapse after a few years, in other words secondary failure. In some a stricter adherence to diet may restore control but in others hyperglycaemia persists and here the addition of metformin is more likely to be successful than changing from one sulphonylurea to another. In this way combined treatment can increase the number of patients who can be controlled without insulin and prolongs the length of time over which control can be maintained.

Some patients maintain adequate control with combined drug therapy in maximum doses and a very restricted diet. If despite this, however, control remains poor or the patient remains unwell and continues to lose weight, insulin must be introduced and drugs stopped without delay. The difficulties which confront the patient with the introduction of insulin are offset in many diabetics by their gratitude at being permitted a more generous dietary allowance. The need to change to insulin occurs most frequently during the first few months, but secondary failure to maintain adequate control can occur at any time even after years of successful treatment. Biguanides have been used in the past in conjunction with insulin in order to obtain smoother control but such a regimen offers no advantage and is not to be encouraged.

Continuing management on OHA may develop in one of three ways.

(1) Not infrequently a patient who has needed OHA for control is found later to maintain normal blood glucose levels on diet alone without drug therapy. Thus, after good diabetic control has been sustained with OHA for at least some months, dosage reduction and/or drug withdrawal while continuing dietary restriction should always be considered. This is a safe procedure and is not accompanied by acute deterioration of diabetes as occurs when insulin is withdrawn. If urine is tested daily or if tablets are stopped 2 to 4 weeks before a visit to the diabetic clinic, a reasonable assessment of the need for OHA can be made. About one-third of patients remain well controlled after withdrawal of tablets, provided that carbohydrate restriction is maintained[33]. If, however, control deteriorates when drugs are withdrawn, then clearly medication must be continued.

(2) Control may remain stable but it will be always apparent that uninterrupted drug administration is essential and will need to continue indefinitely with minor modifications from time to time.

(3) Late or secondary failure may occur, in other words, patients who respond well initially to sulphonylureas subsequently become uncontrolled and this is an indication for a review of therapy, with the introduction of metformin or insulin.

Despite the fact that symptoms are usually mild and easily eliminated by diet and OHA in maturity-onset diabetes, patients are still liable to develop complications over the years with damage to eyes, kidneys, nerves and the arterial tree. It is generally accepted that the more normal the blood glucose levels, the less liable patients are to suffer these complications[34] but, unfortunately, evidence that OHA delay or prevent cardiovascular complications is conflicting. In the American University Group Diabetes Program Trial[35] (UGDP) newly diagnosed maturity-onset diabetics had a higher cardiovascular mortality when treated with tolbutamide or phenformin than when treated with a placebo.

The UGDP was in fact a multicentre study designed to clarify whether control of mild diabetes reduces the incidence of complications. Four different treatment regimes were chosen – diet plus (a) variable insulin doses, (b) fixed insulin dose, (c) fixed dose tolbutamide, and (d) placebo. The results showed that mild diabetics treated with a fixed dose of tolbutamide and diet fared no better than those on diet alone as regards life expectancy, and indeed the mortality from cardiovascular disease was significantly higher in the tolbutamide treated group (12·7%) than other groups (4·9–6·2%) and the trial was stopped[35–37]; patients on phenformin had a mortality similar to that in the tolbutamide group. The statistical analyses and conclusions of this trial have been extensively criticized and have not gained wide acceptance especially as its results are at variance with those of other studies[38,39]. For example, Keen *et al.*[40] concluded that in mild and moderately severe diabetes tolbutamide provided a significant degree of primary protection against cardiovascular events. Nevertheless other studies[41] add some support to UDPG conclusions.

The chief merit of the study is that it has caused specialists in diabetes to recommend now a more cautious use of OHA than before the American trial but it has not been felt that their use should be abandoned as did the US Food and Drug Administration. The UGDP study has not altered practice in the United Kingdom except in a few important regards – no obvious benefit has been shown in the long term in treating mild overt diabetics with OHA routinely – a proper diet is the only treatment necessary in most cases and should be the initial treatment in all cases. The study has emphasized that oral agents are potent and potentially dangerous and should be used with caution only in patients likely to benefit from them and then only in the minimum doses necessary to maintain control. OHA should be reserved for maturity-onset diabetics

Table 3   Oral hypoglycaemic agents

Drug	Proprietary name	Tablet size (mg)	Dose range (mg/day)
Sulphonylureas			
Tolbutamide	Rastinon, Orinase	500	500–2000
Chlorpropamide	Diabinese	100, 250	100–500
Acetohexamide	Dimelor	500	500–1500
Tolazamide	Tolanase	100, 250	100–750
Glibenclamide	Daonil, Euglucon	5	2·5–20
Glibornuride	Glutril	25	12·5–75
Glipizide	Glibenese, Minidiab	5	2·5–30
Sulphonamide			
Glymidine	Gondafon, Lycanol	500	500–2000
Biguanides			
Metformin	Glucophage	500, 850	1000–3000
Phenformin	Dibotin, Dipar	25, 50	25–150

who fail to respond to diet alone and who have marked hyperglycaemia and prominent symptoms requiring a rapid clinical response.
More strenuous attempts at dieting should be made and the dose of
these drugs should never exceed that recommended (Table 3); furthermore attempts should be made to stop the drugs when satisfactory control is achieved and patients may then be maintained on
diet alone.

The sulphonylureas

The sulphonylureas were the first group to be prescribed for the
treatment of diabetes and owe their inception to the use of the early
sulphonamides. In 1942 Janbon and his colleagues[42] in France
traced the deaths of three patients to hypoglycaemia caused by a
sulphonamide. In 1955 the first sulphonamide-derived sulphonylurea, carbutamide, became available and was soon followed by
others which had no antibacterial properties. The general chemical
formula of the sulphonylureas is:

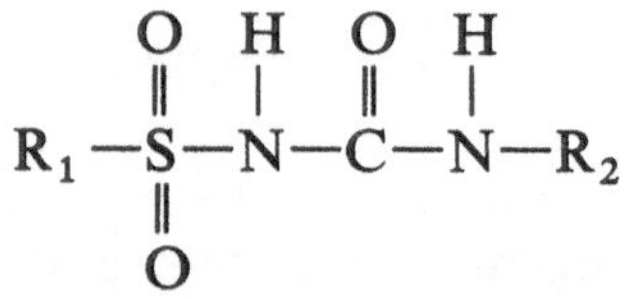

$$R_1 - \overset{\overset{\displaystyle O}{\|}}{\underset{\underset{\displaystyle O}{\|}}{S}} - \overset{\overset{\displaystyle H}{|}}{N} - \overset{\overset{\displaystyle O}{\|}}{C} - \overset{\overset{\displaystyle H}{|}}{N} - R_2$$

and the differences between drugs depend on the 'R' side-chains
(Figure 2). The most commonly used drugs of this group are tolbu-

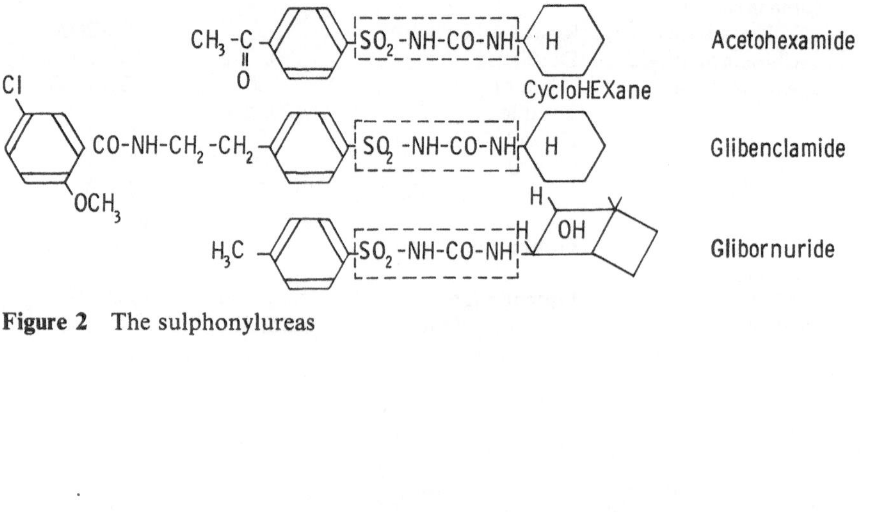

Figure 2   The sulphonylureas

tamide and chlorpropamide but in 1968 it was reported that the addition of a long side-chain in the benzene ring would greatly increase the glucose-lowering effect. The latter resulted in the synthesis of 'second generation' sulphonylureas, such as glibenclamide, which, weight for weight are 100 times or more as potent as the older drugs but not necessarily more effective in the management of diabetes. Indeed, differences between preparations in terms of hypoglycaemic potency are marginal, and there is nothing to be gained by using more than one sulphonylurea preparation at a time and no evidence that if one has failed after maximum doses have been tried, another will be more successful. Most authorities will agree that some 60–70% of adult-onset diabetes benefit from the sulphonylureas.

The sulphonylureas appear to act by both pancreatic and extra-pancreatic effects. There is no doubt that some endogenous insulin must be present for these drugs to be effective. An acute action of sulphonylureas is to stimulate insulin release from the β-cell and the newer sulphonylureas have been reported to stimulate β-cell replication in animals as well as insulin release[43]. It has been confirmed that with chlorpropamide therapy the early phase of insulin secretion usually improves[44], and that in newly treated diabetics there is a transient increase in insulin output[45]. Perkins *et al.*[46] showed that chlorpropamide and glibenclamide given for 4 month periods increased insulin release after oral glucose as well as improving glucose tolerance, and after withdrawal of sulphonylurea both insulin reserve and glucose tolerance deteriorated. Nevertheless, although continued use of the drug may maintain normoglycaemia, the increased output of insulin is shortlived and variable and does not correspond well with blood glucose levels. It appears therefore that the main hypoglycaemic action of the sulphonylureas in long-term therapy may be extrapancreatic[44,46] due possibly to a reduced hepatic glucose output or increased effectiveness of endogenous insulin.

There are eight sulphonylureas (including glymidine which is actually a sulphapyrimidine) available in this country. The effective dose range for most sulphonylureas is very narrow, although the newer preparations, that is the so-called 'second generation' drugs such as glibenclamide, glipizide and glibornuride, have a recommended dose range of approximately 6–12-fold (see Table 3). In general there is no 'best' choice as far as sulphonylureas are concerned; it is best to get used to two or three agents and changes can then be made in the light of the patient's idiosyncrasy.

Chlorpropamide (diabinese) has a prolonged action with a half-life of pharmacological activity of 35 hours and need only be given once daily but is *best avoided in the elderly because of the risk of hypoglycaemia* and is contraindicated in those with renal failure. This precaution particularly applies to new diabetics when drugs are being prescribed for the first time; if, however, treatment is already well established and control satisfactory when the patient is first seen, therapy can be allowed to continue under close supervision. The maximum response to treatment takes about 10 days to become fully manifest after the drug is started or a change in therapy is prescribed.

Tolbutamide (Rastinon, Orinase, Artosin, Pramidex) or glibenclamide (Daonil, Euglucon) are the drugs of choice in the elderly. Tolbutamide is in general a safe drug and is rapidly detoxicated to an inactive carboxy derivative in the liver and excreted in the urine with a half-life of about 3·5–4 hours. Glibenclamide like tolbutamide has an intermediate duration of effective action of 3–24 hours, has few side-effects and is rapidly metabolized in the liver to several different products some of which retain hypoglycaemic activity. Especially where renal failure is present glibenclamide must be used with caution. Tolbutamide is given in divided doses and while glibenclamide may be given in divided doses it is best given as a single daily dose and where the latter is preferred, glibenclamide is the drug of choice. In all cases the initial dose should be low, for example 500 mg twice or thrice daily in the case of tolbutamide and 2·5–5·0 mg daily with glibenclamide until the effect in each individual patient can be assessed. Like tolbutamide, glipizide (Glibenese) also has a short duration of action and should be administered two or three times daily for maximum effect—by virtue of these properties glipizide is also suitable for use in the elderly. Doses may be increased every 4–7 days in the case of short-acting drugs, and in the case of tolbutamide should be by 500 mg/day and with glibenclamide by 5 mg/day. Unless glycosuria persists responses should be confirmed by blood sugar estimations, fasting if possible, before a further dose increase is recommended.

The sulphonylureas are well tolerated and remarkably safe and free from side-effects and although many toxic effects have been reported including rashes, jaundice, leucopenia and antithyroid activity, these are very infrequent. Glymidine does not cross-react with other sulphonylureas if they have caused troublesome rashes. Mild gastrointestinal symptoms including anorexia, nausea, vomiting, diarrhoea and abdominal pain occur in up to 5% of cases but this frequency differs little from that in placebo-treated groups and can usually be overcome by perseverance and taking the tablets with meals. Skin reactions with tolbutamide (0·4–0·8%) are said to be less frequent than with other sulphonylureas (1–5%). Photosensitivity may be induced by all sulphonylureas. Severe toxic effects such as bone marrow depression and exfoliative lesions are rare.

Many patients (up to one-third) taking chlorpropamide may become sensitive to alcohol and develop flushing, headache and nausea within 5–10 min of drinking alcohol. Similar effects are far less common with tolbutamide and avoided if tolazamide or glibenclamide is used instead.

The most serious side-effect to avoid is that of hypoglycaemia. This must be avoided at all costs in the elderly and must be borne in mind constantly as a possible event complicating therapy. Patients may be unable to obtain help or help themselves rapidly enough in this situation to avoid more serious consequences, and the aim, therefore, should always be to err on the side of keeping the patient slightly hyperglycaemic. The fact that clinical presentation may be vague and non-specific, being characterized by features so common in the elderly regardless of diabetes such as confusion, drowsiness and more marked disturbances of consciousness, underlines the need for the highest index of suspicion so that diagnosis is not missed. It must be remembered, furthermore, that typical symptoms and signs may be masked to autonomic neuropathy.

Treatment is carried out on conventional lines by the rapid intravenous injection of glucose (up to 25 g) and the possible need for further injections must be remembered. It goes without saying that blood should be drawn for glucose estimation prior to glucose injection and that the diagnosis should not be accepted on clinical grounds alone however typical the presentation may be. Hypoglycaemia may occur with short- or long-acting drugs but is a more serious hazard with the long-acting chlorpropamide. This drug merits special mention here since the elderly are particularly susceptible to hypoglycaemia especially when the diabetes is very mild. The drug has usually been in use for several weeks allowing a cumulative effect before hypoglycaemia supervenes, and because of the long half-life the hypoglycaemia may continue for 2 or 3 days after the tablets have been stopped necessitating, on occasion, the repeated administration of glucose. The short-acting drugs are not free from danger and occasionally even cause protracted hypoglycaemia. The 'second generation' drugs particularly may produce hypoglycaemia usually within a few hours of their ingestion. A recent study[47] has emphasized the frequency and severity of hypoglycaemic episodes in glibenclamide-treated patients, underlining the potent action of this agent and the care needed in adjusting the dose.

Hypoglycaemia due to sulphonylureas develops more insidiously than with insulin, and broadly can occur in three situations all easily avoided.

(1) The dose may be too large; the initial dose needed to restore normoglycaemia may be unnecessarily high for maintenance therapy and it should be routine to reduce the initial dose to the minimum necessary to maintain a normal blood glucose level. Hypoglycaemia may also be a hazard when renal failure is present since in this situation hypoglycaemic metabolites of the parent compound, such as glibenclamide, may accumulate.

(2) Failure to take an adequate diet, particularly omission of an evening meal, can lead to hypoglycaemia at night and this is of paramount importance, especially in those taking chlorpropamide. Forgetfulness, cerebrovascular disease and the tendency to develop confusion as a non-specific response to even mild intercurrent illness, place the elderly patient at considerable risk in this regard. This danger may be compounded further by the disinclination and lack of motivation to prepare a meal as a result of loneliness and depression.

(3) Drug interactions can dangerously enhance the hypoglycaemic action of the sulphonylureas (see below) – a factor of the greatest importance in the elderly because of the prevalence of polypharmacy in this age group.

The action of OHA may be influenced by a variety of drugs which may either enhance or antagonize the hypoglycaemic effect. In their recent study, Logie, *et al.*[48] found that half of 709 patients in a diabetic clinic were taking drugs with the potential to react with their diabetic treatment. These authors have emphasized that physicians and all staff associated with the care of diabetics should remain aware of possible drug interactions (Table 4) and where relevant, pass on such information to the patients. Copies of information such as that contained in Table 4 should be available for attachment to the case records of each patient taking OHA or insulin.

The most notable interaction is with alcohol which can itself cause hypoglycaemia in starved subjects and this danger is increased greatly in patients taking sulphonylureas. Large amounts of alcohol also increase the risk of lactic acidosis in biguanide-treated patients and diabetics starting treatment with oral agents should be warned

Table 4 Principal drug interactions with OHA and insulin*

Drug group	Interacting drug	Hypoglycaemic effect
Sulphonylureas, biguanides and insulin	Drugs influencing glucose metabolism, such as salicylates, adrenoceptor blocking drugs, monoamine oxidase inhibitors	potentiated
	Thiazide diuretic, glucocorticoids, oestrogens sympathomimetics barbiturates, diazoxide, epanutin	antagonized
Sulphonylureas only	Drugs metabolizing microsomal enzyme inhibitor agents: such as coumarin anticoagulants, monoamine oxidase inhibitors	potentiated
	Displacement from plasma protein drug-binding sites, such as clofibrate, phenylbutazone, sulphonamides, ergotamines	potentiated

* Modified from Logie *et al.*[48]

of these effects. Alcohol may react with chlorpropamide to cause flushing but the latter drug is contraindicated in the elderly, as noted above.

Enhancement of the hypoglycaemic effect of sulphonylureas is reported with aspirin, phenylbutazone, long-acting sulphonamides, oral anticoagulants, clofibrate, fenfluramine, ergotamines, β-blockers and the monoamine oxidase inhibitors, but with the possible exception of the β-blockers there is little danger of severe hypoglycaemia with these compounds. Patients on OHA should not be prevented from using these various drugs and if hypoglycaemia should supervene with any combination, it suggests that the patient may not need OHA at all and should be given a trial with diet alone.

β-Blockers such as propanolol deserve mention in their own right. These drugs antagonize catecholamine-induced responses and not only impair the restoration of normoglycaemia (by increased hepatic glucose output) as blood glucose levels fall, but in addition mask the symptoms and signs of hypoglycaemia. It is particularly this latter effect of the drugs which may make their administration so hazardous in some patients.

Corticosteroids especially in large doses often cause a deterioration of diabetic control but thiazide diuretics have a weak effect in this regard, as have epanutin and sympathomimetics, and rarely necessitate a change in treatment.

Increased susceptibility to lactic acidosis occurs as noted above, with alcohol and with the infusion of fructose or sorbitol and particularly in association with biguanide therapy.

The biguanides
In 1957 Ungar, Freedman and Shapiro[49] published an account of the hypoglycaemic action in several animal species and alloxan-diabetic animals of a new group of compounds chemically unrelated to the sulphonylureas. The active chemical grouping is a condensed diguanidine or biguanide:

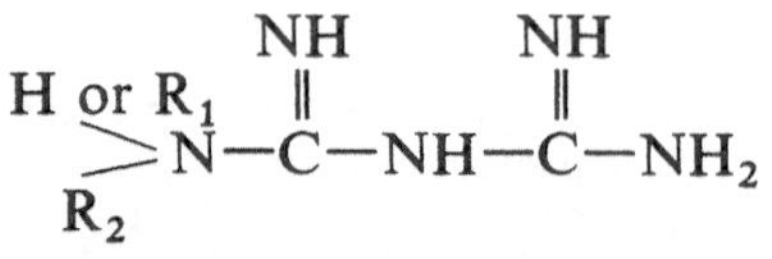

$$\begin{array}{ccc} & NH & NH \\ H\ or\ R_1 & \| & \| \\ {>}N{-}C{-}NH{-}C{-}NH_2 \\ R_2 \end{array}$$

with which several side-chains have been combined to form compounds such as phenethylbiguanide (phenformin) and dimethylbiguanide (metformin) (see Table 3, Figure 3). These drugs resemble the

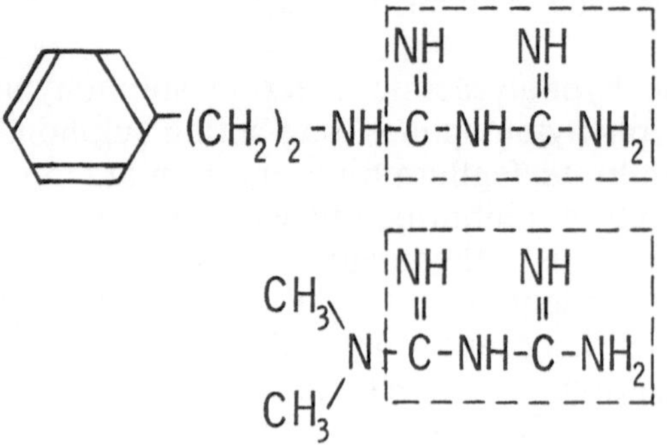

Figure 3 The biguanides

diguanidines of which the best known is decamethylene-diguanidine or synthalin A, a compound used in the oral treatment of diabetes about 30 years ago, but later given up on account of hepatic and renal toxicity.

Biguanides are indicated in two situations. These drugs may be used in obese patients as first-choice treatment as an adjunct to a reducing diet because of the small enhancement in weight reduction which they may effect. Secondly, in other patients the biguanides may be added in combination with a sulphonylurea, when maximum doses of the latter have failed to produce an adequate response. Use of biguanides, however, may be limited by their side-effects (page 188).

Metformin and phenformin are the two commonly available drugs in this group and each have a duration of action of 8–12 hours (buformin is available in Europe but not the United Kingdom). Because of the propensity of phenformin to predispose to lactic acidosis this drug is no longer recommended for patients starting treatment with OHA for the first time. There is a case to be made out, however, for continuing the use of phenformin in patients already safely stabilized on this drug; phenformin must be withdrawn, however, should cardiac, respiratory, hepatic or renal failure supervene, and alternative treatment substituted, such as metformin, sulphonylureas or insulin. Thus, as time passes the use of biguanides will become confined increasingly to taking metformin, unless new preparations emerge on the market. Metformin tablets are manufactured in two doses, 500 mg or 850 mg, and at a dose of 500 mg b.d. the drug will help to reduce blood glucose levels satisfactorily and reduce weight in the majority of maturity-onset diabetics. Nevertheless the prime importance of dietary restriction in these patients must still be stressed and when control is achieved, attempts can be made to reduce or discontinue the tablets altogether; if relapse occurs, therapy can be reintroduced. Since biguanides are short-acting drugs the response to a change in dosage may be assessed within a few days if necessary, but if reassessment cannot wait until the next clinic visit, diabetic control may be reviewed in the community with the help of the general practitioner, district nurse, etc.

The problem of drug interactions must be borne in mind as with the sulphonylureas (see Table 4).

The mode of action of these drugs is uncertain. The biguanides may reduce appetite, reduce intestinal absorption, inhibit hepatic gluconeogenesis or increase glucose uptake by muscle, but do not stimulate insulin secretion and do not lower the blood glucose of non-diabetics. The hypoglycaemic action is less powerful than that of the sulphonylureas.

Gastrointestinal discomfort is more troublesome than with the sulphonylureas and the drugs should be taken with food to reduce these effects. The symptoms are often transient and include nausea, an unpleasant metallic taste in the mouth, indigestion, wind and looseness of the bowels. Some patients develop an insiduous malaise and some taking large doses of metformin have been reported to develop vitamin B_{12} malabsorption[50] but this does not appear to be a serious clinical problem. The most serious side-effect is lactic acidosis and this is discussed in greater detail below.

Lactic acidosis   The fact that this is often fatal has been recognized with increasing frequency in recent years. The diagnosis may be confirmed by finding a large anion gap not accounted for by ketoacidosis, salicylate ingestion or uraemia and by a blood lactate concentration greater than 7 mmol/l. Most cases have occurred in patients on phenformin and buformin (used in Europe but not in the United Kingdom, as noted above), and although some cases have been associated with metformin[51-53] the incidence with the latter is far less than with phenformin. Phenformin differs from metformin in having a long lipophilic side-chain and is more readily taken up and stored by tissues. The mortality in phenformin-associated lactic acidosis is 50% (and may be as high in patients not taking phenformin); the mortality rises even higher in those patients in whom shock supervenes before therapy is instituted.

It seems likely that lactic acidosis develops following excessive accumulation of the drug in blood and/or tissues and may also occur shortly after an increase in the dose of the drug. Both phenformin and metformin are mainly excreted in the urine and only a minor fraction of phenformin is hydroxylated in the liver. Evidence is at present insufficient, however, to clarify whether the difference in lactic acidosis rates for the two drugs is due to pharmacokinetic differences or some important qualitative difference between their modes of action. What is certain is that poor renal function is a major factor precipitating biguanide-induced lactic acidosis. Cardiovascular insufficiency is frequently found in patients with lactic acidosis and even minor degrees of hepatic failure predispose to the complication because of the normally large capacity of the liver for lactate clearance. Even in patients with normal renal function there is often suggestive evidence that some event precipitated lactic acidosis by causing a minor or very transient deterioration in renal function. Whether a defect in renal function explains the finding that about half the cases have occurred in the first 1 to 2 months and the remainder at random intervals over the months or years of treatment, must remain speculative for the present[52].

The Committee on Safety of Medicines[54] has emphasized the unpredictability of lactic acidosis as a complication in patients on phenformin but fell short of recommending complete withdrawal of the drug, saying that this might not be in the interests of selected patients. In the elderly, however, the safest policy to adopt is probably complete withdrawal should there be any doubts at all in the physician's mind.

Although it is known that acute renal failure may precipitate lactic acidosis in patients taking metformin[53] the circumstances under which this complication occurs with metformin are not as yet full characterized. There are at least three recent reports of lactic acidosis in patients receiving metformin[53,55,56], and while in one case lactic acidosis followed a massive overdose of the drug[55] the other patients were receiving normal doses[55], although renal impairment was associated in each case. For the present it seems reasonable to prescribe the drug in the elderly provided that the patient is watched carefully and provided that the serum creatinine is normal; where the latter is elevated, however, or where cardiovascular or hepatic insufficiency is present metformin is clearly contraindicated.

Ethanol impairs lactate uptake by the liver and patients on biguanides should be warned of the danger of excessive alcohol intake which may precipitate lactic acidosis. In the elderly, where nutrition may be poor, it is important to avoid the tendency to use fructose or sorbitol which are rapidly metabolized to lactate.

Clearly prevention is the best method of reducing mortality in lactic acidosis, but once the condition has developed, infusion with hypertonic sodium bicarbonate is the mainstay of treatment and should aim to restore the arterial pH within 2–6 hours. Indeed, patients who have responded best to treatment have been those in whom arterial pH was restored to normal most rapidly, that is within a few hours. In addition to the latter, other principles of treatment are to stop biguanide therapy, treat any hypoxia, correct dehydration and shock and maintain the serum potassium level. A central venous pressure line should be inserted to give an early warning of overload if the patient is not fully alert, and a urinary catheter should be inserted to allow adequate assessment of fluid balance. If there is any doubt about cardiac or renal function, the question of peritoneal or haemodialysis should be considered. In the elderly, unlike the treatment of young patients, a decision may have to be taken at this stage whether or not to proceed with active treatment and consideration of the quality of life and independence of the patient among other considerations will influence the decision. After the pH has been normal for several hours the rate of bicarbonate infusion should be slowed progressively whilst monitoring arterial pH frequently and the infusion should be eventually stopped but increased transiently at any suggestion of relapse.

Insulin

General approach
The use of insulin (Table 5) in the elderly is governed broadly by the same principles which apply to its use in younger patients. Emphasis is again on simplifying treatment as much as possible, that is by the administration of only one injection daily whenever possible, and by erring, if anything, on the side of underprescribing thereby avoiding the danger of hypoglycaemia. In general, patients whose total daily insulin requirement is of the order of 20–30 units can be satisfactorily managed with a single daily dose of intermediate-acting isophane or long-acting lente insulin taken about 30 min before breakfast. Patients with larger daily requirements, for instance 30–80 units/day, whose diabetes is fairly stable (the majority of elderly insulin-requiring diabetics) can be maintained on single daily injections of long-acting insulin. Those patients with marked tendency to ketosis will be better controlled on a regimen containing mixtures of short-acting and intermediate-acting insulin in varying proportions.

The use of lente insulin therefore is particularly indicated in the elderly insulin-requiring diabetic without a propensity to develop ketoacidosis in whom the hyperglycaemia can be controlled satisfactorily with daily injections. The use of short-acting soluble insulin in combination with the intermediate-acting isophane insulin given twice daily half an hour before the morning and evening meals is the most satisfactory treatment for that minority of elderly insulin-dependent patients with unstable diabetes. The injection of isophane insulin means that a smaller dose of the short-acting preparation can be given, thus reducing the risk of hypoglycaemia, while at the same time the duration of insulin action is prolonged until the next injection. The relative proportions and doses of short-acting and intermediate-acting insulin at each injection will vary from patient to patient and can only be decided on the basis of serial glucose estimations in blood and urine at appropriate times during the day (fasting and pre-supper, as a minimum) while the patient is following the prescribed diet. There is little doubt that this regimen provides smoother and more stable control and allows for the frequent and logical adjustment of insulin dosage according to requirements.

Table 5 Highly purified pork insulin

	Onset of action	Peak effect	Duration of action	Manufacturer	Equivalent ordinary insulin
MC Actrapid (monocomponent)	Immediate	1–4 hours	6–8 hours	Novo	Insulin injection BP 'soluble'
MC Semitard (monocomponent)	1 hour	3–8 hours	12–16 hours	Novo	Insulin Zinc Suspension (Amorphous) BP 'Semilente'
MC Monotard (monocomponent)	2–4 hours	6–15 hours	22–28 hours	Novo	Insulin Zinc Suspension BP 'Lente'
Leo Neutral RI (rarely immunogenic)	Immediate	1–4 hours	6–8 hours	Nordisk	Insulin injection BP 'Soluble'
Leo Retard RI (rarely immunogenic)	1–3 hours	6–12 hours	16–28 hours	Nordisk	Isophane injection BP (Neutral Protamine Hagedorn–NPH)

Conversion to a twice-daily regimen of soluble insulin only will often become necessary in patients previously controlled on longer-acting preparations during periods of infection or intercurrent illness, in those undergoing surgery or when the total insulin requirements exceed 60–80 units/day.

Problems of insulin administration may arise in the elderly in terms of forgetfulness and impaired vision; the latter should be specifically searched for and, when found, special arrangements should be made to ensure accurate regular insulin dosage. If a relative or friend is not available to check or take over the insulin administration, then in most settings the district nurse will supervise treatment with daily or twice-daily visits. While not practised in the United Kingdom to the author's knowledge, the possibility has been suggested[19] of leaving a week's supply of filled insulin syringes in the refrigerator with each syringe labelled with the day and time it is to be used; it would seem reasonable, however, to avoid such a practice except in an emergency situation, when in any event alternative arrangements would be considered. Where patients require twice-daily injections of mixtures of soluble and isophane insulin, the two types of insulin may be premixed under sterile conditions in proportions appropriate to morning and evening use so that only one insulin solution need be drawn up for injection – the dose of insulin required and the time to be used may be marked clearly on each bottle thus simplifying the insulin administration to the maximum. With all patients, the exact schedule for insulin should be written out by the physician or district nurse for the guidance of the patient and family and reviewed at each visit.

Diabetic patients who are not ordinarily insulin-dependent may nevertheless require insulin during times of unusual stress, such as surgery or infections. Management of these conditions requires conversion to short-acting insulin and is similar in old people as for any other diabetic and the same principles apply to the management of diabetic ketoacidosis (page 198).

Highly purified insulins
Until recently, most commercial insulin preparations have consisted of mixtures of porcine and bovine insulin, but interest in the purification of insulin has been stimulated by the finding that almost all insulin-treated diabetics, even those treated with apparently pure preparations, have insulin-binding antibodies in their blood (see Table 5).

It was assumed that animal insulins were antigenic in man because their structure differs from human insulin – porcine by one and bovine by three amino acids. This is only partially true in that porcine insulins are less antigenic than bovine but even 'pure' mono-species porcine insulin has resulted in the formation of insulin-binding antibodies, and it is now clear that antibody formation is considerably increased by the impurities contained in the commercial preparation. If commercial crystalline insulin is subjected to Sephadex gel chromatography it can be separated into three fractions 'a', 'b' and 'c'. all of which are in themselves heterogeneous with molecular weights of 20 000, 9000 and 6000 respectively. The 'a' fraction found only in very impure preparations contains various non-insulin pancreatic proteins as well as aggregated and cross-linked insulin and is strongly antigenic. The major component of the 'b' fraction is proinsulin, the precursor of insulin, consisting of A and B chains of insulin linked by a connecting or C-peptide and species differences in C-peptide structure presumably account for its antigenicity. The 'c' fraction is virtually non-antigenic and is predominantly insulin. Thus it is possible to make virtually non-antigenic porcine insulin without removing the 'b' fraction although to make a longer-acting preparation removal of the 'b' fraction (proinsulin-freed insulin) is necessary. Further purification by anion exchange chromatography in order to remove insulin derivatives from the 'c' fraction leaves a highly purified product, in other words 'monocomponent' (MC-insulin) or 'rarely immunogenic' insulin. Pork MC-insulin prepared by recrystallization and chromatography displays only one band on disc electrophoresis and shows little or no immunogenicity in patients[57] but beef MC-insulins are still immunogenic.

At present the transfer of patients previously treated with mixed insulins is indicated in the following situations:

(1) Insulin allergy in the form of severe local skin reactions (provided that faulty injection techniques is not the cause) or, rarely, generalized anaphylactic reactions.

(2) Lipoatrophy – here injections should be given directly into the areas of lipoatrophy. Some degree of fat atrophy is present in about 25% of insulin-treated diabetics.

(3) Insulin resistance where the daily requirement is 100 units or more in the absence of any recognizable cause.

(4) The need for intermittent insulin therapy as in the presence of infections or postoperatively.

It would seem reasonable therefore, in view of the above, to use highly purified insulins for any diabetic requiring insulin for the first time. It should be borne in mind, however, that the cost of highly purified insulin is roughly 3 fold that of currently available commercial preparations.

Insulin requirements usually fall when patients are changed to highly purified insulin but the fall, associated with a reduction in the titre of insulin antibodies, is unpredictable both in magnitude and timing. If the daily requirement exceeds 100 units, the transfer to highly purified insulin should be made in hospital. For outpatients the daily dose should be reduced by 10–20% and the patient instructed about the need for subsequent alterations. Some patients have complained that their warning symptoms of hypoglycaemia are reduced or lost after starting on highly purified insulins which may be due to the rapidity of fall in blood sugar, which again can be corrected by reducing the dose prescribed. It should be re-emphasized that in the elderly the degree of diabetic control ultimately achieved need not attain the level aimed at in the young, and again, if in doubt, the tendency should always be to undertreat so as to avoid the hazard of hypoglycaemia.

From a clinical standpoint the advantages of a lowered incidence of immunological side-effects and a reduction in insulin dose are clear. What is not clear is the extent of the role of insulin antibodies in the development or aggravation of diabetic complications. Insulin antibodies cannot be the cause of retinopathy since the latter is as common in patients who have never had exogenous insulin as in those who have been treated.

There is some evidence that anti-insulin antibodies may play a rôle in the progression of diabetic nephropathy. Thus, in animals immunization with insulin has been shown to cause damage to glomeruli and β-cells and there is hope that the use of highly purified insulins in future will lower the incidence of diabetic complications, especially microangiopathy. There is no obvious correlation between the level of insulin antibodies and the ease of diabetic control – indeed it has been suggested but not confirmed that high levels of antibodies might render diabetics' control somewhat easier.

Long-term supervision of diabetic control

In diabetics, and, particularly in those taking insulin, routine urine testing for glucose offers a useful guide to control. In properly controlled maturity-onset diabetes testing the urine should provide reassurance that all is well, and in poorly controlled patients persistent glycosuria will warn the patient and doctor of the need to improve control and revise treatment.

It is important to determine the renal threshold whenever possible by several estimations of the blood glucose level with corresponding tests for glycosuria on samples passed 15–30 min after the blood is taken, having ensured that the bladder has been emptied shortly before the venepuncture is performed. A high renal threshold means that, although the urine is sugar-free, hyperglycaemia may be present and in such cases monitoring of therapy must depend on more frequent blood sugar estimations. A low renal threshold is much less common in the elderly but again frequent blood sugar estimations will provide a better guide to control than urine tests and would be important information in avoiding overtreatment and hypoglycaemia.

Assuming there is no gross deviation of the renal threshold for glucose from the normal level of 10 mmol/l (180 mg/100 ml) the morning fasting urine test will give a good indication of overnight control. The bladder is emptied on first rising and the specimen discarded; a second specimen is then obtained just before breakfast and is tested for glucose. Testing of fasting urine samples regularly is probably the most important index of control in elderly non-insulin-requiring diabetics and in those insulin-dependent patients stabilized on long-acting insulin. The frequency of urine testing varies with the degree of control and should take place at least once a week even in stable diabetics. Just as important as urine testing, the weight should be taken regularly and recorded in writing, preferably by the patient since this provides a salutary reminder of the importance of adhering to the prescribed diet.

Attendance at the diabetic clinic two or three times a year offers the opportunity for regular assessment and in particular for blood glucose estimations to be carried out. Where possible fasting blood glucose levels should be obtained since these levels represent the most useful indices of diabetic control. While fasting samples are easily obtained from inpatients this is more difficult in those living at home or in residential care and particularly so in insulin-requiring patients, in whom random blood sugar levels will have to suffice. It is true that on occasions a random blood glucose estimation at the clinic is a poor index of the degree of hyperglycaemia during an ordinary day; nevertheless random samples taken about the same time at repeated clinic visits will give a general impression of blood glucose control and the correlation with urine tests as well as the frequency of hypoglycaemic reactions.

If oral therapy has been prescribed the dose can be adjusted according to the response. Where the urine has been free of sugar and the blood sugar normal or near normal, the dose of tablets can either be continued, reduced or even discontinued as a therapeutic trial[33]. On the other hand where control is poor, despite satisfactory weight reduction and adherence to diet, consideration can be given to an increase in the tablets or the introduction of insulin in their place, but sometimes remonstration on the need for more dietary restraint is sufficient in itself. The problem of hypoglycaemia has been dealt with above.

What then constitutes satisfactory control? In addition to little or no glycosuria, reasonable criteria, which would be unacceptable in younger patients, are fasting plasma glucose levels less than 7·8 mmol/l (140 mg/100 ml) and 2 and 3 hour postprandial glucose levels less than 8·9–10·0 mmol/l (160–180 mg/100 ml). The renal threshold for glucose often rises in older diabetics with or without accompanying renal decompensation so that testing for glycosuria may be of little help in monitoring control. Thus although at present control is usually judged by frequent urine tests and occasional blood sugar estimations, both can be notoriously unreliable and may be only crude indices at best for the logical adjustment of therapy. Diurnal blood glucose series carried out on patients at frequent intervals can be much more helpful but can still vary quite markedly even in an asymptomatic patient[58]. Nevertheless, what is reasonably certain is that any patient whose fasting blood glucose levels remain less than 7·8 mmol/l (140 mg/100 ml) is 'safe' in being extremely unlikely to develop severe metabolic deterioration and ketoacidosis.

Patients whose values for glucose tolerance fall in the borderline or probable range should be followed up with regular observations for the development of any clinical evidence of diabetes and for retesting preferably at 6 monthly intervals – at least in terms of a fasting glucose estimation. The only specific advice recommended to such patients in the present state of knowledge should be that regarding weight loss for those who are obese.

Until recently it has not been possible to assess objectively the accuracy of long-term blood glucose regulation but the estimation of glycosylated haemoglobin, that is, haemoglobin Alc (HbAlc), may now provide a solution to this problem[59]. It is known that the presence of haemoglobin and glucose in high concentrations and the relative irreversibility of their ketoamine linkage results in the continuous formation and accumulation of glycosylated haemoglobin (HbAlc) within the red cells – the HbAlc being formed from HbA in a slow, non-insulin dependent reaction. It is also known that HbAlc is increased in diabetes and studies by Koenig *et al.*[60] and Gonen *et al.*[61] have shown that the level of HbAlc correlates closely with the degree of control as assessed by fasting plasma glucose levels or mean daily glucose levels over the previous few weeks. Thus HbAlc levels are high in poorly controlled diabetics and when diabetic patients are admitted to hospital and their blood glucose levels carefully regulated to stay within the optimal ranges, previously high HbAlc levels are reduced to normal with a time lag of 5 to 6 weeks.

These findings suggest that a single HbAlc determination reflects the average blood glucose level in the diabetic patient during the preceding few weeks and is an index of diabetic control over that time. Thus HbAlc measurement which is a simple, rapid, objective procedure should be used to assess diabetic control and may also serve as both a screening test for uncontrolled diabetes and as an indicator of the efficiency of various therapeutic regimens. Serial measurements of glycosylated haemoglobin might allow an objective assessment of blood glucose control over much longer periods.

Two groups[62,63] have recently published their experience with home monitoring of blood glucose, that is with patients measuring their own blood glucose levels in their own homes. The patients are required to prick their own fingers and the glucose content of the blood so obtained is measured by test strips, for example Dextrostix, in combination with a suitable reflectance meter. In these studies no major difficulty was experienced with the patients obtaining their own blood samples and overall the diabetic control was considerably improved. This has had the advantage of enabling diabetic control to be sustantially improved by modification of treatment in the community without the necessity of hospital admission. The admission to hospital of patients with unstable control for blood glucose profiles is wasteful of beds and artificial since life in hospital is unlike day-to-day life outside hospital. Self-monitoring overcomes these problems and saves the patient unnecessary hospital visits since changes in treatment can be made by telephone.

Home blood glucose monitoring can also be used to assess long-term control, and its advantage over HbAlc measurements is that it not only detects poor control but also shows how to correct it. Some patients have found self-monitoring more informative than urine tests and their disease has resulted in better motivation, greater understanding of diabetes and a sustained improvement in control[63].

It is true that far fewer elderly diabetics will be involved in self-monitoring than younger diabetics for several reasons. Firstly, the incidence of insulin-requiring diabetes, where self-monitoring is particularly applicable, is less in the older patients who are predominantly non-insulin-dependent mild diabetics. Secondly, a greater degree of latitude in diabetic control is acceptable in older patients which falls short of the requirements aimed at in younger patients. Finally, the elderly diabetics are generally less able to carry out self-monitoring sufficiently accurately to prove of value in diabetic control. Nevertheless there are a small selected group of patients, possibly those insulin-requiring diabetics presenting only late in life or those in whom the renal threshold for glucose may be increased, where extra efforts are desirable to improve metabolic control. Where such patients have the desire and capability to participate more intensively in their own management, this should receive every encouragement regardless of their age.

Complications of diabetes

Ketoacidosis
Although diabetic ketoacidosis may complicate the clinical course of known diabetics for various reasons, such as failure to take drugs or insulin, stress such as infections or surgical procedures, a small but important group of elderly diabetics present with this complication[64]. Patients with ketoacidosis should be treated in an intensive care unit, yet in spite of advances in intensive care, a mortality of 50% or more is not uncommon in the elderly[65].

The clinical presentation of ketoacidosis has been well described[65] and is similar in all age groups (Table 6). Recently, however, attention has been drawn to the association between diabetic ketoacidosis and hypothermia in the elderly[64]. Indeed in one series of patients hospitalized for hypothermia, ketoacidosis was more common than hypothyroidism[64], and it may be that the occurrence of hypothermia in the course of diabetic ketoacidosis is more frequent than has been recognized hitherto.

The mechanisms of this association are complex. There is evidence that ketoacidosis may affect temperature regulation and predispose to hypothermia by impairing tissue oxygen utilization and heat production[66,67]. Thus fever is uncommon in ketoacidosis even in the presence of infection[68] and several cases in a recent series[64] occurred during the summer months when clearly environmental temperature contributed less to the disturbance.

Conversely hypothermia may aggravate uncontrolled diabetes. At low temperatures insulin secretion is impaired, glucose utilization is reduced, resistance to exogenous insulin develops and the secretion

Table 6 Coma in the elderly diabetic

Clinical and biochemical features	Ketoacidotic hyperglycaemia	Non-ketotic hyperosmolar hyperglycaemia	Lactic acidosis	Hypoglycaemia	Cerebrovascular disease
Kussmaul breathing	+ +	0	+ +	0	0
Dehydration	+ + +	+ + +	0 or +	0 or +	0 or +
Neurological signs focal deficit	0	0 or +	0	0 or +	0 or + + +
Blood glucose	+ + +	+ + +	N or +	0 or +	N or +
Ketosis	+ + +	0	0 or +	–	0 or +
Acidosis	+ + +	0	+ +	0	0

199

of insulin antagonists in the form of cortisol and catecholamines is increased[69–72]. Thus although loss of diabetic control is not inevitable in severe hypothermia, the metabolic disturbance, when it occurs, is characteristically severe.

Accidental hypothermia and diabetic coma carry a high mortality in the elderly and the management of patients with both problems is difficult. Since insulin may be ineffective at low temperatures, rapid rewarming is probably justified. Arterial blood should be used for analysis as stasis and pooling may render venous samples unreliable. Fluid and potassium replacement must be given with caution. Of particular importance is the liability to recurrence in survivors of hypothermic ketoacidosis, and in these patients attention must be paid to potential precipitating factors such as poor housing, alcohol abuse or treatment with barbiturates or phenothiazines.

The prime considerations in the treatment of this medical emergency are correction of acidosis, fluid and electrolyte depletion, insulin deficiency and treatment of the underlying cause where possible. Traditionally insulin has been given in comparatively large doses (80–200 units) by simultaneous intravenous and intramuscular injections at intervals of about 2 hours. The principal dangers of such therapy are late hypoglycaemia, osmotic disequilibrium and hypokalaemia, and it has been recognized that such insulin doses are far in excess of that which is physiologically appropriate. Accordingly, simplified regimes of low dose insulin administration have been introduced successfully in the past few years.

Two approaches have been used: the continuous infusion of insulin and intermittent intramuscular injections of low doses of insulin. Several reports[43,65,73,74] have confirmed the simplicity and effectiveness of these methods. In the first (infusion) method insulin in normal saline is infused at a rate of 4–10 units/hour and adjustment of the infusion rate can easily be made according to the results of frequent (usually hourly) measurements of blood glucose. Sometimes an initial small bolus of 10 units is given intravenously at the beginning of the infusion. Some add albumin to the saline to prevent absorption of insulin onto the infusion apparatus, but many do not. When the blood glucose falls to 10–16 mmol/l (180–288 mg/100 ml) the rate of infusion is lowered and glucose may be added to the infusion to prevent hypoglycaemia. Because of the short half-life of insulin given intravenously, changing the infusion rate will result in the establishment of a new steady-state insulin concentration within 10–15 min. This method of insulin administration is very simple and flexible and is easily applied also to the treatment of hyperosmolar non-ketotic coma.

The second method of low dose insulin treatment employs the intramuscular injection of 5–10 units/hour insulin after an initial dose of 10–20 units. It was suggested that this method was simple particularly outside specialized units and that the time-course of intramuscular injection allowed reasonably swift onset of action without undue prolongation of effect.

The use of both these methods produces a steady fall in blood glucose, ketones, free fatty acids and glycerol. The likelihood of hypokalaemia is lessened and there is some evidence that the amounts of potassium required to maintain normokalaemia are less than with previous high dose insulin regimes. The reason for this is thought to be that small doses of insulin produce lowering of blood glucose mainly by restraining hepatic glucose release (gluconeogenesis) rather than increasing peripheral glucose uptake which is associated with a more rapid rate of potassium uptake[73].

In general there is probably little to choose between these two methods of low dose insulin treatment. In severely ill patients with significant peripheral circulatory insufficiency, the intramuscular route is potentially less satisfactory and failures have been reported[75] so that overall the infusion method is the treatment of choice. The protagonists of the intramuscular method have suggested that in such patients an initial intravenous pulse of insulin may be advisable[74].

Hyperosmolar non-ketotic coma

The serious complication of hyperosmolar non-ketotic coma, increasingly recognized in recent years, is of particular importance as it tends to be found more commonly in the elderly[76]. The condition is about one-sixth as common as diabetic ketoacidosis and the affected patients are almost always mild maturity-onset diabetics controlled by diet alone or diet and OHA or they may be new, previously undiagnosed diabetics who do not require insulin once the disturbance has been corrected. A minority of patients are insulin-requiring diabetics and patients who are actually non-diabetic may be precipitated into hyperosmolar coma by the administration of excessive amounts of carbohydrate. In many patients a precipitating infection or an underlying disease can be implicated in the genesis of the disorder as can a number of drugs including diuretics and steroids.

The condition resembles severe ketoacidosis presenting with increasing weakness, polyuria, polydipsia, dehydration, clinical shock and deepening stupor; the onset may be more insidious than diabetic ketoacidosis, however, and symptoms may be present for as long as 12–14 days. The syndrome differs from ketoacidosis in that acidosis and hence hyperventilation is absent and in the frequency of neurological abnormalities which may be stimulatory (such as seizure) or paralytic. Most patients manifest profound alterations in their state of consciousness but occasionally may be alert and well-orientated. However, the reasons for the severe alterations in central nervous system function are poorly understood but may be due to reduced cerebral perfusion consequent on shock, and this may be especially important in the elderly who might already have areas of compromised circulation. Dehydration is the most striking finding on examination and is due to the osmotic diuresis resulting from glycosuria, vomiting and an inadequate intake of glucose-free water appropriate to the dehydration. The hyperosmolarity is predominantly a consequence of the hyperglycaemia, but also uraemia, which many patients show, and in some cases hypernatraemia. Despite the absence of ketoacidosis, many patients have significant reductions in plasma pH as a result of lactic acidosis, uraemia or unknown factors. The average blood glucose is usually greater than 55·6 mmol/l (1000 mg%) and the plasma osmolarity exceeds 350 mosmol/l. The serum sodium has varied from 118 mEq/l to as high as 188 mEq/l.

The pathogenesis of the syndrome remains poorly understood. Almost all patients have abnormal glucose tolerance and precipitating factors particularly infections, are common. During the period of polydipsia patients often consume large amounts of carbohydrate-containing beverages which contribute significantly to the hyperglycaemia. Renal function, which in many patients is already impaired by underlying cardiovascular and renal disease, is further compromised by dehydration and prerenal uraemia. The development of shock has been an important factor in the high mortality of this condition which in most series has been about 50% but has fallen to 15–25% in more recent studies.

One of the main unsolved aspects of this disorder is the absence of ketosis. In the present state of knowledge it seems likely that decreased mobilization of free fatty acids from adipose tissue may be an important factor contributing to the absence of ketosis and this could be due to the antilipolytic action of insulin which though deficient may be present in significantly higher concentrations than the very low levels which characterize ketoacidosis.

Treatment of this condition should be carried out in an intensive care unit with monitoring of central venous pressure. The most important aspect of therapy is fluid replacement with hypotonic saline (0·45%) and Matz[77] attributed the low mortality rate in his series to the early use of massive amounts of hypotonic, multi-electrolyte solutions at the rate of 1–2 l/hour; he also stressed the vigorous administration of plasma volume expanders, especially in those patients in shock at the time of admission. Insulin should be used in small doses and with extreme caution as these patients are often very sensitive to insulin and too rapid a reduction in the blood glucose level and plasma osmolarity might result in osmotic disequilibrium across the central nervous system and cerebral oedema. It is probably best to give a dose of soluble insulin half that recommended in ketoacidotic coma. A reasonable regimen is the initial administration of 10 units intravenously followed by a constant infusion of 3–4 units/hour (or 5 units/hour by intramuscular injection) with hourly monitoring of blood glucose levels for 2–3 hours before deciding the level of further insulin dosage. In general, patients with hyperosmolar coma require much less insulin than patients with ketoacidosis – in Gerich's series[78] (before low dose regimens were introduced) the former received an average of 133 units compared to 359 units in the latter group. Occasional patients have demonstrated extreme sensitivity or, conversely, resistance to insulin.

Electrolyte status, fluid and acid base balance must be regularly monitored. The rate of fluid administration must be individualized bearing in mind that the patient's cardiovascular status and a urine output of at least 50 ml/hour should be maintained and in view of the significant mortality attributable to shock and dehydration, correction of the latter should receive the highest priority. Similar remarks apply to treatment of the underlying disorder, especially infections with Gram-negative organisms. Of the 34 fatal cases of hyperosmolar coma analysed by McCurdy[79] about half the deaths were due to the pre-existing or precipitating illness while the other half reflected the severe dehydration of the patients.

Lactic acidosis
For discussion and treatment of this condition see page 188.

Care of the feet
This is an aspect of particular importance in the elderly since recent advances in the control of metabolic disorders in diabetes mellitus have led to a considerable increase in their life expectancy. As a result the longer-term diabetic complications are presenting with growing frequency. This is particularly seen in the diabetic foot where the pathology is characterized by vascular disease and ischaemia, neuropathy and sepsis either separately or in combination.

The most important aspect of management of the diabetic foot is one of prevention. A point which cannot be overemphasized to patients and relatives alike and particularly when the patient's eyesight is failing, is that even the *most severe* lesions in the foot may be *painless* – so that normal sensation cannot be relied upon to call attention to trauma, infection or extending disease. All diabetics should have a clear programme of conscious inspection and prophylactic care with foot hygiene in order to reduce the possibility of preventable amputation. Clear instructions should be spelt out to those at risk both verbally and in pamphlets. Minor trauma to the feet can easily lead to sepsis and gangrene since bacteria flourish in an environment of hyperglycaemia and ischaemia.

Feet must be kept clean and dry. Shoes must be comfortable and should be inspected regularly for nails or other areas of roughness. Socks should not be darned and no constricting garters or elastic bands should be worn. Toenails should be cut transversely and, if the patient's eyesight is poor, preferably by someone else; corns and calluses and difficult toenails should be dealt with by a qualified chiropodist. Heating the feet should be avoided – hot water bottles should not be used, the temperature of the bath water should be kept moderate and the feet should not be exposed near a fire or heater. Diabetics should not walk barefoot and any open sore or wound that does not heal rapidly should be seen by the doctor. Any infection of the foot should receive prompt treatment along conventional lines, and fungal infections such as 'athlete's foot' must be prevented or treated early.

Treatment of ischaemia again entails prevention and the heels should be protected by slings which suspend the feet a few centimeters above the bed; sheepskin covers may be used on top of the mattress. Smoking should be actively discouraged at all times. In other respects treatment of vascular disease should follow conventional principles and if arterial reconstruction and amputation become necessary, appropriate rehabilitation will then be required in its own right. Amputees need assistance in getting about and in the use of artificial limbs; patients must be taught care of the stump since the overlying skin may be vunerable to the slightest trauma.

Cramp in the calf muscles at night is a common complaint of the diabetic and may not be associated with neuropathy or ischaemic disease. It can usually be prevented, as in the non-diabetic, by taking a tablet of quinine sulphate before retiring.

It goes without saying that good diabetic control should be maintained at all times and, particularly in the presence of sepsis, it may be necessary to increase the insulin dosage in insulin-dependent patients and to replace OHA with insulin in previously non-insulin-requiring patients.

Disorders of the eye

Present evidence suggests that the development of complications is related to the overall standard of blood glucose control but further studies are needed in this regard[80,81]. Older people with diabetes are potentially subject to the same complications as younger diabetics but in as much as the appearance of complications appears to be related to the duration of diabetes, the actual prevalence of the more serious complications such as retinopathy and nephropathy is not high amongst persons with onset of diabetes late in life.

Diabetic retinopathy is a major cause of blindness affecting 5–10% of diabetics surviving 20 years from diagnosis. The detection and assessment of retinopathy and its management is an essential aspect of the care of the diabetic patient. Good diabetic control offers the best hope of avoiding retinopathy and indeed considerable amelioration of changes already present can occur with improved control[82]. It is true, however, that in many diabetics good control cannot be achieved and, in others, retinopathy develops even when control is apparently satisfactory.

Once retinopathy is established the most hopeful treatment is photocoagulation[80] and reports from England[83] and America[84] have demonstrated convincingly that this treatment is effective in delaying visual deterioration in patients with new vessel formation and maculopathy. To take advantage of this treatment the diabetic clinic should be organized appropriately so that the fundi of all patients are examined at regular intervals with pupils dilated in a dark room; furthermore there must be close cooperation with an eye surgeon with facilities available for fluorescein studies and photocoagulation.

All patients who have retinopathy start with mild background retinopathy which is characterized by dot and blot haemorrhages and microaneurysms never very numerous. Scattered hard exudates and occasional cotton wool spots may also be present. Here loss of vision is minimal or absent with a very rare exception of a haemorrhage of the fovea. The most important duty of any physician caring for patients with mild background retinopathy is to ensure adequate eye follow-up, so that if deterioration supervenes treatment is not long delayed. Once retinopathy is present yearly examination is mandatory.

Maculopathy is the condition in which visual loss is due to macular oedema or a plaque of hard exudate at the macula and the oedema is usually associated with hard exudates, microaneurysms and haemorrhages. In the elderly exudates in the macular area are the commonest cause of defective vision resulting from diabetic retinopathy. Since visual loss in maculopathy is due to leakage from abnormally permeable blood vessels it is reasonable that destruction of these vessels will allow for absorption of the oedema and hard exudates present and that, since no new vessels will form, the retinopathy will improve and vision will be preserved. Photocoagulation using xenon arc or argon laser treatment has significantly improved the prognosis for vision[80,81,85,86] and accordingly is now the recommended therapy for maculopathy.

In proliferative retinopathy new vessels arise from the retinal periphery or from the optic disc and vision remains good until there is a vitreous haemorrhage. Two treatments have been shown to affect the progression of proliferative retinopathy – photocoagulation and pituitary ablation. Results with the latter are no better than with photocoagulation which would always be the treatment of choice in the elderly. There is only one small rare group of patients with rapidly advancing florid retinopathy in whom pituitary ablation would remain the preferred treatment – but this latter would not be indicated in the elderly.

In the last few years vitrectomy has become a widely used method of treatment for vitreous haemorrhage and vitreous membranes. In general the results in diabetes are not as good as in other conditions leading to vitreous haemorrhage as the retina behind the haemorrhage may be too badly damaged by continuing vascular occlusion or retinitis proliferans to have any function. In Great Britain it is unusual to operate until at least 1 year after the vitreous haemorrhage to allow spontaneous absorption to occur.

Diabetic opacities are often associated with senile opacities and the combined effect gives rise to more visual difficulty than either alone so that senile cataract is said to occur at an earlier age in diabetics. This combined effect probably causes operation for senile cataract to be relatively much commoner in diabetics than in others, about $5:1$[87], and indeed a number of elderly diabetics come to diagnosis because of cataract.

A patient going blind should be helped to make adjustments in his/her life and where possible should learn braille and attend a rehabilitation centre. It is important to note that a blind diabetic may be handicapped by diminished sensitivity of his fingertips and should be registered blind as soon as applicable since help may be forthcoming from appropriate authorities. A guide-dog may be useful for mobile, otherwise fit patients and special preset syringes may be used for drawing up insulin or arrangements made for someone else such as a relative or district nurse to give injections.

Urinary tract disease
Infection of the urinary tract is common in diabetics and often difficult to eradicate. Diagnosis by urine examination and treatment with the appropriate antibiotic(s) should follow standard principles. Chronic or recurrent infections are indications for urological examination to rule out an obstructive lesion and this is of particular importance in relation to prostatic hypertrophy in elderly men. The neurogenic and atonic bladder is another occasional predisposing factor that requires attention, but a far more common problem may be the presence of an indwelling catheter. With regard to the latter while antibiotic treatment is useful in the short-term[88], there is no place for long-term therapy, and indeed a recent study[89] has demonstrated the failure of bladder irrigation with antibiotics to reduce the incidence of urinary tract infection.

In terms of the nephropathy itself, therapy is limited to maintaining good diabetic control in the hope that this will either prevent or retard the progression of renal disease. No specific treatment is available and at this moment in time renal transplant has no place in management of the elderly diabetic.

Diabetic neuropathy
Subacute sensory neuropathy improves rapidly, and motor neuropathy more slowly with good metabolic control, although it may initially exacerbate symptoms; in chronic sensory neuropathy signs are unlikely to disappear. Since a specific therapy for neuropathy has not been developed, treatment is confined to general measures and symptomatic relief. Good control of the diabetes should be maintained at all times but there is no evidence of any special virtue in the use of insulin. The diet should be adequate in protein and vitamin content and if there is any doubt about the patient's nutrition, vitamins should be given in full dosage parenterally if necessary, for example as parenterovite. If the patient is wasted it would also be important to add carbohydrate and fat to the diet and modify therapy accordingly to maintain control.

Pain relief may require simple analgesics such as aspirin, but in more severe cases methadone (Physeptone), dihydrocodeine (D.F. 118) or mefenamic acid (Ponstan) are indicated and if pain is very severe in the acute stages even pethidine may be given; carbamazepine (Tegretol), or epanutin is occasionally helpful in severe cases. Adequate sleep is important and the inclusion of a hypnotic in the treatment is usually necessary. Alcohol may aggravate the condition and should be forbidden or at least restricted. In more severe cases, admission to hospital may be the most useful approach to reviewing overall management. If weakness is present, muscle wasting may be diminished by electrical stimulation and intensive physiotherapy should be employed to maintain and improve mobility of the patient. Other measures, such as correction of foot drop may be required. Because of the sensory loss in the legs, care and protection of the feet is vital.

Elderly men with mild diabetes particularly may be affected by diabetic amyotrophy. The condition is usually self-limiting but symptomatically the most important factor is the severe pain which it may cause in affected muscle groups, sometimes resistant to treatment and severe enough to prevent sleep. The condition, often unilateral, typically involves proximal muscles of the limbs especially the quadriceps and pelvic girdle often accompanied by wasting and fasciculation with loss of knee reflexes but little distal involvement.

Autonomic neuropathy with an atonic bladder may present with chronic retention without evidence of obstruction and is more often seen in elderly patients, especially men, in whom it may mimic prostatic obstruction and where catheterization will occasionally be required. Postural hypotension may also prove troublesome in the elderly.

Mononeuropathy may occur acutely in the elderly with involvement of the oculomotor and abducent nerve. Reassurance regarding the likelihood of spontaneous recovery is the only 'therapy' available.

Acknowledgements
I wish to thank Dr J. Wedgwood and Dr J. Nabarro for much helpful discussion and Mrs A. Cooper for typing the manuscript.

References
1 Tattersall, R. B. and Fajans, S. S. (1975). A difference between the inheritance of classical juvenile-onset and maturity-onset type diabetes of young people. *Diabetes*, **24**, 44
2 Cudworth, A. G. (1976). The aetiology of diabetes. *Br. J. Hosp. Med.*, **16**, 207
3 Pyke, D. A. (1968). The incidence and prevalence of diabetes. In W. G. Oakley, D. A. Pyke and K. W. Taylor (eds.) *Clinical Diabetes and its Biochemical Basis*, pp. 181–197. (Oxford: Blackwell Scientific Publications)
4 Butterfield, W. J. H. (1964). Summary of the results of the Bedford Diabetes Survey. *Proc. R. Soc. Med.*, **57**, 196

5 US Department of Health, Education and Welfare (1964). Glucose tolerance of adults: US 1960–62. National Center for Health Statistics, Series 11, No. 2
6 Oakley, W. G., Pyke, D. A. and Taylor K. W. (1978). *Diabetes and Its Management*. 3rd ed., p. 28 (Oxford: Blackwell Scientific Publications)
7 O'Sullivan, J. B. (1974). Age gradient in blood glucose levels. Magnitude and clinical implications. *Diabetes*, **23**, 713
8 Denham, M. J. (1972). The value of random blood glucose determinations as a screening method for detecting diabetes mellitus in the elderly patients. *Age Ageing*, **1**, 55
9 Fitzgerald, M. G. and Keen, H. (1964). Diagnostic classification of diabetes. *Br. Med. J.*, **1**, 1568
10 Royal College of General Practioners (1970). Five-year follow-up report on the Birmingham diabetes survey of 1962. *Br. Med. J.*, **3**, 301
11 Fajans, S. S. (1969). The diagnosis of diabetes. *Gen. Pract.*, **39**, 149
12 Siperstein, M. D. (1975). The glucose tolerance test. *Adv. Intern. Med.*, **20**, 297
13 Andres, R. and Tobin, J. D. (1975). Ageing and the disposition of glucose. *Adv. Exp. Med. Biol.*, **61**, 239
14 Chesrow, E. J. and Bleyer, J. M. (1954). The glucose tolerance test in the aged. *Geriatrics*, **15**, 315
15 West, K. M., Wulff, J. A., Reigel, D. G. and Fitzgerald, D. T. (1964). Oral carbohydrate tolerance tests. *Arch. Intern. Med.*, **113**, 641
16 Gottfried, S. P., Plez, K. S. and Clifford, R. C. (1961). Carbohydrate metabolism in healthy old men and women over 70 years of age. *Am. J. Med. Sci.*, **242**, 475
17 Streeten, D. H. P., Gerstein, M. M., Marmor, B. M. and Doisy, R. J. (1965). Reduced glucose tolerance in elderly human subjects. *Diabetes*, **14**, 579
18 Beck, H., Job, D. and Sebban, C. (1973). Reproductibilité de la mesure de la glycere chez le sujet âge. *Gerontol. Clin.* **15**, 37
19 Williams, T. F. (1978). Diabetes mellitus in the aged. In R. B. Greenblatt (ed.). *Geriatric Endocrinology. Ageing*, **5**, pp. 103–113 (New York: Raven Press)
20 Birmingham Diabetes Survey Working Party (1976). Ten-year follow-up report on Birmingham Diabetes Survey of 1961. *Br. Med. J.*, **2**, 35
21 Tobin, J. D., Sherwin, R. S., Liljenquist, J. E., Insel, P. A. and Andres, R. (1972). Proceedings of the Ninth International Congress of Gerontology, vol. 3, p. 155. (Kiev: USSR)
22 Smith M. J. and Hall, M. R. P. (1973). Carbohydrate tolerance in the very aged. *Diabetologica*, **9**, 387
23 Pozefsky, T., Cocker, J. L., Langs, H. M. and Andres, R. (1965). The cortisone-glucose tolerance test: The influence of age on performance. *Ann. Intern. Med.*, **63**, 988
24 Streeten, D. H. P., Gerstein, M. M., Marmor, B. M. and Doisy, R. J. (1965). Reduced glucose tolerance in elderly human subjects. *Diabetes*, **14**, 579
25 Judd, S. L., O'Leary, E., Read, P. and Fox, C. (1976). The changing role of nurses in the management of diabetes. *Br. J. Hosp. Med.*, **16**, 251
26 Report of the National Commission on Diabetes to the Congress of the United States, 10 December 1975: Long range plan to combat diabetes (1975). *Diabetes Forecast*, **28**, (Suppl. 1), 1
27 Thorn, P. A. and Russell, R. G. (1973). Diabetic clinics today and tomorrow, mini-clinics in general practice. *Br. J. Hosp. Med.*, **16**, 251
28 Ruben, L. A. (1976). Diabetes and the general practitioner. *Br. J. Hosp. Med.*, **16**, 241
29 Burkitt, P. D. and Trowell, H. C. (1975). *Refined Carbohydrate Foods and Disease; Some Implications of Dietary Fibre*. (New York: Academic Press)

30 Report of a Joint Working Party of the Royal College of Physicians of London and the British Cardiac Society (1976). Prevention of Coronary Heart Disease. *J. R. Coll. Physicians*, **10**, 2

31 Tunbridge, R. and Weatherill, J. H. (1970). Reliability and cost of diabetic diets. *Br. Med. J.*, **2**, 78

32 West, K. W. (1973). Diet therapy of diabetes: an analysis of failure. *Ann. Intern. Med.*, **79**, 425

33 Tomkins, A. M. and Bloom, A. (1972). Assessment of the need for continued oral therapy in diabetes. *Br. Med. J.*, **i**, 649

34 Cahill, G. F., Etzweiler, D. D. and Freinkel, N. (1976). Control and diabetes: Editorial. *N. Engl. J. Med.*, **294**, 1004

35 University Group Diabetes Program (1970). A study of the effects of hypogly-caemic agents on vascular complications in patients with adult-onset diabetes. *Diabetes*, **19**, (Suppl. 2), 747

36 University Group Diabetics Program (1971). Effects of hypoglycaemic agents on vascular complications in patients with adult-onset diabetes III. Clinical implications of UGDP results. *J. Am. Med. Assoc.*, **218**, 1400

37 University Group Diabetes Program (1975). A study of the effects of hypogly-caemic agents on vascular complications in patients with adult-onset diabetes V. Evaluation of phenformin therapy. *Diabetes*, **24** (Suppl. 1), 65

38 Keen, H. and Jarrett, R. J. (1970). In R. J. Jones (ed.). Second Symposium on Atherosclerosis, p. 435 (New York: Springer-Verlag)

39 Paasikivi, J. (1970). Long term tolbutamide treatment after myocardial infarc-tion. A clinical and biochemical study of 178 patients without overt diabetes. *Acta Med. Scand.*, **507** (Suppl.), 3

40 Keen, H., Jarrett, R. J., Chlouverakis, C. and Boyns, D. R. (1968). The effect of treatment of moderate hypoglycaemia on the incidence of arterial disease. *Post-grad. Med. J.*, **44**, 960

41 Boyle, D., Bhatia, S. K., Hadden, D. R., Montgomery, D. A. D. and Weaver, J. A. (1972). Ischaemic heart disease in diabetics. A prospective study. *Lancet*, **i**, 338

42 Janbon, M., Chaptal, J., Vedel, A. and Schaap, J. (1942). Accidents hypogly-cémiques graves par un sulfamidothiazol (le VK 57 ou 2254 RP). *Montpellier Med.*, **21–22**, 441

43 Sönksen, P. H. and West T. E. T. (1978). Carbohydrate metabolism and diab-etes mellitus. In J. L. H. O'Riordan (ed.). *Recent Advances in Endocrinology and Metabolism*. pp. 161–186. (Edinburgh: Churchill Livingstone)

44 Hecht, A., Gershberg, H. and Hulse, M. (1973). Effect of chlorpropamide treat-ment on insulin secretion in diabetics: its relationship to the hypoglycaemic effect. *Metabolism*, **22**, 723

45 Barnes, A. J., Garbien, K. J. T., Crowley, M. F. and Bloom, A. (1974). Effect of short and long-term chlorpropamide treatment on insulin release and blood glucose. *Lancet*, **ii**, 69

46 Perkins, J. R., Hay, B. J., Judd, S. L., Quine, K. H., West, T. E. T. and Sönksen, P. H. (1975). Effect of diet, sulphonylurea and placebo therapies on glucose tolerance, blood metabolites and insulin secretion in diabetics. *Diabetologia*, **11**, 369

47 Clarke, B. F. and Campbell, I. W. (1975). Long term comparative trial of gliben-clamide and chlorpropamide in diet-failed, maturity-onset diabetics. *Lancet*, **i**, 246

48 Logie, A. W., Galloway, D. B. and Petrie, J. C. (1976). Drug interactions and long term antidiabetic therapy. *Br. J. Clin. Pharmacol.*, **3**, 1027

49 Ungar, G., Freedman, L. and Shapiro, S. L. (1957). Pharmacological studies of a new oral hypoglycaemic drug. *Proc. Soc. Exp. Biol.*, **95,** 190

50 Tomkin, G. H., Hadden, D. R., Weaver, J. A. and Montgomery, D. A. D. (1971). Vitamin – B12 status of patients on long term metformin therapy. *Br. Med. J.*, **ii,** 685

51 Cohen, R. D. and Woods, H. F. (1976). *Clinical and Biochemical Aspects of Lactic Acidosis.* (Oxford: Blackwell Scientific Publications)

52 Cohen, R. D. (1978). Prevention and treatment of lactic acidosis. In D. W. Vere (ed.). *Topics in Therapeutics,* 4th ed. pp. 191–197. (London: Pitman)

53 Assan, R., Heuclin, C., Ganeval, D., Bismuth, C., George, J. and Girard, J. R. (1977). Metformin-induced lactic acidosis in the presence of acute renal failure. *Diabetologia,* **13,** 211

54 Annual Report for 1977 of the Medicines Commission (1978), p. 22. (London: Her Majesty's Stationery Office)

55 Bismuth, Ch., Gaultier, M., Conso, F., Heuclin, Ch. and Assan, R. (1976). Acidose lactique induite par l'ingestion excessive de metformine. *Nouv. Presse Med.,* **5,** 261

56 Mirouze, J., Mion, C., Beraud, J. J. and Salem, J. L. (1976). Acidose lactique à l'occasion d'insuffisence renale chez deux diabétique traites par metformine. *Nouv. Presse Med.,* **5,** 1004

57 Schlichtkrull, J., Brange, J., Christiansen, Aa. H., Hallind, O., Heding, L. G., Jorgensen, K. H., Munkgaard Rasmussen, S., Sorensen, E. and Volund, Aa. (1974). Monocomponent insulin and its clinical implications. In R. Levene and E. E. Pfeiffer (eds.). *Radioimmunoassay: Methodology and Applications in Physiology and Clinical Studies, Hormone and Metabolic Research,* pp. 134–143 (Stuttgart: Georg Theime)

58 Anderson, J. (1976). Blood sampling and diabetic control. *Lancet,* **ii,** 794

59 Editorial (1976). Glycosylated haemoglobin and diabetic control. *N. Engl. J. Med.,* **295,** 443

60 Koenig, R. J., Peterson, C. M., Jones, R. L., Sandek, C. Lehrman, M. and Cerami, A. (1976). Correlation of glucose regulation and haemoglobin Alc in diabetes mellitus. *N. Engl. J. Med.,* **295,** 417

61 Gonen, B., Rubenstein, A., Rochman, H., Tanega, S. P. and Horwitz, D. L. (1977). Haemoglobin Al: An indicator of the metabolic control of diabetic patients. *Lancet,* **ii,** 734

62 Sönksen, P. H., Judd, S. L. and Lowy, C. (1978). Home monitoring of blood glucose. *Lancet,* **i,** 729

63 Walford, S., Gale, E. A. M., Allison, S. P. and Tattersall, R. B. (1978). Self-monitoring of blood glucose. *Lancet,* **i,** 732

64 Gale, E. A. M. and Tattersall, R. B. (1978). Hypothermia: a complication of diabetic ketoacidosis. *Br. Med. J.,* **2,** 1387

65 Alberti, K. G. M. M. and Hockaday, T. D. R. (1977). Diabetic coma: a reappraisal after five years. *Clin. Endocrinol. Metab.,* **6,** 42

66 Schecter, A. E., Wiesel, B. H. and Cohn, C. (1941). Peripheral circulatory failure in diabetic acidosis and its relation to treatment. *Am. J. Med. Sci.,* **202,** 364

67 Ditzel, J., Anderson, H. and Daugaard, N. (1972). Tissue oxygenation in uncontrolled diabetes mellitus. *Lancet,* **ii,** 818

68 Greenaway, J. M. and Read, J. (1958). Diabetic coma; a review of 69 cases. *Aust. Ann. Med.,* **7,** 151

69 Baum, D., Dillard, D. H. and Porte, D. (1968). Inhibition of insulin release in infants undergoing deep hypothermic cardiovascular surgery. *N. Eng. J. Med.,* **279,** 1309

70 Wynn, V. (1954). Electrolyte disturbances associated with failure to metabolise glucose during hypothermia. *Lancet*, **ii**, 575

71 Young, J. B. and Landsberg, L. (1977). Catecholamines and intermediary metabolism. *Clin. Endocrinol. Metab.*, **6**, 599

72 Sprunt, J. G., Maclean, D. and Browning, M. C. K. (1970). Plasma-corticosteroid levels in accidental hypothermia. *Lancet*, **i**, 324

73 Page, M. McB., Alberti, K. G. M. M., Greehwood, R., Gumaa, K. A., Hockaday, T. D. R., Lowy, C., Nabarro, J. D. N., Pyke, D. A., Sönksen, P. H., Watkins, P. J. and West, T. E. T. (1974). Treatment of diabetic coma with continuous low-dose infusion of insulin. *Br. Med. J.*, **1**, 687

74 Alberti, K. G. M. M., Hockaday, T. D. R. and Turner, R. C. (1973). Small doses of intramuscular insulin in the treatment of diabetic 'coma'. *Lancet*, **ii**, 515

75 Shaw, K. M., Tillyer, C. R., Morgan, P. G. M. and Bloom, A. (1974). Small doses of intramuscular insulin in the treatment of diabetic 'coma'. *Lancet*, **i**, 1115

76 Field, J. B. (1976). Hyperosmolar coma. In S. S. Fajan (ed.) *Diabetes Mellitus* pp. 133–141. (London Department of Health Education and Welfare Publication No. (NIH)) 76–854

77 Matz, R. (1972). Hyperosmolar coma. *Lancet*, **ii**, 1254

78 Gerich, J., Martini, M. M. and Recant, L. (1971). Clinical and metabolic characteristics of hyperosmolar non-ketotic coma. *Diabetes*, **20**, 228

79 McCurdy, D. K. (1970). Hyperosmolar hyperglycaemic non-ketotic diabetic coma. *Med. Clin. N. Am.*, **54**, 683

80 Cheng, H. (1979). Photocoagulation and diabetic retinopathy. *Br. Med. J.*, **1**, 365

81 Kohuer, E. M. (1977). Diabetic retinopathy. *Clin. Endocrinol. Metab.*, **6**, 345

82 Job, D., Eshwege, E., Argenton, C. G., Aubry, J. P. and Tchobroutsky, G. (1976). Effect of multiple daily insulin injections on the course of diabetic retinopathy. *Diabetes*, **25**, 463

83 Interim Report of a Multicentre Controlled Study (1975). Photocoagulation in the treatment of diabetic maculopathy. *Lancet*, **ii**, 1110

84 Diabetic Retinopathy Study Research Group (1976). Preliminary report on effects of photocoagulation therapy. *Ophthalmology*, **81**, 383

85 Patz, A., Schatz, H., Berkow, J. W., Gittlesohn, A. M. and Ticho, G. (1973). Macular oedema, an overlooked complication of diabetic retinopathy. *Trans. Am. Acad. Ophthalmol. Otolaryngol.*, **77**, 34

86 Cheng, H., Kohuer, E. M. and Bailey, J. and others (1977). Photocoagulation in proliferative diabetic retinopathy. *Br. Med. J.*, **1**, 739

87 Caird, F. I., Hutchinson, M. and Pirie, A. (1965). Cataract extraction in diabetes. *Brit. J. Ophthalmol.*, **49**, 466

88 Thornton, G. F., Lytton, B. and Andriole, V. T. (1966). Bacteriuria during indwelling catheter drainage. *J. Am. Med. Assoc.*, **195**, 179

89 Warren, J. W., Platt, R., Thomas, R. J., Rosner, B. and Kass, E. H. (1978). Antibiotic irrigation and catheter-associated urinary tract infections. *N. Engl. J. Med.*, **299**, 570

For further reading

Cudworth, A. G. (1977). The aetiology of diabetes. In M. Besser (ed.). *Advanced Medicine*, 13, pp. 163–172. (London: Pitman Medical)

Alberti, K. G. M. M. and Nattrass, M. (1977). Metabolic disorders of diabetes and their management. In M. Besser (ed.). *Advanced Medicine*, 13, pp. 173–189. (London: Pitman Medical)

Hall, R. and Anderson, J. (1978). Endocrinology and diabetes mellitus. In A. R. Horler and J. B. Foster (eds.). *Progress in Clinical Medicine*, 7th ed., pp. 52–68. (London: Churchill Livingstone)

Watkins, P. J. (1977). Oral hypoglycaemic drugs. *Prescribers J.*, **4**, 76

Pyke, D. A. (1976). Up to date on diabetes. In D. K. Peters (ed.). *Advanced Medicine*, *12*, pp. 236–250 (London: Pitman Medical)

Sönksen, P. H. (1977). New insulins. In M. Besser (ed.). *Advanced Medicine, 13*, pp. 402–412. (London: Pitman Medical)

Tattersall, R. (1978). Highly purified insulins. *Prescribers J.*, **18**, 8

Editorial (1975). Oral hypoglycaemics in diabetes mellitus. *Lancet*, **ii**, 489

Bloom, A. (1977). Some practical aspects of the management of diabetes. *Clin. Endocrinol. Metab.*, **6**, 499

Davidson, M. B. (1979). The effect of aging on carbohydrate metabolism: A review of the English literature and a practical approach to the diagnosis of diabetes mellitus in the elderly. *Metabolism*, **28**, 688

6

Management of Parkinson's disease in the elderly

Marion Hildick-Smith

EPIDEMIOLOGY

Parkinson's disease is one of the commonest neurological conditions in Great Britain and in America but its incidence and prevalence have been little studied. Incidence rates, which measure the number of new cases per unit population per year, are useful for acute onset conditions, but misleading for diseases of insidious onset as many early cases can be missed. Prevalence rates, which measure the number of cases per unit population on a given date, are more useful for more chronic conditions such as Parkinson's disease. In 1952 Garland[1] found a prevalence rate of 59 cases per 100 000 of the general population in the Leeds area, a rate which he regarded as approximate and minimal. Brewis *et al.* in 1966[2] reported an overall prevalence rate of 112·5 per 100 000 in the Carlisle population of 1961, and showed the rates for different age groups. They believed that Parkinsonism was underdiagnosed and therefore that their figure was an underestimate. An American study by Kurland in 1958 in Rochester[3] showed a greater prevalence than that at Carlisle for each age group, and the overall prevalence rate was 187 per 100 000. They believed that their survey, using the facilities of the Mayo clinic, was far more complete than previous ones. A sim·larly complete study in Iceland in 1963 by Gudmundsson[4] gave a figure of 169·5 per 100 000. Official estimates[5] in 1974 suggest there are, at present, 60 000 to 80 000 patients with the disease in Great Britain.

The incidence of Parkinson's disease has been shown to rise with increasing age[2-4]. Its prevalence in people over 50 years old is probably more than 500 per 100 000 while that for those aged 60 or

215

more is probably 1000 per 100 000. Estimates of the percentage of people now alive who, on today's survival rates, might be expected to develop Parkinsonism at some time in their lives might give figures of 1–2%.

Idiopathic Parkinson's disease appears to show a slight, but definite, familial tendency. Gudmundsson found a positive family history in about 20% of his cases in Iceland, while Kurland found one in about 16% in his Rochester cases. The inheritance pattern may suggest an autosomal dominance with incomplete penetrance[1,3].

Not only is Parkinson's disease more common in older people, but there was also a noticeable increase in the proportion of elderly people with the condition attending neurological clinics in the 15 years between 1949 and 1964. In one survey, the mean age of onset rose in those years from 50·9 to 58·3 years[6].

There is no doubt that large numbers of patients are disabled by the disease. Harris in 1971[7] in her survey *Handicapped and Impaired in Great Britain* calculated that there were 22 000 people disabled by Parkinsonism living in the community in Britain, of whom over half were severely handicapped. These figures were calculated before levodopa became available for widespread use in this country. In 1974 it was estimated[5] that there were also 15 000 Parkinsonian patients in institutions such as hospitals or nursing homes. The picture has gradually been changing with the advent of more effective drug treatment during the last 5–10 years. Patients now stay in hospital for shorter periods and survive longer[8]. However, improved survival allows the disease to develop in a manner not previously experienced.

TYPES OF PARKINSON'S DISEASE

Parkinson's disease may be either idiopathic or symptomatic in type.

Idiopathic Parkinsonism

Idiopathic paralysis agitans (or Parkinson's disease proper) results from degenerative changes in the basal ganglia and their connections. There is no known cause, but there are two main theories at present.

(1)   There may be a primary deficiency of specialized cells in the hypothalamus which are responsible for the control of MSH (melanocyte-stimulating hormone) release.

(2) The disease may be due to a virus such as herpes simplex virus. There is a selective increase in humoral antibody response to this virus in some Parkinsonian patients[9].

Symptomatic Parkinsonism

Arteriosclerotic
There is controversy regarding the role of arteriosclerosis in the aetiology of Parkinsonism. Critchley[10] described Parkinson-like features, but without tremor, in elderly arteriosclerotic patients with pyramidal tract signs and dementia. However, there is no real evidence that the disease is due to arteriosclerosis since such patients may show no excess of arteriosclerosis elsewhere. The considerable overlap in the clinical picture between Parkinsonism, cerebral arteriosclerosis and dementia has recently been confirmed by Parkes and his colleagues[11].

Postencephalitic
Postencephalitic Parkinsonism, which accounts for only a small minority of patients today, arose from the epidemic of encephalitis lethargica in 1917–18. Fresh cases have been rare since 1932. Postencephalitic patients are younger than the degenerative group, and their symptoms can appear months or years after the encephalitis. They more frequently show autonomic disturbance, and characteristically may have episodes of oculogyric crises in which the eyes are fixed (usually upwards) for minutes or hours.

Toxic causes
Drug-induced Parkinsonism is seen with increasing frequency. Phenothiazines such as chlorpromazine (Largactil), prochlorperazine (Stemetil), fluphenazine decanoate (Modecate) and butyrophenones such as haloperidol (Serenace) block the postsynaptic dopamine and noradrenaline receptors and cause a Parkinsonian picture. Other drugs such as reserpine (Serpasil) and tetrabenazine (Nitoman) deplete the cerebral stores of dopamine, noradrenaline and 5HT (5-hydroxytryptamine). They prevent dopamine release from the presynaptic neurone, leading to the same result. It is important to be aware of the aetiology as this form of Parkinsonism usually subsides within weeks or months of withdrawing the offending drug. Postsynaptic blockage responds to treatment with anticholinergic agents, but not to levodopa, whereas presynaptic blockage is responsive to levodopa treatment.

A Parkinsonism syndrome has been attributed to manganese poisoning, but in view of the low incidence of the syndrome among the enormous numbers of workers at risk, these cases of so-called manganese poisoning may be cases of idiopathic paralysis agitans occurring by chance in workers in the manganese industry[12].

Carbon monoxide poisoning producing prolonged unconsciousness can cause widespread neuropsychiatric effects, although Smith and Brandon[13] in a study of 206 cases, found long-term extrapyramidal signs in only two patients. Short exposure to carbon monoxide rarely causes lasting damage.

Syphilis has sometimes been advanced as a possible cause of symptomatic Parkinsonism but it is not clear whether this is more than a chance association of two separate conditions.

SIGNS AND SYMPTOMS

The classical description of this condition by James Parkinson in 1817[14] included mention of the tremor, flexed posture, monotonous voice and tendency to falls which are equally characteristic of patients seen today. He did not mention the muscular rigidity nor the immobile masklike facies which are also frequently seen.

It is an old neurological cliché that if you do not recognize Parkinson's disease when the patient first enters the room, you are unlikely to recognize it at all. This is particularly true of old people, who may find that their doctors miss the diagnosis and dismiss their complaints of tiredness, slowness or stiffness as 'just old age'.

There are a number of ways in which the well-known signs and symptoms of the disease may be altered or masked in the elderly. The characteristic, rhythmical four to six per second tremor may be completely absent, or absent when the patient's arms are supported in his lap. The best chance to observe the tremor may be when it is increased by walking, excitement or anxiety, as when the patient first enters the room. Tremor may be a presenting symptom in 50–70% of cases[6], but is less often present in the elderly.

The characteristic flexed posture of head, shoulders and thorax may be overlooked in an elderly patient, or assumed to be due to osteoarthritis of neck and spine; the possible flexion and adduction of the arms may be missed if the patient is manipulating a walking frame. An immobile facies may be assumed to be the result of depression or deafness. The characteristic lead-pipe or cog-wheel rigidity of Parkinsonism, which may often begin unilaterally, must be distinguished from spasticity due to pyramidal tract disorder, or from passive resistance to movement because of stiff or painful joints.

The symptoms resulting from bradykinesia (slowness of voluntary movement) may be accepted by the patient as part of the ageing process. He may not realize that his inability to do up buttons, cut up meat, or sign his pension book quickly and legibly is the result of a treatable disease process. Similarly difficulty in getting in and out of bed or chair, or turning over in bed may be accepted as due to arthritis, so specific questions must be asked about these characteristic disabilities.

If a patient is suspected of having Parkinson's disease, it is essential to see him walk, turn and if possible negotiate an obstacle such as a doorway. The characteristic early loss of arm-swing, short length of steps, appearance of turning 'all in one piece' and hesitation, 'freezing', or 'stuttering' steps when negotiating the doorway may make the diagnosis clear.

Disturbance of autonomic function in Parkinsonism can cause constipation, undue sweating or seborrhoea and the excessive salivation which is aggravated by infrequent swallowing and the flexed head posture of the condition. It is worth asking about difficulties with swallowing; as some experts believe there is a specific disturbance involving the lingual, pharyngeal and primarily the lower oesophageal components of swallowing[15,16] which may be present at a quite early stage in the disorder. 'Giddy turns' or falls may be due to postural hypotension as a result of poor autonomic regulation of blood pressure.

Though mentality is unaffected in some Parkinsonian patients, others will exhibit gradual retardation of thought processes or impaired concentration and memory, which they attribute to ageing. Depression or obsessional or demanding behaviour may enhance the increasing social isolation of some elderly patients, while others may exhibit episodes of acute confusion during infections, etc., and may later show frank dementia.

USEFUL CLINICAL TESTS

As the diagnosis of Parkinsonism is a clinical one it is useful to have a number of further tests which can be used as objective evidence (such as a timed signature) or which can be used to monitor progress, such as the Webster timed test[17] (see appendix, page 252) or repeated evaluation of ventilatory function[18]. One test which measures rigidity in the neck muscles is the so-called 'psychic pillow test'[19]. For this test the patient lies on the bed without a pillow and with his head resting on the physician's left hand. The patient's head is then lifted by the physician's right hand and is allowed to fall. In Parkinsonism the head will descend slowly and perhaps remain above the physician's left hand.

No assessment of an elderly patient is complete without a functional assessment. This should include questions and practical ADL assessment of kitchen, toilet and bathroom activities. A special note should be made of those problems which cause the patient most concern.

As multiple pathology can be expected in elderly Parkinsonian patients[20], careful note should be made of any further conditions likely to affect choice of drug treatment, such as glaucoma, prostatism, postural hypotension, myocardial infarction or cardiac arrhythmia. Specific questioning about past medication with phenothiazines such as prochlorperazine (Stemetil) is often rewarding.

MENTAL SCORE TEST

The most important part of the further examination is to assess the patient's mental capacity. This is important both from the point of view of likely response to treatment and of compliance in taking the drugs prescribed. The abbreviated mental test[21] gives a convenient and reliable method of assessment (Table 1). For alert patients it is tactful to introduce the questionnaire, explaining that it is a means of testing how good the patient's memory is.

Table 1   Abbreviated mental test*

---

1. How old are you?
2. What time is it? (to nearest hour)
3. Address for recall at end of test – this should be repeated by the patient to ensure it has been heard correctly:
   42 West Street
4. What year is it?
5. What place is this? Name of institution or address
6. Recognition of two people (doctor, nurse, etc.)
7. Day and month of birth
8. Year of start of the First World War
9. Name of present monarch
10. Count backward 20 to 1
Total number of correct answers = mental score

---

* Make sure patient is not dysphasic, depressed, deaf or drugged

DIFFERENTIAL DIAGNOSIS

It is important to distinguish patients with Parkinsonism from those who suffer from other causes of mental confusion, rigidity or tremor, and from those with more rapidly progressive neurological disorders.

Cerebral arteriosclerosis and/or dementia may overlap with Parkinsonism[11]. In addition to the flexed posture, shuffling steps, and festinant gait these patients may show a variety of tremors, and have poor mental scores. They may show primitive reflex responses (such as a grasp reflex) characteristic of frontal lobe involvement. Supranuclear (pseudobulbar) palsy from past bilateral pyramidal tract damage gives rise to emotional lability, explosive speech and some Parkinson-type signs and symptoms. Depressed or myxoedematous patients may show slow responses and a poor mental score.

Symptoms of widespread arthritis, or rheumatism, may be very like the 'prodromal' symptoms which often precede the characteristic tremor in Parkinsonism. Alternatively Parkinsonism may lead to leg muscle cramps, mimicking intermittent claudication, or hand cramp, mimicking a writer's cramp or mild stroke.

Benign (hereditary) essential tremor is absent at rest and most prominent when the patient tries to maintain a fixed posture. Cerebellar tremor is an intention tremor and worsens as the hand nears the object.

Metabolic disorders give rise to a variety of tremors, those of liver disease flapping, and that of alcohol violent and variable, while hyperthyroidism/anxiety may cause a rapid fine tremor. Some Parkinsonian patients with motor overactivity (akathisia), weight loss and excessive autonomic involvement (wide-eyed facies, heat intolerance and seborrhoea) are difficult to distinguish from patients with hyperthyroidism.

There are a number of conditions which may be indistinguishable from Parkinson's disease for months or years before developing their characteristic signs or symptoms. Olivopontocerebellar degeneration may look like Parkinsonism at first, but later pronounced cerebellar signs develop, and there may be a family history of the condition. Nigrostriatal degeneration, lacking the tremor of Parkinsonism but otherwise very similar, is a remorselessly progressive disease, which cannot be diagnosed with confidence during life. Supranuclear palsy (Steele – Richardson syndrome) is a condition where Parkinsonian signs or a generalized akinesia may be accompanied by progressive palsy of conjugate ocular movements. Shy–

Drager syndrome has some characteristics of Parkinsonism, but autonomic failure leading to severe postural hypotension is a prominent feature. Jacob – Creutzfeld syndrome may have some similarity with Parkinsonism, but later development of myoclonic jerks and progressive dementia usually lead to death within a year. All these latter conditions tend to pursue a relentless downhill course, and there is little response to any treatment, even to levodopa or bromocriptine.

PATHOLOGY

The exact site, extent and nature of the lesions responsible for the varied clinical manifestations of Parkinsonism remain controversial. Loss of melanin-containing cells from the substantia nigra has long been recognized as characteristic of Parkinson's disease. Greenfield and Bosanquet in 1955[22] found that, when brains from Parkinsonian patients were cut open, the substantia nigra lacked pigment. Further investigation in this region showed that the melanin-containing neurones particularly in the pars compacta had undergone a variety of changes from cytoplasmic inclusions (so-called Lewy bodies) to complete dissolution.

Although the most prominent changes were in the substantia nigra there were also changes in the globus pallidus, putamen and caudate nucleus. Changes less severe, but of almost equal constancy were found in the locus caeruleus and in the pigmented cells of the dorsal nucleus of the vagus. Damage to these vagal nuclei might result in the autonomic symptoms of Parkinsonism.

Latterly the clinical overlap between Parkinsonism and Alzheimer's type dementia has been confirmed by overlap of pathological findings. Some generalized cerebral atrophy, greater than the patient's age would suggest, is common in advanced cases of Parkinsonism. A recent review[23] quotes studies showing a high prevalence of neurofibrillary tangles, senile plaques, and cerebral atrophy in disproportionate quantity in brains of Parkinsonian patients.

NEUROCHEMISTRY

Although understanding of the underlying mechanisms of Parkinson's disease is far from complete, progress in neurochemistry has begun to provide some answers. In 1960, Ehringer and Hornykiewicz[24] reported a striking deficiency in dopamine (3HT) in the corpus striatum and substantia nigra of the brains of six Parkinsonian patients. Bernheimer *et al.*[25] showed that there was a correlation between the degree of cell loss in the substantia nigra and the level of dopamine deficiency in the striatum. Birkmayer and Hornykiewicz[26] gave an intravenous injection of levodopa, the immediate metabolic precursor of dopamine, to 20 patients with Parkinson's disease and reported dramatic short-term improvement in their symptoms. The picture of dopamine deficiency leading to Parkinsonian symptoms appeared complete[27].

Evidence gradually accumulated of a constant deficiency in striatal dopamine in Parkinsonism, together with deficiencies of its synthesizing enzymes tyrosine hydroxylase and dopa decarboxylase, and of its metabolite homovanillic acid (Table 2). Moreover the severity of akinesia in Parkinsonism correlated significantly with the degree of dopamine deficiency in the caudate nucleus, while in patients with predominantly unilateral signs the dopamine deficiency was greater in the contralateral striatum. Drugs that blocked presynaptic or postsynaptic transmission of dopamine often caused Parkinsonian symptoms, whereas levodopa or such dopamine agonists as bromocriptine sometimes relieved them (Table 3).

Table 2   Influences on dopamine synthesis

Inhibitors		Enzymes
	Tyrosine	
alpha-Methyltyrosine	↓	Tyrosine hydroxylase
	Levodopa	
RO4-4602 Benserazide	↓	DOPA decarboxylase
MK 486 Carbidopa	Dopamine	
	↓	
	(Noradrenaline)	
	↓	
	(Homovanillic acid)	

The role of anticholinergic drugs in treatment suggested that one feature of Parkinson's disease was a relative excess of cholinergic transmission leading to an imbalance between the cholinergic-excitatory and dopaminergic-inhibitory mechanisms in the brain. The increased ratio of acetylcholinesterase to dopamine in the brains of Parkinsonian patients tended to confirm this[28]. According to one hypothesis, as dopaminergic neurones fail and abandon the receptors in the striatum, cholinergic neurones sprout and innervate these vacant sites.

Table 3   Regulation of dopamine

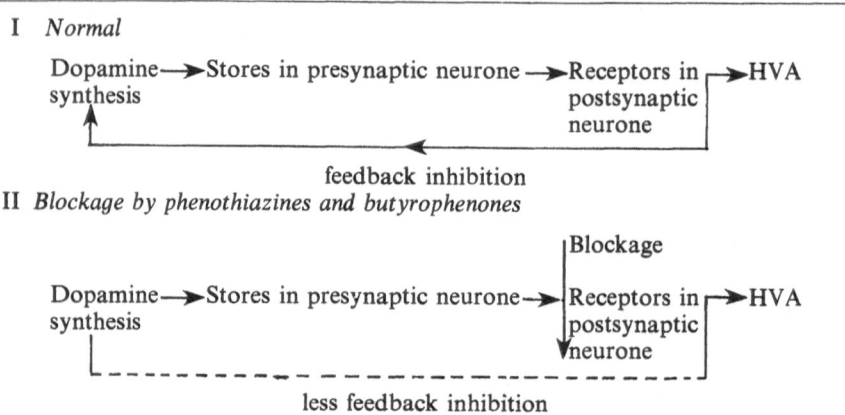

I *Normal*

Dopamine——▶Stores in presynaptic neurone ——▶Receptors in ┌─▶HVA
synthesis   postsynaptic
                                                                                 neurone

feedback inhibition

II *Blockage by phenothiazines and butyrophenones*

Blockage

Dopamine——▶Stores in presynaptic neurone——▶Receptors in ┌─▶HVA
synthesis   postsynaptic
                                                                              neurone

less feedback inhibition

III Reserpine causes reduction in amine stores (particularly dopamine) in presynaptic neurones

All the manifestations of Parkinson's disease cannot, however, be explained by dopamine deficiency. Some patients, for example, fail to respond to levodopa treatment; and the underlying progress of the disease is unaltered by dopamine replacement. The decreasing response to levodopa during prolonged treatment may be explained on the basis of chronic denervation leading to hypersensitivity at the receptor site – clinically apparent as levodopa-induced dyskinesia.

Although dopamine deficiency is the most important and constant biochemical lesion in Parkinson's disease, the roles of other neurotransmitters may be of some importance. The concentration of the inhibitory agent GABA (gamma-aminobutyric acid) and of its synthesizing enzyme GAD (glutamic acid decarboxylase) is reduced by half in patients dying of Parkinson's disease[23]. Unfortunately treatment of Parkinsonian patients by GABA analogue makes them worse, so it seems likely that the GABA depletion is a secondary effect and not a cause of Parkinson's disease. Similarly, though there is deficiency of another transmitter serotonin (5HT) in Parkinsonian brains, treatment with serotonin-augmenting agents has not produced clinical improvement. The importance of the widespread reduction of noradrenaline in many parts of the brains from Parkinsonian patients is not clear, nor is the role of the peptide angiotensin.

Further work is hampered by such difficulties as

(1) The post-mortem studies required are technically difficult because of the minute quantities of the neurotransmitters involved.

(2) The biochemical investigations which can be made in the living subject are limited.

(3) There are unfortunately major restrictions on the interpretation of data on specimens of cerebrospinal fluid obtained during life.

(4) There is no adequate animal model of the disease.

So far as the elderly are concerned, recent work suggests that choline acetyltransferase (CAT) activity in the brain may decline with normal ageing[29], as may receptor binding of acetylcholine (ACh). There is no evidence so far of the effect of ageing on dopamine production or receptors in the brain. If ACh activity is reduced in ageing, theoretically it seems likely that levodopa might be even more effective in the elderly in restoring the balance between ACh and dopamine in Parkinson's disease – though the contribution of other neurotransmitters has not yet been evaluated.

Similar research interest in neurotransmitters is occurring in the field of dementia. One recent double-blind trial was completed in 14 patients with senile dementia using small doses of levodopa. Ten of the 14 cases showed evidence of intellectual improvement, though other aspects of behaviour were largely unaltered[30]. Improved knowledge of neurochemical balance may produce more specific therapy in this field, as in Parkinsonism, in the next few years.

NATURAL HISTORY OF PARKINSON'S DISEASE

The prognosis in this condition is variable but on the whole the disease progresses insidiously. It has long been recognized[6] that a small group of patients who are not severely disabled for 20 or more years may still be said to have benign Parkinsonism (Figure 1). Another group who have a better prognosis than the rest are those with drug-induced disease, where symptoms may resolve rapidly when the responsible drug is withdrawn.

The picture for the majority of Parkinsonian patients is, however, less optimistic. Data collected on 802 patients in the 15 years prior to levodopa treatment[6] indicated that the disease disabled two-thirds of its victims within 5 to 9 years of onset, and 80% of its victims within 10 to 14 years. Parkinsonism significantly shortened lifespan; the patients having a mortality rate almost three (2·9) times that of the general population of the same age, sex and colour. Bronchopneumonia and urinary infections were causes of death more frequently than in the general population.

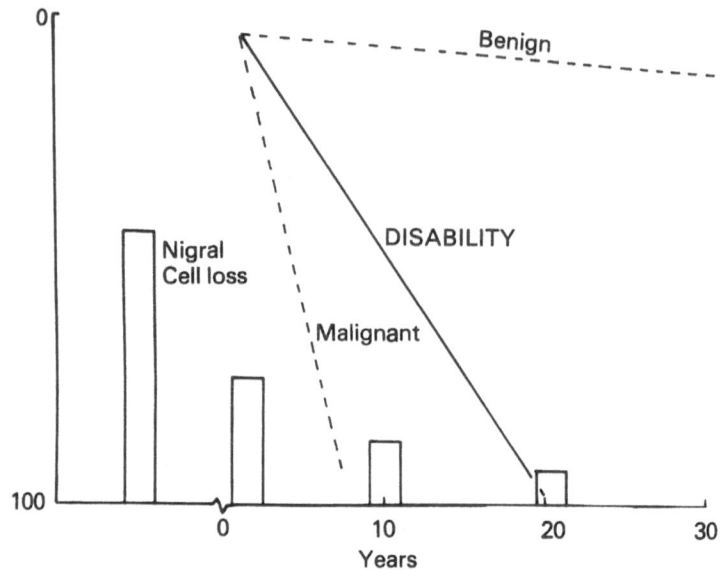

Figure 1 Natural history of Parkinson's disease. The severity of disability and degree of loss of substantia nigra neurons are shown on a 0 to 100% scale against time (year). The onset of symptoms (at 0 year) is prefaced by a period of progressive but asymptomatic nigral cell loss (and consequent striatal dopamine depletion). The solid line indicates the average progression of disability. The dotted lines highlight the variable course in individual patients, from a rapidly progressive 'malignant' disease to a slowly advancing 'benign' condition

This excess mortality of the disease has been reduced by levodopa treatment. One study of 100 patients treated for 5 years[8] shows an excess mortality of 1·9; while another, where 349 patients were treated for 7 years, shows an excess mortality of 1·85[9]. Birkmayer[31], in a study of 1450 patients treated for 12 years found that levodopa therapy prevents a high death rate in the early years of their disease. For the elderly this was of great significance; for example for those aged 80 to 90 years at the onset of their disease the likely year of decease extended from 2 to 6 years after onset, and during this time levodopa treatment improved disability by almost 50%. It will be easier to make clear comparisons in 5 or 10 years' time when a significant proportion of patients will have been treated with levodopa preparations from the start of their disability.

Not only is the length of survival increased, but the quality of life during these years has improved. Instead of a downward progression, many patients experience an increasing improvement in their disability over the first months or year of treatment, followed by a

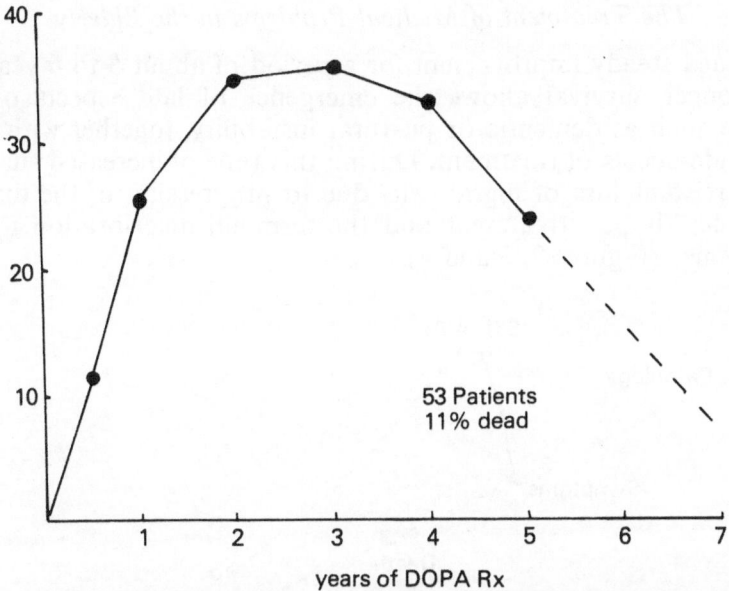

Figure 2 Average outcome of long-term levodopa treatment. The mean percent improvement in total disability scores from pretreatment values for the group (ordinate) is shown against duration of therapy (abscissa) over a 5 year period. The dotted extension predicts subsequent events

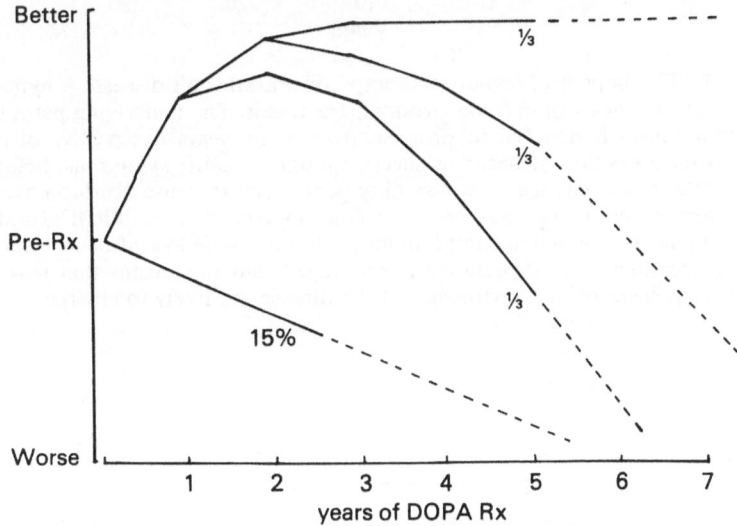

Figure 3 Subgroups of response to long-term levodopa therapy. Based on the data in Figure 2, 85% of patients showed an initial response to therapy; 15% did not and have subsequently declined or died. Of those who did respond, a third held their initial improvement, a third have lost some of the benefit, and a third are worse off than before starting treatment 5 years previously. The dotted lines predict subsequent events

227

continued steady improvement for a period of about 5 to 6 years in all. Longer survival allows the emergence of late aspects of the disease such as dementia or postural instability, together with long term side-effects of treatment. During this time of increased survival the persistent loss of nigral cells due to progression of the disease continues despite treatment and the terminal deterioration finally supervenes (Figures 2, 3 and 4).

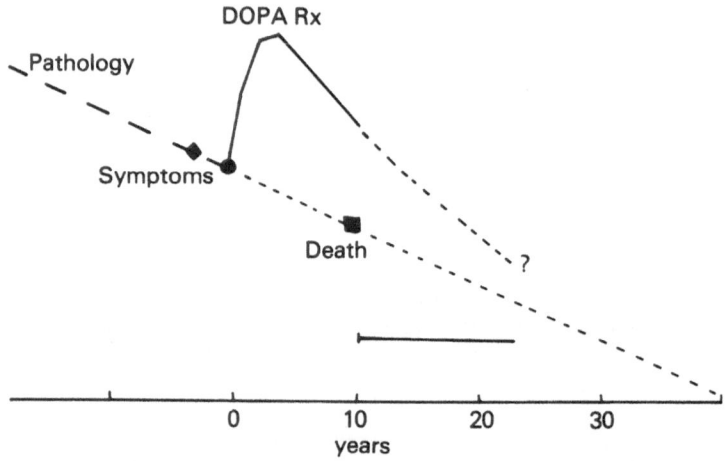

Figure 4 The impact of levodopa therapy on Parkinson's disease. A hypothetical concept of the effects of chronic levodopa treatment. The underlying pathology (of unknown cause) is believed to progress over many years irrespective of therapy. After an initial period, it becomes severe enough to cause symptoms. Before levodopa, pathological changes and disability progressed to cause death on average 10 years after onset. Levodopa therapy results in considerable initial symptomatic improvement, but no change in pathology. Despite some loss of benefit after a few years of treatment, life expectancy is prolonged, but this means that new aspects and consequences of the progression of the disease are likely to emerge

DRUG THERAPY

Solanaceous alkaloids

The first drugs which were used in 1867 to give symptomatic relief in Parkinson's disease were the solanaceous alkaloids, such as hyoscine, atropine and other members of the belladonna group. Although these were effective in decreasing rigidity, the large doses required led to unpleasant side-effects such as paralysis of accommodation and dryness of the mouth.

Synthetic anticholinergic and antihistamine drugs

The synthetic drugs which superseded the solanaceous alkaloids from about 1950 onwards, were chiefly anticholinergic, but in some cases also antihistamine in action. These drugs may relieve rigidity but usually have no effect upon the tremor of Parkinson's disease. The antihistamine drugs such as orphenadrine (Disipal) are used for their atropine-like (anticholinergic) effect and not for their ability to antagonize histamine. The anticholinergics may produce troublesome drowsiness, and can cause mental confusion and hallucinations in about 20% of patients[32].

All drugs with anticholinergic effects may aggravate prostatism with danger of urinary retention, may worsen constipation, cause blurred vision and aggravate glaucoma. They are helpful in sialorrhoea. There is probably little to choose in effectiveness between the drugs in this group, though individual patients may tolerate one better than another. Overall it is likely that this group of drugs may give 20–30% improvement in symptoms to patients who can tolerate them (Table 4). Postencephalitic patients sometimes tolerate unusually high doses with benefit.

In general, the anticholinergic drugs, especially procyclidine and orphenadrine, are useful in drug-induced Parkinsonism and in the early stages of idiopathic or symptomatic Parkinsonism before the disability is sufficient to need levodopa therapy. There is some disagreement whether it is beneficial to continue these agents once levodopa is started. An additive effect was claimed by Hughes[33] but subsequent workers found an increase in neuropsychiatric side-effects rather than additional benefits[34,35]. There is some suggestion that anticholinergics (though possibly only in larger doses) can delay gastric emptying time, giving time for degradation of levodopa in the stomach and reducing its effect. If it is decided to withdraw anticholinergics, this is best done slowly to avoid a withdrawal crisis.

It has been argued that older patients should be started on anticholinergic drugs rather than levodopa, since levodopa is less well tolerated in the elderly. However Caird and Williamson point out that anticholinergics are also less well tolerated in the old, particularly in confused patients[36]. They feel strongly that elderly patients should, equally with young ones, receive levodopa as the drug of first choice. This would seem a reasonable view once the patient is disabled, but there is an earlier stage at which selected anticholinergics might be valuable, and might delay the moment when levodopa needs to be started.

Table 4   Anticholinergic-type drugs for Parkinsonism

Approved name	Trade names	Dose range in the elderly
Benzhexol	Artane or Pipanol	start 1–2 mg. o.d. or b.d. usual maximum 10–12 mg/day
Procyclidine	Kemadrin	start 2.5–5 mg o.d. usual maximum 10–30 mg/day
Benztropine	Cogentin	start 0.5–1 mg nocte usual maximum 6 mg/day
Ethopropazine HC1	Lysivane	250 mg i.m.
Benaprizine	Brizin	start 50 mg o.d. or b.d. usual maximum 200 mg/day
Orphenadrine HC1	Disipal	start 50 mg o.d. or b.d. usual maximum 300 mg/day

Benzhexol (Artane or Pipanol)
This drug may be more likely than other anticholinergics to cause visual hallucinations and confusion in the elderly, who can rarely tolerate more than 10 to 12 mg/day in divided dosage. It develops its peak action in 2 to 3 hours, so should be given 4 hourly, and the dosage built up slowly from 1 to 2 mg once or twice daily at first.

Procyclidine (Kemadrin)
This is less likely to cause mental side-effects so may be more suitable in the elderly. It is best given after meals, with slow increase in dosage. It was shown to be more effective than placebo or piribedil (a new antiparkinsonian agent) in controlling phenothiazine-induced Parkinsonism in 16 schizophrenic patients. It was well-tolerated, and the trial counteracted previous suggestions that anticholinergics might be ineffective in this situation[37].

Benztropine (Cogentin)
This drug is excreted slowly so once-daily dosage is sufficient. It may cause drowsiness, so is best given at night starting with a quarter or half a tablet. Other side-effects, which are uncommon, include an allergic rash.

Ethopropazine (Lysivane)
In its intramuscular preparation (dosage 250 mg) this drug is said to be useful in the treatment of the uncommon oculogyric crises of the postencephalitic patients.

Benaprizine (Brizin)
This is a newer preparation having maximal central and minimal peripheral action, and is said to produce less side-effects than benzhexol but possibly is also less effective. Dosage is from 50 to 200 mg/day.

Orphenadrine (Disipal)
This drug should be given after meals to avoid gastric irritation. It has a definite euphoric effect which is often helpful.

Amantadine (Symmetrel)
In contrast to the logical development of the treatment of Parkinson's disease with levodopa or its derivatives, the origin of amantadine treatment resulted from a fortunate chance. In 1968 a 58-year-old woman with Parkinson's disease noticed a remarkable remission in her symptoms during the previous three months, when she had been taking amantadine hydrochloride 100 mg twice daily to prevent influenza. Her symptoms relapsed within 6 weeks of stopping the drug[38]. Further testing of the drug with ten, and later with 163 patients confirmed an improvement in akinesia rigidity and tremor in 66%. Of those showing improvement, benefits were sustained in about half for 3–8 months. However, about one-third of the patients who experienced benefit at first found a slow but steady reduction in benefit in 4–8 weeks, though medication at 200 mg b.d. was continued exactly as before. This fading of effect has been confirmed repeatedly and is a major drawback to amantadine treatment.

Amantadine is rapidly and completely absorbed from the gut, and probably acts by releasing dopamine from the intact dopaminergic terminals that remain in the basal ganglia.

Side-effects
Side-effects are not common on the usual dose of 100–200 mg/day. Mental side-effects of importance in the elderly include insomnia, confusion and restlessness and sometimes hallucinations. The appearance of livedo reticularis, often on the thighs, is usually of cosmetic importance only. Ankle oedema is sometimes a worrying side-effect, subsiding only slowly after the drug is withdrawn.

Amantadine can be given with levodopa and is used by some workers as an additional treatment in patients who can tolerate only suboptimal doses of levodopa.

L-dopa (levodopa)

History of L-dopa

The most encouraging advance in the medical treatment of Parkinsonism has been the introduction of L-dopa (L-34-dihydroxyphenylalanine) a precursor of dopamine which can cross the blood-brain barrier, whereas dopamine cannot. The steps which led up to its use were logical and have been briefly described. They culminated, in 1961, in the first treatment by Birkmayer and Hornykiewicz of 20 Parkinsonian patients by intravenous L-dopa[26] which was reported as showing short-term dramatic results. Subsequent therapeutic trials led to controversial reports but in 1967 Cotzias, van Woert and Schiffer[39] succeeded in giving large doses of oral dopa for longer periods than in any previous study. They used DL-dopa as it was cheaper than the L-isomer. Although ten out of their 16 patients showed striking improvement, four out of the 16 developed transient granulocytopenia, so they felt that a similar long-term investigation of pure L-dopa would be the next step.

Numerous workers were able to show the effectivness and relative freedom from haematological problems, of treatment with pure L-dopa[40–43]. Reports of short-term use over a few months gave way to those in which the drug had been successfully used for increasing numbers of years. The characteristic side-effects of the drug became clearer, as did the proportion of patients able to benefit. So far as the elderly were concerned, levodopa had a bad start. In a widely quoted review of 90 patients showing mental symptoms on L-dopa treatment[44], it was found that a particular small subgroup of elderly patients (average age 70·6 years) had become suicidal or psychotic. The dosages, where quoted, proved to be high, usually more than 3·5 g/day of L-dopa. Godwin-Austen *et al.*[45] studied the effect of age and arteriosclerosis in the response of Parkinsonian patients to levodopa. Based on a study of ten patients aged under 65 and 12 aged 65 or over, they concluded that the younger patients showed a better response (61 % versus 28 % improvement) than the older groups after 12 months dosage. They had previously found[46] that those over 65 tolerated slightly lower doses of levodopa, and that slow introduction of treatment offered no advantage in the maximum dosage tolerated.

Peaston and Bianchine[47], in a primarily metabolic study, drew conclusions about the relationship between degree of improvement on levodopa and age of the patients, although their numbers were small and the differences also small. They reported seven cases aged 50–59 years showing 75 % improvement; nine cases aged 60–69 years showing 63% improvement, and six cases aged 70+ years showing 55% improvement. They concluded on this basis that improvement tended to be inversely related to the age of the patient. Although their average total dose over the 6 month treatment period was 3 g/day, they do not show the doses tolerated by the different age groups. Their conclusion was that, as all patients had actually improved, L-dopa was the treatment of first choice.

These papers have had long-lasting effects. The British National Formulary 1976–78, states 'levodopa is least valuable with elderly people. . . who rarely tolerate a dose big enough to overcome their deficit'. A recent authoritative leader in the Lancet[48] suggests that 'one approach is to reserve the most powerful drugs for the most disabled patients irrespective of age; another is to start young people on levodopa and older people on anticholinergics or amantadine, since levodopa is better tolerated in the young'. Most physicians working with the elderly would favour the first alternative. Their experience[36,49,50] is that, in suitable dosage, levodopa is effective in the elderly; whereas anticholinergics and amantadine are relatively ineffective and have confusional side-effects of their own.

In general levodopa has proved a great advance in treatment, being effective both for bradykinesia and for rigidity. Tremor was slow to respond, if at all. After about 6 years' use it was clear that about 75% of patients, including the elderly, showed a significant response[49,50] and essentially all symptoms, including defects in posture, sialorrhoea and increased sebum secretion, could respond. The mean decrease in disability in those who responded was 40–50%.

Effects in treatment
Dosages used for elderly patients should be smaller than those for younger adults, and built up slowly. A usual initial levodopa dose for younger patients would be 250 mg up to three times daily, building up to a total of 2–4 g/day or more. Sutcliffe[49], who studied 50 elderly patients, recommended a starting dose of 125 mg twice daily, increasing cautiously by 125 mg/week to a usual level of 1 g/day at 12 weeks. Vignalou and Beck[50], in a study of 122 patients aged 70 years or more, found an average daily dosage by the end of treatment of 2.4 ± 0.84 g. Patients prescribed larger doses in another study were found later to have reduced their own drug dosages to 1.75–2.0 g/day because of nausea and vomiting[51].

After taking the drug, the peak serum value occurs in 1–2 hours, with gradual decrease over 3–4 hours. These values may be altered by sluggish gastric emptying time or slow intestinal transit time.

Absorption is normally rapid from the small intestine and insignificant amounts are excreted in the stools. It is unlikely that absorption is affected in the elderly. About two-thirds of the dose of levodopa is excreted in the urine in 8 hours[47], as dopamine and as a number of active metabolites of the drug, which can stain underwear brown.

Side-effects of treatment
Side-effects vary from one series to another, depending on the dosages of levodopa used. Vomiting has been a problem in most series, occurring in 70–90% of cases on large doses, but reducing to 57%[50] or even 10%[49] if very slow cautious increases were made. Patients are advised always to take the drug with or after food. There is some disagreement about which antiemetic agents should be used. Many authors advocate metoclopramide (Maxolon) 10–20 mg/day, but this drug can itself cause extrapyramidal dyskinesias and is better avoided. An alternative antiemetic would be cyclizine (Valoid) 50 mg, which has some anticholinergic activity.

Dyskinetic movements (orofacial, or choreiform involving head, trunk or limbs) are a problem in 26–60% of cases on treatment. Usually they coincide with maximum improvement in mobility, and the milder forms are well-tolerated by patients, although they cause anxiety to the relatives. Treatment consists of reduction of levodopa dosage, but this may be accompanied by a recurrence of Parkinsonian rigidity.

Mental symptoms are usually the most important side-effects in series involving elderly patients. Vignalou[50] found 'psychic intolerances' in 31% of his elderly patients, while average incidence of confusion, delirium or hypomania in younger patients would be 10–15%. A few cases of increased libido have occurred and have given rise to disproportionate interest. Postural hypotension, occurring as a result of levodopa treatment in 2–8% of cases is a perplexing finding in view of the known central effect of catecholamines (including dopamine) in raising the blood pressure. Cardiac side-effects, including arrhythmias, result from the stimulating effect of dopamine on the cardiac beta-adrenergic receptors.

Contraindications to treatment
There are a number of contraindications to levodopa treatment. The drug must not be given within 4 weeks of a monoamine oxidase inhibitor, because interaction between the drugs could give rise to a dangerous hypertensive crisis. Drugs which block dopamine receptors or deplete stores such as phenothiazines and reserpine will inactivate part of the action of levodopa. Vitamin B_6 (pyridoxine) enhances the

extracerebral metabolism of levodopa to dopamine, and leaves less levodopa for intracerebral action, causing the Parkinsonian symptoms to reappear suddenly. Fortunately there are some multivitamin preparations (Vitavel[52] (GB), Larobec (USA)) which contain no pyridoxine and can safely be taken by patients on levodopa.

Patients with recent myocardial infarction or with cardiac arrhythmias are probably best admitted to hospital if introduction of levodopa is essential to control their Parkinsonian disability[53]. Patients with narrow-angle glaucoma run some risk of worsening their eye condition, as levodopa can cause pupillary dilation.

Patients undergoing general anaesthesia with cyclopropane or halothane should discontinue levodopa 12 hours preoperatively, as these anaesthetic agents sensitize the heart to the action of sympathomimetic amines. When oral fluids are permitted postoperatively dosage can be restarted at 50–75% of previous doses, and built up again.

Sinemet and Madopar
One of the problems of treatment with levodopa alone is that perhaps 95 percent[54] of ingested levodopa is metabolized by extracerebral dopa decarboxylase. To overcome this wastage high doses of levodopa are given but the metabolites which are produced in the intestines, liver and kidney, as well as in the brain, contribute to the toxicity of the drug. Slow buildup of dosage is necessary to avoid nausea and vomiting, and improvement is delayed.

The combination of peripheral dopa decarboxylase inhibitors with levodopa was an important advance[55] since now the formation of dopamine could be prevented at the extracerebral sites. Consequently lower doses were needed and the incidence of vomiting was cut from about 80% to 15% of patients. Two main inhibitors were used: α-methyldopa hydrazine (carbidopa) and Ro4-4602 (benserazide) in Sinemet and Madopar respectively. It was found that neither inhibitor resulted in any antiparkinsonian action nor ill-effect when used alone, and the results of combined treatment with carbidopa and levodopa or with benserazide and levodopa were found to be similar, though some patients fared better on the one than on the other[56,57]. Either type of combined treatment resulted in a 4-fold or 5-fold reduction of levodopa dosage[58] and clinical response occurred within 1 or 2 weeks rather than months[59,60].

Cardiac arrhythmias, caused by levodopa metabolism in the heart, were reduced or avoided[61], and postural hypotension minimized[62], while the risk of glaucoma was lessened. The response to combined therapy was unaltered by pyridoxine[63].

As neither carbidopa nor benserazide can cross the blood–brain barrier, the intracerebral effects of the levodopa treatment are not altered by combined treatment. Thus the dose-limiting involuntary dyskinetic movements occur at the same plasma dopa levels and the incidence of neuropsychiatric problems is similar to that with levodopa. The 'on–off' phenomenon, an abrupt onset of akinesia followed by equally sudden return of therapeutic response to levodopa, was first reported by Cotzias[39]. It had proved an increasing problem and occurred eventually in up to 50 % of patients after some years of levodopa treatment. It seemed likely that this problem would occur on combined treatment, but might arise even earlier in the course of combined treatment.

By 1973–74 there were numerous satisfactory reports of the value of combined treatment[54,59,64], and Sinemet or Madopar had become the drug of first choice in treatment of Parkinsonism, giving benefit in up to 85 % of patients, and reducing disability by up to 50 % of its previous level.

As for levodopa alone, so for combined treatment the dosages used in the elderly should be lower, and for this reason the smaller tablet sizes are likely to prove more useful, as shown below:

Sinemet 110   containing carbidopa   10 mg and levodopa 100 mg
Sinemet 275   containing carbidopa   25 mg and levodopa 250 mg
Madopar 125   containing benserazide   25 mg and levodopa 100 mg
Madopar 250   containing benserazide   50 mg and levodopa 200 mg

Only the fixed combinations of a 1 : 10 (Sinemet) or a 1 : 4 (Madopar) ratio of inhibitor to levodopa are available, but the dosages provided have been flexible enough to meet most patients' needs. It is important to quote the number as well as the drug name in prescribing these tablets to ensure that the patient receives the same dosage.

Doses are often quoted in terms of the amount of levodopa; starting doses in the elderly would be the equivalent of 50–100 mg levodopa (plus inhibitor) given once or twice daily. This dose would be increased every 4 or 5 days till a satisfactory improvement is obtained, or till side-effects supervene. An average maintenance dose might be 500 mg levodopa combined with 50 mg carbidopa a day, the tablets being given in divided doses, always with food[36,65]. The success rate of such a regime in elderly patients seems comparable to that in younger patients[49].

Side-effects of treatment
Common minor side-effects include temporary nausea (perhaps best relieved by cyclizine 50 mg), abnormal taste in the mouth, abnormal

sweating and sleep disturbances including nightmares. Drugs which are contraindicated with Sinemet include levodopa, monoamine oxidase inhibitors, and general anaesthetic agents, while hypotensive drugs have to be used with care. Occasional reports have been made of haemolytic anaemia, transient neutropenia and stimulation of activity of malignant melanomas during long-term treatment.

Opinion now differs whether dosage should be pushed to the maximum or maintained at 600–750 mg/day levodopa for patients of average age. The normal geriatric practice of using the lowest effective dosage seems likely to result in less patients with later 'on–off' complications.

Long-term effects of levodopa treatment
After the early enthusiasm for levodopa treatment, reports began to be made of fading of response[66] at roughly the same time as combined treatment was coming into prominence. There are now authors who have experience of using levodopa over periods up to 12 years[31], and it is becoming clear that the main dose-limiting effects are the central dyskinetic ones. These effects occur whether or not the levodopa is administered in combined form, and they have been reported in many countries[67,68]. Most physicians in those countries where higher dosage regimes have been used, such as in the United States, report higher incidences of the 'on–off' phenomenon, ranging from 20–47%, while those from countries like Finland and Britain, who use lower dosages, report incidences of 2·8–15%.

Marsden in a review article[69] has described five variants of the 'on–off' phenomenon.

(1) Early morning akinesia results from low morning plasma levels of dopamine, as the half-life of present levodopa preparations is 3–4 hours.

(2) 'Freezing' episodes; sudden immobility of unknown cause, when confronted with a difficult task, such as going through a doorway. These may last seconds or minutes and be released by a sharp command or surprise.

(3) End-of-dose deterioration – the commonest variant – occurs in up to 50% of patients after 3 years' therapy. Benefit from each dose shortens from 4 hours to 3 hours or less, and the same doses have to be given at shorter intervals. The physician later attempts to decrease the size, but not the frequency, of the doses, in order to avoid peak-dose problems.

(4) Peak-dose dyskinesias: In these, 'on' corresponds to high or increasing serum dopamine levels, and 'off' corresponds to low or decreasing ones.

(5) There is a rare peak-dose akinesia, and a form of wildly fluctuating dyskinesia which he has called 'yo-yoing'.

Some authorities believe that these problems are the result of underlying progress of the disease, others that long-term toxic effects of levodopa dosage may be involved, and others that a combination of these two factors occurs[70].

Apart from the dyskinesias and 'on–off' phenomena, two other long-term conditions have emerged on prolonged treatment. Postural instability leading to increasingly frequent and severe falls are an early feature of loss of long-term benefit, and usually indicate a downward turn in the prognosis. Dementia, together with other mental changes, is increasingly seen, perhaps as a result of longer survival.

Bromocriptine (Parlodel)

This drug (2-Br-α-ergocryptine, CB 152) was first introduced in 1972 to reduce serum prolactin, later proved to be useful in acromegaly and now proves to be a valuable dopamine agonist. It, therefore, has a place in the treatment of Parkinson's disease, though its exact role remains to be determined. Theoretically a dopamine agonist, stimulating the dopamine receptors directly, could have a number of advantages over levodopa. For example it could still act late in the disease when the enzyme machinery required to convert levodopa to dopamine might have been exhausted, and hence levodopa response might have faded.

Clinical studies with bromocriptine followed the observation that this drug stimulated striatal dopaminergic receptors in the rat. Early investigations were performed with relatively low doses of bromocriptine (10–30 mg/day), comparable to those used to reduce plasma prolactin[71], and established a weak antiparkinsonian action, similar to that of amantadine or anticholingergics. Subsequently, using higher doses (30–150 mg/day) it has been found that bromocriptine can induce a therapeutic response similar to that of levodopa[72–74], with benefit in bradykinesia, akinesia and often in tremor. However, patients do not benefit from bromocriptine if they have already failed to respond to levodopa.

Bromocriptine at 100 mg/day is probably roughly equivalent to 1 g levodopa[73]. Bromocriptine is rapidly absorbed with a peak serum level (therapeutic range 2–15 ng/ml) 2 hours after oral dosage, but its half-life is three or four times that of levodopa, giving a smoother response, and hence less likelihood of 'on – off' phenomena. Although dyskinesias are less common with bromocriptine than with levodopa psychiatric reactions (hallucinations and delusions) are commoner – possibly due to the lysergic-acid-amide part of the molecule. The reactions may also be more florid, can occur even at low dosage, and can take several weeks to resolve after stopping the drug.

Erythromelalgia (tender, red, oedematous feet) can be induced by high doses of bromocriptine and occasionally patients have suffered from digital vasospasm[75], and increased angina. Some patients had diplopia or nasal congestion.

It is not yet known whether long-term treatment with bromocriptine will give rise to 'on–off' symptoms, as the longest reported trial is for 30 months[76]. If it does not do so, bromocriptine may replace levodopa as treatment of choice in many patients, as the 'on – off' phenomenon is now the major complication of long-term levodopa treatment. A present use for bromocriptine is to enable patients with this distressing complication to reduce their levodopa dosage (by an average of 41%)[76] by adding bromocriptine to their drug regime. The dosage of bromocriptine is started at a low level. Calne[76] and his colleagues, for example give a test dose of 1 mg in case the patient is very sensitive to the hypotensive effect of the drug, followed by 2·5 mg two or three times daily. Increases should be slow, to a range of 50–90 mg/day, while the levodopa is concurrently reduced. For elderly patients a dosage of 3·5 to 10 mg/day is about equivalent to levodopa 100 mg plus inhibitor – an average dose.

Contraindications to treatment
Contraindications to bromocriptine therapy, which include a history of confusion or dementia, severe ischaemic heart disease or peripheral vascular disease, appear to rule out its use in many elderly patients with Parkinsonism. At the same time the problem of 'on – off' effects has been less in the elderly, possibly because of the smaller dosages of levodopa used, so the need for bromocriptine in this age group is perhaps less. It could be useful in selected patients unable to tolerate even combined treatment without unacceptable nausea. Few series have referred specifically to the elderly, but since improvement on the drug shows itself rapidly, it would be worth a cautious trial in slowly increasing doses in suitable cases. Those already satisfactorily stabilized and showing continued response to combined levodopa therapy should not however be changed to this relatively untried and expensive treatment.

Other new drugs for Parkinsonism

Of the synthetic dopamine agonists which have been tried, bromocriptine is probably the most promising. Piribedil unfortunately is unpredictable in action and may precipitate vomiting and cause psychiatric reactions[71]. Apomorphine causes severe vomiting and renal damage. Lergotrile can give rise to change in liver functions which may limit its use.

Oxiperomide, a new dopamine receptor antagonist has been found to decrease dyskinesias in six Parkinsonian patients receiving levodopa or other therapy, without necessarily increasing the Parkinsonian symptoms[77]. This finding provides evidence that more than one population of dopamine receptors exists in the extrapyramidal system. Unfortunately oxiperomide itself causes unacceptable drowsiness.

Deprenyl is an inhibitor of monoamine oxidase type B, the enzyme predominantly concerned with degradation of dopamine. This drug, pioneered in Hungary, has no antiparkinsonian action of its own but can enhance and prolong the action of levodopa. Thus it can be effective in end-of-dose akinesia, and has been used together with levodopa with promising results by Birkmayer[78] to combat the 'on–off' effect. The drug is at present only in very limited supply.

The recent history of the drug treatment of Parkinsonism has been one of rapid change, and there is every indication of further advances in treatment in the future. While this causes difficulty for the prescribing physician in balancing the claims of newer preparations against those well-tried, it gives good hope for improved drug treatment in the future for all groups of Parkinsonian patients of whatever age.

SURGICAL TREATMENT

This type of teatment which had its greatest vogue in the 1960's, is much less used now that drug treatment has advanced, and its current role is limited. The patient with severe unilateral tremor who has failed to respond to medical treatment may be greatly helped by stereotactic thalamotomy. In such cases the risk of morbidity, about 5%, is justified. The operation has no effect on hypokinesia and gait and speech disturbance can be made worse especially if bilateral operations are performed[79,80]. Dementia and arteriosclerosis are contraindications to surgery. In geriatric practice the place of surgery is now virtually nil, and Greer found that not one of 200 patients was referred for surgery[81]. Though few operations are now carried out, many patients are being followed up who have had operations in the past. Selby[80] in a study of 148 patients found that the operation inhibited dopa-induced dyskinesias on the affected side, and suggested operation for selected severe cases where dyskinesias prevented the use of optimal doses of levodopa.

USEFUL SUPPORTING DRUGS
FOR PARKINSONIAN PATIENTS

Antidepressants
Tricyclic drugs are valuable, especially as their anticholinergic effects are useful. Imipramine (Tofranil) up to 30–90 mg/day for retarded depression, or amitryptiline (Tryptizol) 50–100 mg at night for agitated depression probably remain as effective as newer preparations. Monoamine oxidise inhibitors are contraindicated with levodopa. A single case study of a patient who had a hypertensive crisis while on normal doses of Sinemet, amitryptiline and metoclopramide has been reported[82], though any two of these drugs alone seem safe. Cyclizine would perhaps be a good substitute for metoclopramide in depressed patients who were nauseated while on sinemet.

Psychotropic drugs
Confused patients should first have their antiparkinsonian drugs tailed off, and restarted at low dosage only if it is clear that they are necessary, and not causing the confusion. One particular and common hallucination consists of seeing numerous people going about their business in the house or ward. Such hallucinations may be mistaken by the patients for familiar characters from, say, the television screen. These delusions may disappear slowly when all drugs are gradually withdrawn. A non-phenothiazine drug such as L-tryptophan can be useful in mild confusion. If more severe, the drug which is most likely to be useful is thioridazine (Melleril)[83]. This drug has a low affinity for postsynaptic dopamine receptor binding sites in the corpus striatum, so is least likely to block the action of levodopa. In addition thioridazine possesses useful anticholinergic properties and may exhibit 'its own inbuilt antiparkinson-

ian activity'. Pigmentary retinopathy can however occur on large doses, and T wave changes on the ECG and occasional agranulocytosis are reported.

Laxatives
After ensuring that the patient has adequate roughage and bran in the diet, and adequate fluids and exercise, stool-bulking agents can be added if constipation continues. The patient should be persuaded not to take liquid paraffin, because of the danger of aspiration pneumonitis or lipoid pneumonia, especially if any dysphagia is present. There is sometimes a problem, too, with anal leakage of paraffin.

Hypnotics
Every attempt should be made to prevent the patient adding a hypnotic to his already powerful drug regime. If this fails, dichloralphenazone (Welldorm) or chlormethiazole (Heminevrin) would be suitable hypnotics.

Drugs for aching and restless legs
Anticholinergic drugs may be more useful for this symptom than levodopa. Some members of the Parkinson's Disease Society reported being helped by a hand-held vibrator which can be purchased for use at home; others are helped by sitting in a rocking chair. Analgesics such as aspirin or distalgesic are also sometimes of benefit.

Drugs for tremor
Occasional patients who are not helped by levodopa benefit from propranolol up to 10 mg three times daily.

Miscellaneous drugs
Patients on treatment for cardiac failure with digitalis and diuretics, can continue these drugs while on levodopa. A patient who has a fresh myocardial infarct is best advised to omit levodopa (or Sinemet) for the first 24 hours. If hypertension does not respond to rest or thiazides, a beta-blocker or small doses of α-methyldopa (Aldomet) can be given. Analgesics and antibiotics can be given as necessary to patients on levodopa.

As for all medication in the elderly, dosages should be small, increments cautious and the final dose titrated to the patient's need. Clearly labeled and easily opened (not childproof) containers should be used if the patient is to open them himself.

PARKINSON'S DISEASE AND DEMENTIA

James Parkinson concluded the opening paragraph of *An Essay on the Shaking Palsy* with the phrase 'the senses and intellects being uninjured'. About 70 years later a contrary opinion appeared in the French literature when Ball wrote 'Paralysis agitans is accompanied more often than is thought by intellectual difficulties'[84]. Many attempts have since been made to resolve this controversy, using various tests of intellectual function on patients with Parkinsonism. Unfortunately there was a lack of norms, making it impossible to correct for the intellectual decline which may occur with normal ageing. A good study in 1972[85], before levodopa became widely available, used the Wechsler Adult Intelligence Scale, which is the best standardized and most widely used test for general intelligence, and compares an individual with others of his own age. Results in 63 patients who had a mean age of 64·4 years showed that intellectual impairment was present in over 36% of patients. The patient's greatest difficulty lay in comprehending and analysing new stimuli, and in recent memory span. Loranger and his colleagues[85] concluded that this decline could not be explained on the basis of accompanying depression alone, nor on the motor slowing of the disease nor on anticholinergic nor prior surgical treatment. There was no relationship between the intellectual impairment and the patients' age or length of illness. Their conclusion was in agreement with Ball's statement in 1882 that 'a slight degree of intellectual disturbance is almost the rule in this disease'. In 1972 a study[86] of psychiatric disturbances in 153 Parkinsonian patients gave an incidence of 40% suffering from varying degrees of dementia. Every type of Parkinsonian syndrome, whether postencephalitic, arteriosclerotic or idiopathic, appeared to give a similar range of psychiatric sequelae.

Though there is overlap between Parkinsonism and arteriosclerosis there is a poor correlation between the two conditions[87]. It has been found that cortical atrophy occurs more frequently in Parkinsonian patients than in normal individuals of the same age, and the increasing use of computerized axial tomography (CAT scanning) will enable this to be further investigated[88]. The dementia and cortical atrophy of Parkinsonism may well be caused by an Alzheimer-type condition, resulting from the same degenerative process as that which produces the nigrostriatal lesions which are characteristic of the disease. While the frequency and extent of cortical changes in untreated Parkinsonism remain unclear, it is difficult to judge the effect of treatment on mental aspects of the disease.

There is some controversy over whether pre-existing confusion or dementia should preclude treatment with levodopa. The results of Jenkins and Groh showing poor treatment response have already been mentioned[44]. Sacks and Messeloff later reported alarming reactions in three demented patients who were given 4 g/day of levodopa[89]. These patients, whose ages were not mentioned, developed an agitated hallucinatory delirium which took a month to resolve after the levodopa was stopped. Wolf and Davis also reported a single case of permanent dementia following levodopa[90]. The strong impression was left that levodopa frequently produces adverse effects in confused patients. However a study[34] of 21 elderly patients, of whom 18 were demented, showed significant benefit when they were treated with levodopa using an average maintenance dose of 1·7 g. Mental function improved in nine of the 13 demented patients who completed 6 months of treatment. Broe and Caird[34] suggested, as a result of this study, that dementia was not a contraindication to a trial of levodopa in small doses.

A similar disagreement has continued about whether patients with arteriosclerosis and Parkinsonism should receive levodopa. Godwin-Austen *et al.* in 1971[45] found no improvement in symptoms in two patients with 'arteriosclerotic Parkinsonism' treated with levodopa for a year. Parkes *et al.* in 1974[11] and Pearce in 1974[88] confirmed the overlap between Parkinsonism, arteriosclerosis and senile or presenile dementia, and emphasized the lack of response to levodopa. However, Drachmann and Stahl in 1975[91] reported a useful degree of improvement (both intellectual and motor) in five of the nine patients with 'extrapyramidal dementia' in whom levodopa 1–3·75 g/day was tried. They concluded that 'even if only an unpredictable minority of patients with extrapyramidal dementia can benefit from levodopa therapy, the size of the problem would justify further therapeutic trials'. In another study of 50 elderly patients, about half of whom had idiopathic and half arteriosclerotic Parkinsonism, Sutcliffe[49] found benefit with levodopa in 75% of cases (from both groups).

Both the mental and the physical aspects of Parkinsonism cause problems. In a large survey by Pollock and Hornabrook[92], about 25% of patients with Parkinson's disease were a burden to their families from dementia rather than from physical disability. This survey emphasizes the problem of mental symptoms in this disease, and lends support to suggestions that a trial of combined levodopa treatment in small doses in such patients would be worthwhile.

THE ROLE OF THE THERAPIST
IN PARKINSON'S DISEASE

Therapy programmes

Now that there are effective drugs available for treating this condition, patients are surviving longer and at a higher level of mobility. Their increased activity is, however, constantly at risk. Any prolonged break from physical activity because of intercurrent infection, other illness or injury can prove disastrous. Many patients will need instruction how best to keep their muscles active by simple exercises at home, perhaps using the exercises they have been taught during a period of day-hospital rehabilitation.

A very detailed report on the regime employed by therapists at Sinai hospital, Baltimore as a result of 7 years' experience with Parkinsonian patients, has been written by Davis[93]. The work of this unit, though perhaps directed towards elderly patients at an earlier stage of disability than those seen in hospital in the United Kingdom, nevertheless contains many helpful guidelines and ideas which can be modified for use by those who are more disabled. Judith Davis' programme of therapy covers 2 hourly sessions a week for 4 weeks, which can be modified to half-hourly sessions once or twice weekly for 16 or 8 weeks respectively to avoid overtiring the patients. Her evaluation at the start of treatment is a detailed one carried out by occupational therapists and physiotherapists and includes a number of timed activities such as dressing, etc. In British practice when there are often fewer skilled staff available, one or two simple timed tests such as timed name and address, or the Webster timed test for walking and turning is all that is possible. Data from these tests form part of weekly progress reports at case conferences. Each patient, after assessment in Baltimore, goes into a cycle of activities in the gymnasium which are very similar to those used in some British Parkinson classes, although Davis' sessions can be longer so she can therefore develop a structured sequence of exercises. Commonly used warm-up exercises include matwork with rolling over, sideways movements and leg-raising, often done to music, and during this time the therapist can give individual treatment, passively stretching the hamstring muscles which are often rigid. Parallel bar work can include practice in stepping over the rungs of a 'walking ladder' placed on the floor, or this can be replaced by chalk marks or by a series of small obstacles, as has long been good geriatric practice[94]. Exercise-bicycle work which Davis uses, is probably beyond most elderly patients' ability, but arm-pulley sessions are helpful and not too tiring.

Group exercises, in which patients sit in a ring in armless chairs, are a good way of encouraging a full range of movement of arm and shoulder muscles, combined with deep breathing and facial muscle exercises. They have the further advantage of giving the patients social contact with each other, as can easy games such as ball-throwing or baton-passing, and one therapist and helper can treat six or eight patients at a time. Davis' groups consisted of 12 or 15 patients, but they were able to join in musical games, and some could even hop, so she was obviously able to cope with larger numbers at one time as they needed less individual help. Taking off shoes and loosening clothing for the exercises also provides the patients with good practice in self-care.

Much of the work as described by an occupational therapist in America would be carried out by a physiotherapist in Britain, though there should be a fair amount of flexibility in the two roles. Further practice in walking in the gymnasium can include practice in turning in a large semicircle which is easier for Parkinsonian patients than truning on the spot. A trial of a wheeled walking-aid is worthwhile, as many patients can achieve smoother progress with this aid than with a Zimmer Frame. Rollators with hand-operated brakes are now coming onto the market, and should help the patient who cannot stop when moving forward with the aid.

Another useful innovation is a 'falling-down class' for patients and relatives. Confidence and morale can improve if relatives have practical instruction in how best to help the patient get on his feet again.

Occupational therapists in this country have long advised doctors and patients about suitable heights for chairs and beds, handles beside the bed to aid rolling over, etc. Firm mattresses on solid bases also help in this manoeuvre, and grab-handles at strategic places in bedroom, bathroom and kitchen, together with raised toilet seats if needed, can all help in independence. Suitably designed garments are now available in which hooks and eyes and buttons are replaced by velcro bands and zips. Patients disagree about spring-loaded forward hinged seats as an aid to standing. Some confident patients find them helpful, others fear them and leave them unused in the corner of the room.

As a result of a grant from the Parkinson's Disease Society, the role of the occupational therapist in this disease is being investigated at Glasgow, where therapists are visiting 41 patients in their own homes. This study, under the guidance of Professor Francis Caird, is still in progress. An early finding is that relatively inexpensive aids such as non-slip mats, special cutlery, suctioned cups, special bath-rails and raised toilet seats can all help considerably in making life easier for the patient. The Society also has details of a Hodge seat, a swivel seat fitted to a car, which can be provided by the DHSS to help a disabled patient to get out of a car more easily.

The role of the social services departments

The social services departments have a considerable part to play in supporting Parkinsonian patients in their own homes. Services like those of the home help and meals-on-wheels help district nurses and family doctors in their task of treating the patients and avoiding unnecessary admission to a hospital or a home. The psychological and medical help given by a good family doctor can make all the difference to a patient, and to the family. In the complex and inter-locking network of services for the elderly, geriatric day-hospitals have a vital role, and many of them have Parkinsonian patients accounting for up to 10% of their attenders. Money spent on these services is well spent compared with the millions of pounds previously used up on long-term hospital care for Parkinsonian patients.

Social workers can play a vital advisory role such as giving advice about selling a home and moving into a warden-assisted flat or old people's home, either private or state-provided. Similarly they can often 'match' a suitable local vacancy with a patient ready for discharge from hospital. Occasionally it is necessary, perhaps because of increasing frailty, for a patient to allow a relative Power of Attorney to manage his financial affairs, and doctor, solicitor and social worker will usually work together over this issue. Sometimes, if the patient is too confused to understand and give informed consent for a Power of Attorney, a Court of Protection application must be completed instead, and will usually take many months to resolve. A further legal aspect of Parkinson's disease concerns the occasional patient who refuses hospital treatment because of confusion or eccentricity and who then becomes a danger to himself and to others. Such patients under Section 45 of the National Assistance Act 1948 can be taken into a designated hospital for 3 weeks if a magistrate and the district community physician agree.

The majority of patients do not need such legal constraints and are happy to accept treatment. Many find that, against their will, they suffer from the 'social costs of Parkinson's disease', studied by Singer[95]. This was a multicentre American study of 169 Parkinsonian patients prior to the time of levodopa treatment. Singer's social study found that patients with this condition had less social contacts, pursued more solitary leisure activities, such as reading or watching television and spent more of their time idle or dozing than others of similar age. Her early study highlighted again the potential benefit of effective drug therapy.

TREATMENT OF MILD OR EARLY PARKINSONISM

It is becoming clear that, with the newer antiparkinsonian drugs such as dopa plus an inhibitor, benefit can be obtained for most patients in the form of increased mobility and independence, for a period of about 5 years. After this time the underlying progress of the disease and the long-term side-effects of the drugs may make treatment less and less effective and the terminal phase of the disease gradually supervenes. It seems, as previously discussed, that the 5 year benefit period may relate to the total levodopa dosage over the years, so there is a tendency now to put off the start of dopa treatment until significant disability makes this step necessary. Thus mild or early cases, with little disability are probably best treated with a regime of steady exercise (say 1 mile a day, with deep breathing exercises), accompanied by a course of physiotherapy instruction. Later either an antihistaminic agent such as orphenadrine (Disipal) 100–300 mg/day, or amantadine (Symmetrel) 50–300 mg/day may be tried. Advice about raising the height of chair or bed, and about suitable clothing and fastenings may also be very useful at this stage, as well as later in the condition. No strict rules can be made, however, and some patients may need levodopa soon after the onset of their symptoms.

In geriatric practice such patients are referred under a variety of non-specific labels: slowing down, unable to live alone, generalized muscular aches and arthritis. It is worth checking the patient's drug regime, as drug-induced Parkinsonism should subside in weeks or months if the drug is slowly withdrawn. The underlying diagnosis may well have been missed, particularly as the characteristic tremor may not be evident in some elderly patients. Once the diagnosis is sure, it is probably better to tell the patient and the family, at the same time providing them with as much information as possible. The leaflets written for the Parkinson's Disease Society[96,97] are very useful as they are informative, up to date and presented in a reasonably optimistic tone. If there is a local branch of the Society (and by 1979 there will be 45 branches in the United Kingdom), some patients and relatives find the meetings helpful and supportive. Other patients, however, prefer not to identify themselves in any way with fellow-sufferers, but to keep their interests and friendships among the healthy – and this attitude must, of course, be respected. It is important to encourage patients and families not to hide disabilities within a restricted circle. This policy can lead to over protection and to overdependence on one individual, and the supporting relative may find the responsibility and care impossible to bear. As far as possible the patient must continue to take part in family discussions and decisions and to maintain his social contacts and activities. It takes courage, for example, to eat in public when one has a tremor, or is very slow and in need of some help, but it can be beneficial not only to the patient and relatives, but also to society which must come to terms with the increasing numbers of aged and disabled in its midst.

The geriatrician may some times be asked to advise younger patients. These patients should remain at work as long as possible. Professional people may have to reduce their additional commitments in order to achieve their essential workload without undue fatigue. Some patients who have to appear or speak in public find a beta-blocker such as propanolol (Inderal) helpful. Tiring physical work has to be limited and a longer time allowed to complete a task.

The question of when a patient with Parkinson's disease stops driving a car is a matter for careful consideration in each case, and the hospital physician may be asked to advise on this matter by the family doctor. Parkinson's disease is now specifically mentioned as one of the diseases which constitute a 'prospective disability' and should be declared once the patient is aware of the diagnosis. Patients over 70 years of age have to apply for renewal of driving licence every 3 years and must declare their condition then, or when applying for driving insurance. Taking drugs such as levodopa or amantadine is not by itself a reason for stopping driving. However, once the patient's actions are significantly slowed by the disease, he should stop driving.

TREATMENT OF MODERATE PARKINSONISM

In moderately disabled patients, particularly those who show bradykinesia and difficulty in self-care, combined treatment with Sinemet or Madopar is now the treatment of first choice. The author tries to explain to patients, particularly at this stage, that treatment by drugs is a matter of their own choice and that there is no such thing as a drug which is fully effective and fully safe from side-effects. Patients should realize that side-effects can be expected as the drug dose is built up, but that a balance is being sought between the best effective dose and the lowest incidence of these side-effects. The aim is not total eradication of all symptoms and signs of Parkinson's disease (although that can sometimes be achieved in fortunate cases). Usually the aim is for a satisfactory control of symptoms and regaining of independence, combined with the least incidence of side-effects which can be achieved. If time is taken to explain this balance, the patient is less likely to have impossibly high expectations of cure.

Now that many general practitioners use Sinemet or Madopar, the patient may often be referred to the specialist because dosage has been started too high, or increased too fast. Commonly the patient may have choreiform or athetoid dyskinetic movements which are thought to be a natural progression of the Parkinson's disease. These results of overdosage are often improved by cutting the daily dose by half. On other occasions the patient may be reported to have become prejudiced against one of the combined preparations after too high a dosage has caused vomiting or dyskinetic movements. The author's policy in these patients is to start again, after explanation, with the alternative combined preparation, building up dosage at an even slower rate than usual.

Another problem which often arises at this stage is the patient who has faith in an older antiparkinsonian preparation such as an anticholinergic, which he has taken for years, but is dissatisfied with his response to it. Fortunately it is not necessary to stop the patient taking an anticholinergic or amantadine, though it might be advisable to reduce the dosage before building up the dose of a combined preparation. It is sometimes important to retain the patient's confidence by keeping him on his old preparation. The only exception to this rule is where the patient is on levodopa, as this must be discontinued, preferably for 12 hours, before a combined preparation is started. It may sometimes be necessary, at a later stage, to simplify any overcomplex drug regime, when the patient is well-settled on the new medication.

A starting dose in the elderly would be Sinemet 110, one tablet once or twice a day, or Madopar 125, one tablet once or twice a day. Dosage should be increased slowly, and stopped at any level where the patient is satisfied with his improvement. It might have been expected that, in a slowly progressive condition, the dose would have to be increased gradually over the months or years. In fact, this is not so, and the majority of physicians find that patients can remain on their chosen dose with benefit for a period of years.

After this period the patient may begin to experience side-effects at a drug level which had previously been satisfactory, such as dyskinetic movements and end-of-dose deterioration, which necessitate very vareful alterations in timing and dosage of drugs. Subsequently the side-effects may re-emerge at lower and lower dosages, and the patient then enters the stage of the disease which requires most skill to achieve any measure of control.

It is probably worth while to keep newer drugs such as bromocriptine (Parlodel) in reserve for this stage when all changes of drug dosage, timing, additional drugs, etc. have been exhausted. Although the place of bromocriptine is not yet fully established, it does seem likely that it is most effective in those patients who were previously responsive to levodopa or its derivatives, as previously discussed, and who suffer from 'on–off' phenomena. Doses should start low, 2·5 mg/day and slowly build up while levodopa can be reduced. Doses ranging from 50–90 mg/day of bromocriptine are quoted by various authors but probably a range of 10–20 mg is more suitable for the old. In view of the side-effects of hallucinations and postural hypotension, bromocriptine is at any rate unlikely to be a very successful drug for use in the elderly.

TREATMENT OF SEVERE OR TERMINAL PARKINSONISM

In severe or terminal patients with Parkinson's disease, the disease has progressed beyond the stage where drugs are effective, but it is still necessary to use every care and skill to ensure that the symptoms of the last months are relieved and that death will be as peaceful and dignified as possible. Many patients and families will value the help of their own clergyman or the hospital chaplain. Sometimes patients are referred to the geriatric physician for the first time at this stage perhaps following a fall or a fracture; they may be very confused and on numerous drugs. Probably the best line of treatment in hospital at this stage is to withdraw all the drugs since some of them (dopa derivatives, tricyclic antidepressants or phenothiazines in particular) may be the cause of the confusion and agitation. After ensuring good general nursing care, fluid intake, bladder and bowel care, it is possible to reassess the patient's true mental and physical state and determine what drug therapy is essential. Sometimes small doses of a combined preparation may lessen rigidity sufficiently to allow the patient to be moved in bed or sat in a chair with less strain on the nursing attendants. Sometimes a change to a different antidepressant (such as L-tryptophan) may improve the mental state if there was paradoxical agitation on the tricyclic compound. Sometimes noisy and restless behaviour will necessitate use of phenothiazines such as Melleril. The slight danger of worsening the Parkinsonism with this drug is worth taking at this stage of the disease.

Patients with severe Parkinson's disease may well be incontinent of urine and need catheterization. The multiple causes of the incontinence may include immobility, confusion, faecal impaction, incomplete bladder emptying and drug effects. Urinary infections often result and are a cause of death more frequently than in the general population.

A number of terminal patients with Parkinsonism present a picture very suggestive of carcinoma of the oesophagus. They are wasted and cachectic, and have dysphagia, which may be caused by deficiency of dopamine in the brainstem control mechanism for swallowing, possibly in the nucleus of the vagus nerve. Studies of oesophageal motility in these patients have, as mentioned earlier, shown abnormal muscular contractions in the lower part of the oesophagus, and a barium swallow examination, if attempted, may show a holdup of the contrast medium. If this complication of Parkinsonism occurs early in the disease it is necessary to investigate by barium studies, oesophagoscopy, etc. to exclude local lesions in the oesophagus which may need treatment. Where this complication occurs in the latest stages of the disease, it is not the author's normal practice to investigate (though treatment with Sinemet or Madopar is sometimes beneficial). Sooner or later the patient will probably have an aspiration bronchopneumonia worsened by poorly acting respiratory muscles. This infection should, in the author's view, be allowed to proceed in terminal Parkinsonism to its natural fatal outcome without antibiotic treatment, but with all full nursing care.

APPENDIX

Further clinical tests – Details

(1) Watch patient walk for 20 feet or so. Observe for armswing, length of stride, appearance on turning.

(2) Time patient signing name and address. Observe for tremor, size of handwriting, slowness. (If written in clinical notes, this information provides a permanent record for later comparison).

(3) Watch patient tapping repeatedly on the back of his other hand.

(4) Watch patient pronating and supinating forearm repeatedly for 20 seconds.

(5) Watch patient touching thumb to each finger of same hand in turn, as fast as possible.

(6) Glabellar tap. Patient blinks when base of nose is tapped gently. Normal patient stops blinking after first few taps, but Parkinsonian patient persists. Not so useful in the elderly as in younger patients, as cerebral arteriosclerosis may also cause a persistent glabellar tap reflex.

(7) Webster timed test[17] (useful to monitor progress). Let patient rise from sitting in a chair (note if helped), walk 15 feet forward, turn around, sit down. Time with stopwatch in seconds, and count the number of steps taken by the patient's right leg during the entire test. These two numbers when multiplied give a value in step-seconds. Normal persons score 50 to 100 step-seconds, early Parkinsonians 100 to 200, moderate cases 200 to 400, and severe cases more than 400 step-seconds.

(8) Webster rating scale. (Time-consuming but useful for research evaluations). Score from 0 (no involvement) to 3 (severe involvement) for each of ten items: bradykinesia of hands, rigidity, posture, armswing, gait, tremor, facies, seborrhoea, speech, self-care.

(9) Ventilatory function by Wright's peak flow-meter may also be a useful means of monitoring response in first weeks of drug treatment[18].

Acknowledgement
The author is grateful to Professor Marsden for permission to use Figures 1 to 4, originally published in a review in *Lancet* (1977) **1**, 345.

References
1 Garland, H. G. (1952). Parkinsonism. *Br. Med. J.*, **1**, 153
2 Brewis, M., Poskanzer, D. C., Rolland, C. and Miller, H. (1962). Neurological disease in an English city. *Acta Neurol. Scand.*, 24 (Suppl.) **42**, 31
3 Kurland, L. T. (1958). In: W. S. Fields (ed.). *Pathogenesis and Treatment of Parkinsonism*, p5. (Springfield, Ill.: Charles C. Thomas)
4 Gudmundsson, K. R. (1967). A clinical survey of Parkinsonism in Iceland. *Acta Neurol. Scand.*, 33 (Suppl.), **43**,
5 *Parkinson's Disease* (1974). Studies of Current Health Problems No. 51. (London: Office of Health Economics)
6 Hoehn, M. M. and Yahr, M. D. (1967). Parkinsonism: onset, progression and mortality. *Neurology*, **17**, 427

7 Harris, A. I. (1971). *Handicapped and Impaired in Great Britain* (London: HMSO)

8 Sweet, R. D. and McDowell, F. H. (1975). Five years treatment of Parkinson's disease with levodopa: therapeutic results and survival of 100 patients. *Ann. Intern. Med.*, **83**, 456

9 Rinne, U. K. (1978). Recent advances in research on Parkinsonism. *Acta Neurol. Scand.*, 67 (Suppl.) **57**, 77

10 Critchley, M. (1929). Arteriosclerotic Parkinsonism. *Brain*, **52**, 23

11 Parkes, J. D., Marsden, C. D., Rees, J. E., Curzon, G., Katamaneni, B. D., Knill-Jones, R., Akbar, A., Das, S., and Kataria, M. (1974). Parkinson's disease, cerebral arteriosclerosis and senile dementia. *Q. J. Med.*, **43**, 49

12 Locket, S. (1957). *Clinical Toxicology.* (London: Kimpton)

13 Smith, J. S., and Brandon, S. (1970). Acute carbon monoxide poisoning – three years' experience in a defined population. *Postgrad. Med. J.*, **46**, 65

14 Parkinson, J. (1817). *An Essay on the Shaking Palsy.* (London: Sherwood, Neely and Jones)

15 Nowack, W. J., Hatelid, J. M. and Sohn, R. S. (1977). Dysphagia in Parkinsonism. *Arch. Neurol.*, **34**, 320

16 Logemann, J. A., Blonsky, E. R. and Boshes, B. (1970). Dysphagia in Parkinsonism. *J. Am. Med. Assoc.* **231**, 69

17 Webster, D. D. (1968). Critical analysis of the disability in Parkinson's disease. *Mod. Treatment*, **5**, 257

18 Mehta, A. D., Wright, W. B. and Kirby, B. J. (1978). Ventilatory function in Parkinson's Disease. *Br. Med. J.*, **1**, 1456

19 Wartenberg, R. (1952). Head-dropping test. *Br. Med. J.*, **1**, 687

20 Hildick-Smith, M. (1976). Assessing dementia in the older Parkinsonian patient. *Mod. Geriatr.*, **6**, 33

21 Hodkinson, H. M. (1972). Evaluation of a mental test score for assessment of mental impairment in the elderly. *Age Ageing*, **1**, 233

22 Greenfield, J. G. and Bosanquet, F. D. (1953). The brainstem lesions in Parkinsonism. *J. Neurol. Neurosurg. Psychiatry*, **16**, 213

23 Pearce, J. M. S. (1978). Actiology and natural history of Parkinson's disease. *Br. Med. J.*, **4**, 1664

24 Ehringer, H. and Hornykiewicz, O. (1960). Verteilung von Noradrenalin und Dopamin im Gehirn des Menschen und ihr Verhalten bei Erkrankungen des extrapyramidalen Systems. *Klin. Wochenschr.*, **38**, 1236

25 Bernheimer, H., Birkmayer, W., Hornykiewicz, O., Jellinger, K. and Seitelberger (1965). Zur Differenzierung des Parkinsön – Syndroms. *Proceedings of 8th International Congress of Neurology*, p. 145 (Vienna: Medical Academy)

26 Birkmayer, W. and Hornykiewicz, O. (1961). Der L-3, 4 dioxyphenylalanin (= DOPA) Effekt bei der Parkinsonakinese. *Wien. Klin. Wochenschr.*, **73**, 787

27 Barbeau, A., Sourkes, T. L. and Murphy, G. F. (1962). Les catecholamines dans la maladie de Parkinsonism. In J. de Ajuriaguerra (ed). *Monoamines et Système Nerveux Centrale*, p. 247. (Paris: Masson)

28 Rinne, U. K., Riekkinen, P., Sonninen, V. and Laaksonen, H. (1973). Brain acetylcholinesterase in Parkinson's disease. *Acta Neurol. Scand.*, **49**, 215

29 Bowen, D. M. and Davison, A. N. (1978). Biochemical changes in the normal ageing brain. In B. Isaacs (ed). *Recent Advances in Geriatric Medicine*, p. 54. (Edinburgh, London and New York: Churchill Livingstone)

30 Lewis, C., Ballinger, B. R. and Presly, A. S. (1978). Trial of levodopa in senile dementia. *Br. Med. J.*, **1**, 550

31 Birkmayer, W., Ambrozi, L., Neumayer, E. and Riederer, P., (1974). Longevity in Parkinson's disease treated with L-dopa. *Clin. Neurol. Neurosurg.*, 1, 15

32 Duvoisin, R. C. (1969), In Crane, G. E. and Gardiner, R. Jr. (eds.). *Psychotropic Drugs and Dysfunction of Basal Ganglia.* p. 134 (Washington: US Public Health Services)

33 Hughes, R. C., Polgar, J. G., Weightman, D. and Walton, J. N. (1971), L-dopa in Parkinsonism – the effects of withdrawal of anticholinergic drugs. *Br. Med. J.*, 2, 487

34 Broe, G. A. and Caird, F. I. (1973). Levodopa for Parkinsonism in elderly and demented patients. *Med. J. Aust.*, 1, 630

35 Caird, F. I. (1974). Parkinsonism. In Anderson W. F. and Judge T. C. (eds.). *Geriatric Medicine*, pp. 171–183 (London and New York: Academic Press)

36 Caird, F. I. and Williamson J. (1978). Drugs for Parkinson's disease. *Lancet*, i, 986

37 Mindham, R. H., Lamb, P. and Bradley, R. (1977). A comparison of piribedil, procyclidine and placebo in the control of phenothiazine-induced Parkinsonism. *Br. J. Psychiatry* 130, 581

38 Schwab, R. S., England, A. C., Poskanzer, D. C. and Young, R. R. (1969). Amantadine in the treatment of Parkinson's disease. *J. Am. Med. Assoc.*, 208, 1168

39 Cotzias, G. C., van Woert, M. H. and Schiffer, L. M. (1967). Aromatic amino-acids and modification of Parkinsonism. *N. Engl. J. Med.*, 276, 374

40 Calne, D. B., Spiers, A. S., Stern, G. M., Lawrence, D. R. and Armitage, P. (1969). L-dopa in idiopathic Parkinsonism. *Lancet*, ii, 973

41 Godwin-Austen, R. B., Tomlinson, E. B., Frears, C. C. and Kok, H. W. L. (1969). Effects of L-dopa in Parkinson's disease. *Lancet*, ii, 165

42 Yahr, M. D., Duvoisin, R. C., Hoehn, M. M., Schear, M. and Barrett, R. E. (1968). L-dopa, its clinical effects in Parkinsonism. *Trans. Am. Neurol. Assoc.*, 93, 56

43 Mawdsley, C. (1970). Treatment of Parkinsonism with Laevodopa. *Br. Med. J.*, 1, 331

44 Jenkins, R. B. and Groh, R. H. (1970). Mental symptoms in Parkinsonian patients treated with L-dopa. *Lancet*, ii, 177

45 Godwin-Austen, R. B., Bergmann, S. and Frears, C. C. (1971b). Effect of age and arteriosclerosis on the response of Parkinsonian patients to levodopa. *Br. Med. J.*, 4, 522

46 Godwin-Austen, R. B., Frears, C. C. and Bergmann, S. (1971a). Incidence of side-effects from levodopa during the introduction of treatment. *Br. Med. J.*, 1, 267

47 Peaston, M. J. T. and Bianchine, J. R. (1970). Metabolic studies and clinical observations during L-dopa treatment of Parkinson's disease. *Br. Med. J.*, 1, 400

48 Leader (1978). Drugs for Parkinson's disease. *Lancet*, i, 754

49 Sutcliffe, R. L. G. (1973). L-dopa therapy in elderly patients with Parkinsonism. *Age Ageing*, 2, 34

50 Vignalou, J. and Beck, H. (1973). La L-dopa chez 122 Parkinsoniens de plus de 70 ans. *Gerontol. Clin.*, 15, 50

51 Hildick-Smith, M. (1973). The patient's view of L-dopa after one year's therapy. *Gerontol. Clin.*, 15, 74

52 Hildick-Smith, M. (1973). Pyridoxine in Parkinsonism. *Lancet*, ii, 1029

53 Hunter, K. R., Hollman, A., Laurence, D. R. and Stern, G. M. (1971), Levodopa in Parkinsonian patients with heart disease. *Lancet*, i, 932

54 Marsden, C. D., Parkes, J. D. and Rees, J. E. (1973). A year's comparison of treatment of patients with Parkinson's disease with levodopa combined with carbidopa versus treatment with levodopa alone. *Lancet*, ii, 1459

55 Cotzias, G. C., Papavasiliou, P. S. and Gellene, R. (1969). Modification of Parkinsonism – chronic treatment with L-dopa. *N. Engl. J. Med.*, **280**, 337

56 Diamond, S. G., Markham, C. H. and Treciokas, L. J. (1978). A double-blind comparison of Levodopa, Madopa and Sinemet in Parkinson's Disease. *Ann. Neurol.*, **3**, 267

57 Korten, J. J., Keyser, A., Joosten, M. G. and Gabreels, F. J. M. (1975). Madopar versus Sinemet. *Eur. Neurol.*, **13**, 65

58 Martin, W. E., Toloso, E. S., Loewenson, R. B., Lee, M. C., Resch, J. A. and Baker, A. B. (1976). Safer drug treatment for patients with Parkinson's disease. *Mod. Geriatr.*, **6**, (no. 2) 11

59 Marsden, C. D., Barry, P. E., Parkes, J. D. and Zilkha, K. J. (1973). Treatment of Parkinson's disease with levodopa combined with L-alpha-methyldopahydrazine, an inhibitor of extracerebral DOPA decarboxylase. *J. Neurol. Neurosurg. Psychiatry*, **36**, 10

60 Critchley, 'E. (1975). L-dopa and carbidopa (sinemet) in the management of Parkinsonism. *Postgrad. Med. J.*, **51**, 619

61 Mars, H. and Krall, J. (1971). L-dopa and cardiac arrhythmias. *N. Engl. J. Med.*, **285**, 1437

62 Calne, D. B., Petrie, A., Rao, S., Reid, J. L. and Vakil, S. D. (1972). Action of L-alpha-methyldopahydrazine on the blood pressure of patients receiving levodopa. *Br. J. Pharmacol.*, **44**, 162

63 Klawans, H. L., Ringel, S. P. and Shenker, D. M. (1971). Failure of vitamin B6 to reverse the L-dopa effect in patients on a dopa decarboxylase inhibitor. *J. Neurol. Neurosurg. Psychiatry.*, **34**, 682

64 Barbeau, A., Mars, H., Botez, M. I. and Joubert, M. (1972). Levodopa combined with peripheral decarboxylase inhibition in Parkinson's disease. *Canad. Med. Assoc. J.*, **106**, 1169

65 Hildick-Smith, M. (1976). Alternatives to levodopa. *Br. Med. J.*, **1**, 1406

66 Hunter, K. R., Laurence, D. R., Shaw, K. M. and Stern, G. M. (1973). Sustained levodopa therapy in Parkinsonism. *Lancet*, ii, 929

67 Barbeau, A. (1976). Six years of high-level levodopa therapy in severely akinetic Parkinsonian patients. *Arch. Neurol.*, **33**, 333

68 Sweet, R. D., and McDowell, F. (1974). The 'on – off' response to chronic L-dopa treatment of Parkinsonism. In McDowell, F. H. and Barbeau, A. (eds.). *Advances in Neurology*, **5**, p. 331. (New York: Raven Press)

69 Marsden, C. D. and Parkes, J. D. (1976). 'On – off' effects in patients with Parkinson's disease on chronic levodopa therapy. *Lancet*, i, 292

70 Yahr, M. D. (1977). Longterm levodopa in Parkinson's disease. *Lancet*, i, 706

71 Calne, D. B., Teychenne, P. F., Claveria, L. E., Eastmann, R., Greenacre, J. K. and Petrie, A. (1974). Bromocriptine in Parkinsonism. *Br. Med. J.*, **4**, 442

72 Kartzinel, R., Teychenne, P., Gillespie, M. M., Perlow, M., Gielen, A. C., Sadowsky, D. A. and Calne, D. B. (1976). Bromocriptine and levodopa (with or without carbidopa) in Parkinsonism. *Lancet*, ii, 272

73 Parkes, J. D., Debono, A. G. and Marsden, C. D. (1976). Bromocriptine in Parkinsonism: longterm treatment, dose response and comparison with levodopa. *J. Neurol. Neurosurg. Psychiatry*, **39**, 1101

74 Marsden, C. D. and Parkes, J. D. (1976). Bromocriptine in Parkinsonism. *Lancet*, ii, 419

75 Wass, J. A. H., Thorner, M. O. and Besser, G. M. (1976). Digital vasospasm with bromocriptine. *Lancet*, **i**, 1135
76 Calne, D. B., Plotkin, C., Williams, A. C., Nutt, J. G., Neophytides, A. and Teychenne, P. F. (1978). Longterm treatment of Parkinsonism with bromocriptine. *Lancet*, **i**, 735
77 Bédard, P., Parkes, J. D. and Marsden, C. D. (1978). Effect of new dopamine-blocking agent (oxiperomide) in drug-induced dyskinesias in Parkinson's disease and spontaneous dyskinesias. *Br. Med. J.*, **1**, 954
78 Birkmayer, W. (1976). Medical treatment of Parkinson's disease: General review, past and present. In Birkmayer, W. and Hornykiewicz, O. (eds). *Advances in Parkinsonism*, pp. 407–424 (Basle: Roche)
79 Quaglieri, C. E. and Celesia, G. G. (1977). Effect of thalamotomy and L-dopa therapy on the speech of Parkinsonian patients. *Eur. Neurol.*, **15**, 34
80 Selby, G. (1976). The influence of previous stereotactic thalamotomy on L-dopa treatment in Parkinson's disease. *Proc. Aust. Assoc. Neurol.*, **13**, 55
81 Greer, M. (1976). How to achieve maximum benefit for the patient with Parkinson's disease. *Geriatrics*, **31**, 89
82 Rampton, D. S. (1977). Hypertensive crisis in a patient given sinemet, metoclopramide and amitryptiline. *Br. Med. J.*, **2**, 607
83 Hausner, R. (1976). Drugs that reduce efficacy of levodopa. *N. Engl. J. Med.*, **295**, 1538
84 Ball, B. (1882). De l'insanité dans la paralysie agitante. *Encéphale*, **2**, 22
85 Loranger, A. W., Goodell, H., McDowell, F. H., Lee, J. E., and Sweet, R. D. (1972). Intellectual impairment in Parkinson's syndrome. *Brain*, **95**, 405
86 Celesia, G. C. and Wannamaker, W. M. (1972). Psychiatric disturbances in Parkinson's disease. *Dis. Nerv. Syst.*, **33**, 577
87 Eadie, M. J. and Sutherland, J. M. (1964). Arteriosclerosis in Parkinsonism. *J. Neurol. Neurosurg. Psychiatry*, **27**, 237
88 Pearce, J. (1974). Mental changes in Parkinsonism. *Br. Med. J.*, **2**, 445
89 Sacks, O. W., Messeloff, C., Schartz, W., Goldfarb, A. and Kohl, M. (1970). Effects of L-dopa in patients with dementia. *Lancet*, **i**, 1231
90 Wolf, S. M. and Davis, R. L. (1973). Permanent dementia in idiopathic Parkinsonism treated with levodopa. *Arch. Neurol.*, **29**, 276
91 Drachman, D. A. and Stahl (1975). Extrapyramidal dementia and levodopa. *Lancet*, **i**, 809
92 Pollock, M. and Hornabrook, R. W. (1966). The prevalence, natural history and dementia of Parkinsonism. *Brain*, **89**, 429
93 Davis, J. C. (1977). Team management of Parkinson's disease. *Am. J. Occup. Ther.*, **31**, (no. 5) 300
94 Hurwitz, L. J. (1964). Improving mobility in severely disabled Parkinsonian patients. *Lancet*, **ii**, 953
95 Singer, E. (1973). Social costs of Parkinson's disease. *J. Chron. Dis.*, **26**, 243
96 Godwin-Austen, R. B. (1971). *Parkinson's Disease*. A booklet for patients and their families, published and distributed by the Parkinson's Disease Society, 81 Queen's Road, London
97 *Parkinson's Disease Day to Day*. A further booklet published by the Parkinson's Disease Society, London

Reviews
Jewesbury, E. C. O. (1970). Parkinsonism. *Br. J. Hosp. Med.*, **4**, 825
Leader (1974). Mental changes in Parkinsonism. *Br. Med. J.*, **2**, 1

Bianchine, J. R. and Sunyapridakul L. (1974). Individualisation of levodopa therapy. *Med. Clin. N. Am.,* **58,** 1071

Davison, W. (1974). Management of Parkinsonism. *Mod. Geriatr.,* **4,** 102

Hornekiewicz, O. (1975). Parkinson's disease and its chemotherapy. *Biochem. Pharmacol.,* **24,** 1061

Barbeau, A. (1975). Longterm assessment of levodopa therapy in Parkinson's disease. *Canad. Med. Assoc. J.,* **112,** 1379

Yahr, M. D. (1975). Levodopa. *Ann. Intern. Med.,* **83,** 677

Calne, D. B. (1976). Developments in the treatment of Parkinsonism. *N. Engl. J. Med.,* **295,** 1433

Bianchine. J. (1976). Drug therapy of Parkinsonism. *N. Engl. J. Med.,* **295,** 814

Leader (1976). Alternatives to levodopa. *Br. Med. J.,* **1,** 1169

Curzon, G. (1977). The biochemistry of the basal ganglia and Parkinson's disease. *Postgrad. Med. J.,* **53,** 719

Godwin-Austen, R. B. (1977). The treatment of Parkinson's disease. *Postgrad. Med. J.,* **53,** 729

Marsden, C. D. and Parkes, J. D. (1977). Success and problems of longterm levodopa therapy in Parkinson's disease. *Lancet,* **i,** 345

Duvoisin, R. C. (1977). Problems in the treatment of Parkinsonism. In Messiha, F. S. and Kenny, A. D. (eds.). *Parkinson's Disease,* pp. 131–149. (New York and London: Plenum Press)

Stern, G. M. and Lees, A. J. (1978). Choice of treatments in Parkinson's disease. *Practitioner,* **219,** 537

Pearce, I, and Pearce, J. M. S. (1978). Bromocriptine in Parkinsonism. *Br. Med. J.,* **1,** 1402

7

Drugs acting on the central nervous system

M. Impallomeni and F. M. Antonini

Drugs acting on the central nervous system (CNS) are the most widely prescribed drugs in this country. This trend is particularly evident in older patients, where diseases affecting the central nervous system are so common.

Gibson and O'Hare in 1968[1] found that 28% of 273 consecutive patients seen at home on behalf of the Glasgow Geriatric Service were on psychotropic drugs. Shaw and Opit in 1976[2] found that about 20% of people over the age of 70 in a Birmingham practice were on long-term treatment with drugs acting on the central nervous system. This finding was confirmed by similar observations by Law and Chalmers in 1976[3]. Williamson in 1978[4] found in a multicentre survey of patients newly admitted to geriatric departments in the United Kingdom that out of 1998 admissions 81·3% were on drug treatment, and 12·5% had adverse drug reactions; the commonest offenders were sedatives, muscle relaxants and anticonvulsants. Learoyd in 1972[5] showed that 16% of all admissions to a psychogeriatric department were due to adverse drug reactions to psychotropic drugs.

Despite the high incidence of side-effects, drugs acting on the central nervous system can greatly improve the quality of life of the older patient. None of these drugs is curative, although a few, such as the antiepileptic drugs, may be life-savers. The great majority provide only symptomatic relief, and may have to be administered for a long period of time as the diseases for which they are used tend to have a rather protracted course in the elderly.

Several types of mental illness occur in old age. Functional disorders such as anxiety and hysteria are not so common, being seen

259

more in the 60–70 age group than in older patients; they tend to improve with advancing age. These patients tend to have a long history of such disorders, usually dating back to their youth, punctuated by improvements and relapses. Depression, on the other hand, is increasingly common with increasing age; the commonest form is reactive. Schizophrenia may present for the first time in old age though this is rare; it usually takes the benign form of paraphrenia. Acute confusional states are particularly common in the elderly and may be precipitated by any disease or drug administration. Dementia is rare before the age of 60. More than half the cases occurring in those over the age of 60 are due to senile or Alzheimer-type dementia while arteriosclerotic or multi-infarct dementia accounts for a small proportion; the remainder are mostly mixed senile and vascular types.

All these mental disorders can be ameliorated with prudent use of psychotropic drugs. As a general guideline most psychotropic drugs are given in doses varying between half and two-thirds of those used for younger patients, spaced at longer intervals and increased more slowly. All these drugs can cause unpleasant side-effects in the elderly, in particular excessive sedation, drowsiness, lethargy or the opposite, restlessness, agitation and severe confusion. At times it may be difficult to judge whether the patient's acute confusional state is due to the physical disease being treated or to the psychotropic drugs being used.

Old people seem to be particularly sensitive to the effect of psychotropic drugs. This is due to changes in drug handling which occur in old age and changes in target organ sensitivity. Standard doses of drugs may cause higher blood levels in the elderly that last longer. This is usually the result of a combination of decreased volume of distribution of drugs following the progressive loss of lean body mass, decreased liver metabolism and urinary excretion.

ANATOMICAL AND BIOCHEMICAL CHANGES IN THE BRAINS OF OLD PEOPLE

In normal old people there is a progressive loss of brain weight with thinning of the gyri and widening of the sulci affecting mainly the frontal and parietal lobes. Histologically, there is an increase of fibrillary astrocytes, with characteristic alterations of nerve cell bodies, including lipofucsin deposition, granulovacuolar degeneration, neurofibrillary tangles and senile plaques. These, most commonly found in the cerebral cortex, the hippocampus and the limbic system, increase steadily with age and are thought to be associated with the deposition of amyloid. There is no convincing evidence that in normal old people there is loss of nervous cells with the exception of Purkinje cells in the cerebellum[6]. There is, however, a progressive loss of neuronal dendritic processes and synapses.

Recently biochemical changes have been shown to occur in the brain of normal old people[7]. There is an accumulation of aluminium in the neurones but the significance is not known. Changes in neurotransmitter metabolism occur with a progressive decrease of catecholamine synthesis, as well as an increase in monoamine oxidase activity in various parts of the brain, including the basal ganglia. The cholinergic neurone system, which is thought to be involved in memory function and in higher mental activity is less affected. Acetylcholine production decreases between the age of 20 and 50, remaining unchanged thereafter. There is however a progressive loss of postsynaptic cholinergic muscarinic receptor sites after the age of 60. This or some other mild, as yet unidentified, defect in the cholinergic system is thought to be the cause of loss of memory in old age.

In senile or Alzheimer-type dementia the same histological changes seen in normal old age occur, but in greater quantity. Specific biochemical changes have been recently demonstrated in this disease in the cerebral cortex. Choline acetyltransferase, an enzyme that synthetizes acetylcholine, and acetylcholinesterase that degrades acetylcholine, have been found consistently decreased[8-10]. This fall parallels the severity of the histological changes, especially senile plaques, and the severity of the intellectual impairment, as measured by a mental test score[11]. The noradrenergic and dopaminergic systems appear to be spared and the gamma-aminobutyric acid (GABA) content does not seem to be affected.

These findings would support a cholinergic hypothesis in senile dementia, attributing the functional impairment to inadequate cholinergic transmission. This would make senile dementia a neurotransmitter deficiency disease similar to Parkinson's disease and Huntington's chorea. As there seems to be no loss of postsynaptic cholinergic receptors in comparison with age-matched control subjects, restoring acetylcholine levels in the brain of senile dementia patients should restore normal mental function. Unfortunately, no safe way of achieving this has yet been found. These findings would explain the clinical observation that drugs with anticholinergic effects may aggravate confusion in patients suffering from senile dementia.

THE ACTION OF PSYCHOTROPIC DRUGS

There are now many drugs capable of altering mood, feeling, behaviour, or level of consciousness (Table 1). Anxiolytic drugs or minor tranquillizers produce sedation when given in small doses, and sleep in larger doses. Minor tranquillizers have general cerebral depressant and anticonvulsant properties; they do not produce extrapyramidal side-effects. On the other hand the neuroleptic drugs or major

Table 1   Psychotropic drugs

1. Anxiolytics, sedatives, hypnotics or minor tranquillizers
   Barbiturates
   Benzodiazepines
   Chloromethiazole
   Chloral hydrate and allied drugs
   Paraldehyde
   Ethyl alcohol
   Carbromal
   Promethazine
   Meprobamate
   Gluthetimide
   Methaqualone
2. Neuroleptics, antipsychotics or major tranquillizers
   Phenothiazines
   Butyrophenones
   Thioxanthines
   Tetrabenazine
3. Antidepressant or thymoleptic drugs
   Monoamine oxidase inhibitors
   Tricyclic and tetracyclic drugs
   Flupenthixol
   Tofenacin
   L-tryptophan
   Lithium
4. Psychostimulants
   Caffeine
   Amphetamines

tranquillizers are more selective, acting mainly on the hypothalamus and reticular activating system. They commonly produce extrapyramidal side-effects. Psychostimulants increase alertness and motivation but are seldom indicated in old age.

ANXIOLYTICS, SEDATIVES, HYPNOTICS OR MINOR TRANQUILLIZERS

Barbiturates

These drugs have been in medical use for over 70 years being first introduced in 1903. They were originally used as hypnotics, later as antiepileptics, and later on as sedatives.

They are rapidly absorbed when administered by mouth. They are mostly metabolized by the liver, and only partly excreted unchanged by the kidney. Phenobarbitone (Luminal) and barbitone (soluble barbitone) have the longest plasma half-life, between 60 and 90 hours. The shorter-acting barbiturates, amylobarbitone (Amytal), pentobarbitone (Nembutal), quinalbarbitone (Seconal), butobarbitone (Soneryl), cyclobarbitone (Rapidal) have a half-life of 30–40 hours. Phenobarbitone is only partly metabolized by the liver and 30% is excreted unchanged by the kidney. The ultra-short acting barbiturates such as thiopenthone (Pentothal) are used for general anaesthesia.

The barbiturates have a limited use in geriatric practice, being safe only for anaesthesia and at times for the control of epilepsy. Old people are particularly intolerant of these drugs[12], often developing restlessness and confusion instead of sedation. Some insight into the problems of short-term administration of barbiturates may be derived from the study by Irvine and colleagues in 1974[13], where it was shown that an oral dose of amylobarbitone produced in elderly people higher plasma levels lasting much longer than in younger people. Chronic intake of barbiturates has been shown to cause a syndrome of impaired mental function, slurred speech, nystagmus and ataxia.

All barbiturates are powerful enzyme inducers; this can cause severe drug interactions, especially dangerous with oral anticoagulant drugs, corticosteroids and tricyclic antidepressants. The plasma levels of some tricyclic antidepressants may be reduced by as much as a half. Prolonged administration of barbiturates may interfere with vitamin D metabolism causing osteomalacia, with folate metabolism causing folate deficiency and rarely megaloblastic anaemia. Alcohol and any other drug which causes depression of the central nervous system have additive depressant effects when given together with barbiturates. Barbiturates may precipitate hypothermia. They are particularly contraindicated in untreated myxoedema and liver failure, where they can precipitate coma. They are also contraindicated in respiratory failure as they depress the respiratory centre, and in porphyria. Their prolonged use may lead to tolerance, due to liver enzyme induction, chemical tolerance at cellular level, and drug dependence. Sudden discontinuation of therapy induces a withdrawal syndrome in which epileptic fits may occur.

Barbiturates are still used by some physicians as sedative/hypnotic drugs in the elderly. Fortunately, the number of prescriptions issued every year for this purpose has been steadily falling at the rate of about 10% a year over the past decade.

Overdose with barbiturates is not commonly seen in the elderly, but may present with barbiturate coma, respiratory depression, hypotension and hypothermia.

Benzodiazepines
These drugs were introduced in medicine in the early 1960s and have quickly become the most widely prescribed of all psychotropic medications. It is claimed that they have a selective effect on that part of the central nervous system which controls emotion, the limbic system, and are the closest to the ideal tranquillizers, reducing anxiety without sedation. Others, however, believe that their central action is similar to that of the barbiturates, but that they have a greater safety margin, as even massive overdoses seldom kill. Recently a specific receptor has been described for diazepam (Valium) in astrocytic cells.

Benzodiazepines do not affect monoamine receptors in the nervous system. They are not effective against psychoses, and have no autonomic or extrapyramidal side-effects. They have anticonvulsant and some central muscle-relaxant effects. This group of drugs includes chlordiazepoxide (Librium), oxazepam (Serenid), diazepam (Valium), medazepam (Nobrium), lorazepam (Ativan), nitrazepam (Mogadon), fluorazepam (Dalmane), temazepam (Normison), clonazepam (Rivotril). Clonazepam is marketed as a broad spectrum antiepileptic, nitrazepam, fluorazepam and temazepam as hypnotics, the others as sedatives, although these drugs are chemically similar and have similar pharmacological actions. Some produce active metabolites – diazepam is a metabolite of medazepam, oxazepam of diazepam – and a number of benzodiazepines produce the same active metabolites; desmethyldiazepam is a common active metabolite of diazepam, medazepam and chlorazepate, which has a long half-life and may attain a higher plasma concentration than the parent drug when this is administered for a prolonged period of time. The metabolites are conjugated to glucuronide and finally excreted by the kidney. With the exception of temazepam the benzodiazepines have a long half-life. Short-term administration of diazepam and chlordiazepoxide was shown to be followed by drowsiness almost twice as commonly in people over the age of 70 as in those under the age of 40[14]. Diazepam has been shown to have a longer half-life in older people[15]. On the other hand nitrazepam was shown to have the same half-life in older as in younger subjects, about 33 hours, but its short-term administration was shown to cause deeper and more prolonged hangover effects in the elderly[16]. Chronic administration of nitrazepam in old age has been shown to cause a syndrome characterized by progressive confusion, lack of initiative and falls[17].

When given as an hypnotic the benzodiazepines have been shown to suppress rapid eye movement (REM) sleep although contrary claims have been made as well. They may also cause vivid nightmares. They may cause hypothermia, and respiratory depression, although this is rare.

There are some conditions, however, in which intravenous diazepam can be safely used in the elderly: as premedication before endoscopy or minor operative procedures, to control sudden bursts of aggressive behaviour in demented or acutely confused elderly patients, and in status epilepticus where it is the drug of choice. A dose of 10 mg is usually sufficient, and this can be repeated after a few minutes if necessary.

Chlormethiazole (Heminevrin)
This drug has a molecular structure similar to vitamin B_1 or thiamine; it is widely used as a sedative and hypnotic in the management of the confused, agitated, restless elderly patient in whom it is claimed to be particularly safe. Chlormethiazole is now thought to be an 'intermediate' tranquilliser, having a potency halfway between the minor and the major tranquillisers. The plasma half-life is short, about 4 hours. It possesses antiepileptic properties, but does not cause extrapyramidal side-effects, nor does it affect blood pressure or the respiratory centre. It is the only tranquillizer that depresses prolactin blood levels, and it is a liver enzyme-inducer.

Side-effects are rare, the most common being a tingling sensation in the nose, sneezing and at times conjunctival irritation. It can, however, cause drowsiness, excessive sedation or even confusion in the elderly, but this is rare if started in small doses and slowly built up. It should not be used in patients already on phenothiazines or butyrophenones whose action it potentiates. It also has an additive effect with barbiturates and alcohol.

Restless patients suffering from acute confusional states, or dementia are usually treated with 250–500 mg three times a day in tablet or capsule preparation. The dose can then be gradually increased until adequate sedation is achieved. The majority of patients are well controlled on this dose, but doses up to 1 g three times a day may have to be used. The hypnotic dose is 0·5–1 mg at night-time. There is also a syrup preparation, but some elderly people find this unpalatable. Chlormethiazole is also available as an aqueous solution for intravenous infusion, at a concentration of 0·8% (8 mg/ml). This is highly effective in status epilepticus, but it is also used in some centres for the treatment of the very agitated, aggressive confused elderly patient. The effect of this infusion is immediate, but it should be administered slowly as too rapid an infusion may produce unconsciousness with even hypotension and respiratory depression. Chlormethiazole is also used in a short course to control acute withdrawal symptoms in alcoholics.

Chloral hydrate and allied drugs mainly used as hypnotics
Chloral hydrate was the first synthetic hypnotic drug to be introduced in medicine (1869). It is rapidly absorbed from the gut and induces sleep in about half an hour with little hangover the following morning. It is rapidly metabolized by the liver, kidneys and red blood cells into trichloroethanol, the active metabolite, which is finally conjugated to glucuronide in the liver. It is only available in suspension form. The dose is 0·5–2 g. This drug is not widely used nowadays because it is too irritant on the gastric mucosa, and may be dangerous in severe renal or liver failure. It also interacts with oral anticoagulants potentiating their effect by displacing them from their binding sites in the plasma proteins.

Dichloralphenazone (Welldorm) is obtained by combining phenazone, a powerful enzyme-inducer, with chloral hydrate, a bond which is split in the liver; it is not irritant on the gastric mucosa. The dose is 650–1300 mg. It is very safe in the elderly, although it can cause skin rashes, and rarely agranulocytosis.

Trichlorophos (Trichloryl) is a stable ester of chloral hydrate which is transformed in the body to trichloroethanol; the dose is 0·5–1·5 g.

Paraldehyde is a cyclical ether which is a very effective sedative/hypnotic drug, and particularly free from side-effects once it reaches the blood. Unfortunately it has a very unpleasant flavour, and is therefore not given by mouth; it is seldom used nowadays. When administered intramuscularly it is painful, sometimes causing sterile abscesses, and it may also dissolve some of the modern disposable plastic syringes. It is partially eliminated by the lungs, but mostly by the liver.

Ethyl alcohol is a naturally occurring drug with pleasant taste, but very addictive when used for prolonged periods of time. It is beneficial as a nightcap, but tolerance occurs rapidly. It is a liver microsomal enzyme-inducer. It potentiates virtually all other cerebral depressant drugs, and may precipitate epileptic fits in predisposed patients. It stimulates diuresis which may counteract the beneficial effects it has as a natural hypnotic.

Carbromal is chemically related to the barbiturates and is combined with pentobarbitone in Carbrital which contains bromine as well. This product is now obsolete.

Promethazine (Phenergan) is a phenothiazine drug mainly used as an antihistamine but sometimes as a hypnotic. The dose is 25 mg at night-time. It is claimed by some to be safe in the elderly, but by others to cause hangover, drowsiness and confusion.

Meprobamate (Equanil, Miltown) was introduced as a tranquillizer about 20 years ago. It is not now thought to be of much value as a daytime tranquillizer; it is, however, a useful and safe hypnotic drug, particularly when there is difficulty in getting off to sleep[12], the dose is 400–800 mg at night. It has a short half-life and seldom causes hangover effects.

Gluthetimide (Doriden) is chemically similar to the barbiturates, with similar pharmacological action and adverse reactions. It is also a powerful enzyme-inducer. Drowsiness and confusion are a common occurrence when given to old people.

Methaqualone in combination with diphenhydramine, an antihistamine (as Mandrax), is a powerful hypnotic drug, and has an action similar to the barbiturates. Confusion is unfortunately particularly common when the drug is given to the elderly.

Management of insomnia
Most old people sleep just as many hours as when they were young, but take more time to fall asleep, wake up more often and take more time to fall asleep again[19]. Some old people sleep shorter hours at night, but generally make this up by taking more naps during the daytime[20]. Consequently old people may underestimate the number of hours slept, mistaking the change of sleep pattern with lack of sleep. Some argue that having a 'snooze' in the afternoon actually decreases the amount of sleep needed at night. It is thus the pattern and not the quantity or quality of sleep that changes in old age. Electrophysiological studies in 'sleep laboratories' have shown that stage 4 sleep is virtually non-existent over the age of 70, and stage 3 much reduced. Rapid eye movement (REM) sleep is not affected by age[19].

Sleeplessness is a complaint which may be due to a number of causes very few of which require treatment with a hypnotic. Thus environmental factors, such as sleeping in a different bed after admission to hospital, or pain, shortness of breath, urinary frequency, anxiety, depression, or hallucinations may cause insomnia. Treatment of the disease causing the symptoms usually makes hypnotic drugs unnecessary.

There are other reasons for reluctance in prescribing hypnotics. Chemically induced sleep is physiologically abnormal; hypnotics alter brain function, most suppress REM sleep, which is thought to be necessary for normal mental health, and dreaming. Hangover is particularly common in the elderly. Accumulation when the next dose is taken before the previous one has been eliminated easily occurs as most hypnotic drugs have a long half-life. Dependence, overdosage and self-poisoning are dangers common to all age groups.

When all treatable causes of insomnia have been excluded, some patients may need a hypnotic drug usually to tide them over a short crisis such as bereavement. The drugs most commonly used in the elderly are chlormethiazole, trimipramine, dichloralphenazone, meprobamate and trichlorophos. However, some physical activity before retiring to bed, and a warm milky drink at night may work just as well as a hypnotic.

MAJOR TRANQUILLIZERS, ANTIPSYCHOTICS OR NEUROLEPTICS

Phenothiazines

Phenothiazines were introduced in medicine just over 25 years ago when chlorpromazine (Largactil) was introduced from France. Their main use in mental illness in old age are:

(1)   To reduce agitation and excessive motor activity in some elderly patients with dementia or toxic confusional states.
(2)   To treat hallucinations and delusions.
(3)   To control anxiety states and psychosomatic disorders; usually low doses are adequate.
(4)   To control psychoses such as schizophrenia which, however, are not very common in old age.

Phenothiazines are also used in non-mental disorders. The effect of analgesic agents can be potentiated and consequently the dose of narcotic drug reduced. Phenothiazines may be helpful in the treatment of nausea and vomiting, persistent hiccup or pruritus.

Chemically phenothiazines have a tricyclic structure similar to some of the antidepressant drugs, but they contain a sulphur atom in the middle ring. They can be subdivided into three groups according to the side-chain on the phenothiazine nucleus (Table 2). They are metabolized in the liver and are enzyme-inducers.

Table 2   Classification of phenothiazines

Group 1	Aliphatic side-chain derivatives (dimethylaminopropyl derivatives) for example chlorpromazine (Largactil), promazine (Sparine).
Group 2	Piperazine derivatives such as fluphenazine (Modecate), perphenazine (Fentazin), trifluperazine (Stelazine), thiopropazate (Dartalan), prochlorperazine (Stemetil), thiethylperazine (Torecan).
Group 3	Piperidine derivatives, for example thioridazine (Melleril), pericyazine (Neulactil).

All phenothiazines have a wide number of actions on neurotransmitters within the central nervous system, blocking dopaminergic, cholinergic, triptaminergic receptors within the system. They also have peripheral alpha-adrenergic blocking properties, as well as antihistamine properties. Groups 1 and 2 have strong alpha-adrenergic blocking properties and weak anticholinergic effects, whereas Group 3 has strong anticholinergic and weak alpha-adrenergic blocking properties. It is the strong anticholinergic action of the piperidine derivatives which is thought to be the reason why Parkinsonian side-effects are seldom seen. Their mode of action is thought to be due to their effect on the brainstem reticular formation, the hypothalamus, and limbic systems, all structures rich in monoamines. Indeed, their tranquillizing qualities and their extrapyramidal side-effects correlate well with their dopamine receptor blocking actions. Two pathways are particularly rich in dopamine: the mesolimbic system ascending from the brainstem to frontal limbic structures, and the nigrostriate pathway that ascends from the substantia nigra to the corpus striatum. The tranquillizing effect is thought to be due to blockade of the first system, and extrapyramidal complications to blockade of the second.

The adverse side-effects of phenothiazines on the central nervous system are mainly due to their interference with monaminergic transmission[21]. Extrapyramidal syndromes are often seen when these drugs are given in large doses for the long-term treatment of diseases such as schizophrenia. Some authorities believe that the dosage is inadequate until some mild extrapyramidal side-effects are seen. Parkinsonism is especially common with piperazine and aliphatic side-chain phenothiazines. This does not respond to L-dopa as the dopaminergic receptors are blocked, but is easily controlled by anticholinergic drugs, such as orphenadrine (Disipal), 50–100 mg t.d.s. Dystonic reactions involving the trunk, neck and limbs may occur and respond to withdrawal of the drug and administration of antihistamine medications, such as orphenadrine. Late or tardive dyskinesias, which are focal choreiform movements of the face, tongue, lips with lip-smacking and grimacing may occur after prolonged phenothiazine treatment. Treatment is by stopping the drug and giving tetrabenazine (Nitoman) or thiopropazate (Dartalan), but results may be disappointing. Akathisia or motor restlessness may be seen.

Phenothiazines may cause confusion, drowsiness, or even profound unconsciousness. They can precipitate epileptic fits and potentiate all other cerebral depressant drugs, including alcohol. Hypothermia may occur due to their effect on the thermoregulating centres and inhibition of piloerection and shivering. Dopaminergic blockade increases prolactin blood levels and may cause gynecomastia. Depression may occur with prolonged administration of phenothiazines but it is very rare.

Due to their alpha-receptor blocking and anticholinergic effects, phenothiazines can cause postural hypotension due to peripheral pooling of blood; but tachycardia, constipation, and dryness of the mouth may also occur.

Phenothiazines have other side-effects. Lens and corneal opacities are seen mainly with chlorpromazine, while pigmentary changes in the retina occur mainly due to thioridazine. These changes occur when the drugs are given in very high dosages for long periods of time, but they are fortunately fairly rare. Skin rashes sometimes develop; cholestatic jaundice is particularly associated with the use of chlorpromazine, the chlorine in the molecule being thought to be responsible. Phenothiazines may have a quinidine-like action on the myocardium with ECG changes.

Chlorpromazine (Largactil) is a very powerful tranquillizer and has a strong sedative effect. Some physicians consider this the drug of choice in old patients, but others believe that its capacity to cause excessive sedation, drowsiness and hypotension make it unsuitable for its regular use. If it is used it is advisable to start with small doses such as 10–25 mg orally as tablets or elixir, three times a day, and to increase the dose slowly. It can be given intramuscularly in the very acutely disturbed patient. Seldom more than 300–400 mg/day are necessary.

Dose for dose promazine (Sparine) has one-third the potency of chlorpromazine, and causes less sedation and hypotension than chlorpromazine. It has no hepatotoxicity. For these reasons it is preferred to chlorpromazine by a large number of physicians dealing with the elderly. Initial dose is 25–50 mg orally, as tablets or suspension, three times a day; there is also a parenteral preparation. The dose can be gradually built up until the required effect is achieved.

Weight for weight thioridazine (Melleril) has two-thirds the potency of chlorpromazine. It has few extrapyramidal and hypotensive side-effects, causes less sedative effects, but it has a strong atropine-like action. It is considered by a number of geriatricians as the drug of choice in the elderly. Initial dose is 10–25 mg as tablets or syrup three times a day; an extra 50 mg can be added at night-time in those patients in whom the confusion is worse at night. The dose is then gradually increased until adequate sedation is achieved. It is seldom necessary to give more than 300 mg/day, but doses up to 800–1000 mg can be safely given; such high doses if given for a prolonged period of time may be associated with the eye changes already described.

Drugs of the piperazine group have no special advantage over the other two groups in the treatment of the agitated elderly patient with dementia or acute confusional state. Some can, however, be very useful in some specific situations.

Fluphenazine decanoate (Modecate) was first introduced as a depot injection for the control of schizophrenia in patients unwilling to take oral therapy with shorter-acting drugs. In the elderly, besides the treatment of schizophrenia, this preparation can be used to control physically fit but agitated and confused patients suffering from dementia. Here 12·5 mg every 3–4 weeks, roughly half the dose used in younger patients, is usually sufficient. The most common complication is Parkinsonism, but some old patients may also go off their feet, and have frequent falls even without excessive sedation.

Thiopropazate (Dartalan) is at times used for dyskinesias which are relieved by the development of extrapyramidal rigidity induced by that drug. Prochlorperazine (Stemetil), trifluoperazine (Stelazine), thiethylperazine (Torecan) are widely used as antiemetic drugs. They are effective in controlling vertigo of Ménière's disease and other labyrinthine disorders, but are not usually effective in controlling giddiness of non-labyrinthine origin so often seen in old age. They very consistently produce Parkinsonian rigidity. Pericyazine (Neulactil) recommended for character disorders in younger patients does not appear to be superior to other phenothiazines in old patients.

Other major tranquillizers
Butyrophenones have pharmacological actions very similar to those of the phenothiazines, but lack alpha-adrenolitic and anticholinergic effects. They do not cause postural hypotension. Extrapyramidal complications are however relatively common such as dystonia and Parkinsonism, which respond to orphenadrine. Butyrophenones are said to be less likely to cause sedation and drowsiness than the phenothiazines. They are more popular among psychiatrists dealing with the elderly than among geriatricians.

Haloperidol (Serenace) is given as 0·5 g orally three times a day for the relief of anxiety and tension, and 1–3 mg three times a day for severely agitated patients. Larger doses can be given, up to 10 mg three times a day plus 30 mg at night in emergency situations such as sudden outbursts of violent behaviour[22]. This drug is very effective in the control of schizophrenia and in manic psychosis. The liquid oral preparation is odourless and tasteless and can be added to drinks or food.

Trifluperidol (Triperidol), benperidol (Anquil) belong to the same group. Benperidol has been used to treat antisocial behaviour. However, depression may occur after prolonged therapy with these drugs.

Thioxanthines are chemically and pharmacologically similar to the phenothiazines with comparable therapeutic effect and adverse drug reactions. Chlorprothixene (Taractan) is comparable to chlorpromazine in its action but is said to have moderate antidepressant properties as well. Flupenthixol decanoate (Depixol) 20–40 mg intramuscularly every 3–4 weeks has similar indications to fluphenazine. In smaller doses this drug has been used as a mild antidepressant.

Tetrabenazine (Nitoman) resembles reserpine in its mode of action causing depletion of monoamines (noradrenaline, dopamine, 5HT) in the central nervous system. Although it has tranquillizing properties, its main use is for Huntington's and senile chorea, and dyskinesias. Its recommended dose is 12·5 mg b.d. orally, increasing by 25 mg/day every third day up to a maximum of 200 mg/day. Adverse effects include drowsiness, confusion, depression and Parkinsonism.

ANTIDEPRESSANT DRUGS

Depression is the most common form of mental illness in the elderly, its prevalence rising with increasing age. Modern antidepressant drugs have revolutionized the management of this disease in recent years. But like any other psychotropic drug, the use of these drugs is beset by a high incidence of adverse drug reactions.

Neurotransmitters and depression
The limbic system which is mainly associated with emotional behaviour is particularly rich in two monoamines, noradrenaline and serotonin. These amines have been found to be consistently decreased in the brains of depressed patients[23]. The elderly brain shows a progressive loss of monoamines with increasing age which may account for the high prevalence of depression in old age.

Reserpine depletes central nervous system stores of monoamines, and often leads to depression. This can be reversed by L-dopa or L-tryptophan which replete such stores, by monoamine oxidase inhibitors (MAOI) or tricyclic antidepressants which increase the amount of monoamines available at the nerve terminals. Methyldopa, by inhibiting the synthesis of noradrenaline, often produces depression.

Monoamine oxidase inhibitors (MAOI)
These drugs introduced in the late 1950s were the first really effective agents for the treatment of depression. They antagonize the action of monoamine oxidase, the enzyme widely distributed in the brain which causes intracellular degradation of noradrenaline, adrenaline, dopamine and 5-hydroxytriptamine (5HT), thus increasing the concentration of monoamines within the brain. Their action on mood takes 2–4 weeks to become manifest. This effect persists for 2–3 weeks after discontinuation of therapy.

MAOI are divided in two groups: hydrazines which include iproniazid (Marsilid), isocarboxazid (Marplan), phenelzine (Nardil), nialamide (Niamid); and non-hydrazines, such as pargyline (Eutonyl), tranylcypromine (Parnate). They have gradually gone out of fashion because of the frequency of adverse drug reactions and they are no longer marketed in some countries. Tranylcypromine 10–30 mg/day in divided doses is the only drug still in some use in this country. This drug also possesses direct stimulant effect, similar to amphetamine, and can cause insomnia; the last dose should not be given later than early afternoon. It has a quicker onset of action than other MAOI drugs, but its efficacy as a true antidepressant is unpredictable.

MAOI may cause two types of adverse reaction. The first is due to interaction with other drugs. When patients on MAOI treatment take substances such as ephedrine, amphetamines, and tyramine, which release noradrenaline from its stores in adrenergic nerve ter-

minals, severe hypertensive crises resembling those of phaeochro-
mocytoma may occur. Ephedrine is a common ingredient of cough
mixtures that can be bought over the counter, while tyramine is
found in foods such as cheese, beer, wines, yeast products and game.
These hypertensive crises should be treated with α- and β-blockers,
such as phentolamine and propanolol. Patients on MAOI should be
given specific diet instructions.

Central nervous system depressants and alcohol are potentiated
by MAOI. Pethidine in the usual therapeutic doses can cause severe
respiratory depression, and at times even coma. This is due to inhibition of liver enzymes that desmethylate pethidine. The same may
occur with other narcotic drugs.

Tricyclic antidepressants in combination with MAOI[24] may cause
agitation, psychotic episodes and more rarely epileptic fits and
coma. Some centres however have successfully used them in conjunction for the treatment of some cases of severe depression.

The metabolism of sulphonylureas is decreased so that hypoglycaemia may occur in the diabetic patient previously well stabilized
on these drugs. Increased sensitivity to insulin may also occur.

Secondly, there are the reactions due to the drugs themselves.
Atropine-like side-effects cause constipation, dry mouth, retention of
urine and postural hypotension. Water retention, oedema and
epileptic fits may develop, while hydrazine drugs can cause serious
hepatocellular damage.

Tricyclic antidepressants
These are the drugs of first choice in the treatment of depression in
the elderly. They were originally synthesized through a chance
discovery during the development of phenothiazines, which they
resemble chemically. They are thought to act by inhibiting the reuptake of monoamines from the synaptic cleft into adrenergic nerve
terminals, so prolonging their effect on the receptor sites. Other
actions may, however, be responsible for their effect on mood, as
experimental inhibition of monoamines reuptake can be shown to
occur within an hour or two of administration, whilst their effect on
depressed mood does not become clinically manifest for 10–15 days
after commencement of therapy. When given by mouth tricyclic
drugs are readily absorbed and rapidly attain high levels in the
brain. These drugs prolong and potentiate the pressor effects of
ingested or injected directly acting sympathomimetics; hypertensive
crises have been observed especially following local anaesthesia in
oral surgery. Ephedrine and tyramine do not cause hypertensive
crises as stores of monoamines are not increased. Tricyclic antide-

pressants block the neuronal uptake of some adrenergic blocking drugs, such as guanetidine (Ismelin), bethanidine (Esbatal) and debrisoquine (Declinax), interfering with their hypotensive action. They also have anticholinergic, antiserotonin, and antihistamine effects.

The standard tricyclic antidepressant drugs are imipramine (Berkomine, Tofranil) and amitriptyline (Tryptizol, Domical) which have been shown to be superior to placebo in the treatment of depression by a large number of double-blind trials. All the more recently introduced antidepressant drugs have been compared to either amitriptyline or imipramine for reference, but have not been found to be consistently superior to them although they may have fewer side-effects.

Both imipramine and amitriptyline are desmethylated in the liver to active metabolites, desipramine and nortriptyline, which can attain plasma levels higher than the parent drug. Desipramine and nortriptyline are in fact available as separate drugs (desipramine = Pertofran, nortriptyline = Aventyl). They are bound to plasma and tissue proteins, and are slowly eliminated from the body. Steady state occurs after about 10 days and it takes approximately a similar period of time for these drugs to be completely eliminated. For this reason imipramine, desipramine, amitriptyline and nortriptyline can be given as a once-daily dose. Once steady state has been reached, plasma levels are a good guide to therapy as it has been shown that giving the same dose to elderly patients, matched for age, weight and sex, can produce plasma levels with a 10-fold difference from toxic to subtherapeutic. Optimum effect occurs with intermediate plasma levels[25] since at low levels the concentration of the drug in the brain is inadequate, while at high levels the therapeutic action may be neutralized by its atropine-like effect, the onset of an acute confusional state or ataxia. Even at high plasma levels some patients remain depressed without any clinical signs of overmedication[26]. Under and overtreatment are very difficult to distinguish clinically. If monitoring of plasma levels becomes routine, then it would be advantageous to use desipramine or nortriptyline, as only one substance would need to be measured.

Tricyclics can be clinically divided into those with mainly sedative action, such as amitriptyline, trimipramine, and doxepin, which are useful when agitation and anxiety accompany depression; those with mainly stimulant action such as imipramine, nortriptyline and protriptyline, useful in the apathetic and withdrawn patient; and the remainder which are 'neutral' in effect. Chemically tricyclics can be divided into four groups (Table 3).

Table 3 Classification of tricyclic drugs

---

1. Imidodibenzyl subgroup of the dibenzazepines, for example imipramine (Berkomine, Tofranil), desipramine (Pertofran), trimipramine Surmontil), iprindole (Prondol).
2. Dibenzocycleheptones – for example amitriptyline (Tryptizol, Domical) nortriptyline (Aventyl), protriptyline (Concordin)
3. Dibenzoxepines – for example doxepin (Sinequan)
4. Dibenzothiepines – for example dothiepine (Prothiaden)

Adverse effects to tricyclics are unfortunately common, including drowsiness, ataxia with falls, confusion, agitation and insomnia. They may precipitate strokes and cause epileptic fits. The autonomic side-effects are mainly due to the anticholinergic properties and include constipation, retention of urine, tachycardia, postural hypotension.

The cardiovascular side-effects include fluid retention with oedema, precipitation of cardiac failure, tachycardia, dysrhythmias, ECG changes with ST segment and T wave depression, prolongation of QT interval, and sudden death in patients with cardiac disease. Other adverse drug reactions include skin rashes, photosensitization, nausea, vomiting, gynecomastia, bone marrow depression, increased ADH secretion. They may also cause hypothermia and precipitate myxoedema coma.

Tricyclics interact with other drugs in addition to antihypertensive drugs, MAOI, and directly acting sympathomimetics. They generally enhance cerebral depression due to alcohol, tranquillizers, and other depressants. They can decrease the effectiveness of antiepileptic medication, while the effect of anticholinergic drugs is potentiated to the extent that paralytic ileus may occur. Tricyclics potentiate the pharmacological effect of L-dopa in Parkinson's disease and if these are given together cardiac dysrhythmias and postural hypotension may develop. Oral anticoagulants may be potentiated through inhibition of enzymes involved in their metabolism.

Treatment of depression in the elderly should therefore be commenced in small doses, increasing at weekly intervals according to the therapeutic effect. The commonly used tricyclic drugs such as imipramine, amitriptyline are started in dosages of 30–75 mg/day, and slowly increased up to 150 mg/day, according to the patient's response. Sudden cessation of therapy with tricyclic drugs may unleash a withdrawal syndrome within one or two days with nausea, vomiting, diarrhoea, fatigue, muscle pains. They should be restarted and tapered off over a period of 2–4 weeks.

Non-tricyclic drugs

Tetracyclic compounds have a similar pharmacological action to the tricyclics, inhibiting the reuptake of monoamines in the adrenergic nerve terminal. They may cause the same adverse drug reactions but have fewer atropine-like side-effects. Benzoctamine (Tacitin) is given in an oral dose of 10–20 mg three times a day. It has a sedative effect. Maprotiline (Ludiomil) is chemically similar to benzoctamine, but the dose is 75–100 mg/day orally and is said to act more rapidly. Unfortunately epileptic fits are more likely to occur than with other antidepressants. Mianserin (Bolvidon) is used in an oral dose of 10–20 mg three times a day, and is said to possess 5-hydroxytryptamine (5HT) receptor-blocking activity. It causes sedation, and can affect glucose metabolism and decompensate diabetes mellitus. Viloxazine (Vivalan), 100–150 mg in divided doses, lacks sedative effect and is said not to be potentiated by alcohol. It has anticonvulsant properties, and also inhibits enzymes that metabolize phenytoin which may precipitate phenytoin toxicity. Unfortunately it can cause gastrointestinal side-effects, such as nausea and vomiting. It is entirely excreted unchanged in the urine.

Other antidepressant drugs

Flupenthixol (Fluanxol), a thioxanthine drug, is given in an oral dose of 0·5 mg/day in the morning, and in the early afternoon, increasing the dose by 0·5 mg/day up to 3 mg. This drug is said to have a rapid onset of action; if depression has not been relieved within 7 days it should be discontinued. Since it may cause insomnia, the last dose should not be given after 4.0 pm. At this low dosage it seldom causes Parkinsonism. No drug interaction has been reported with tricyclic antidepressants.

Tofenacin (Elamol), a derivative of orphenadrine, is given in a dose of 80 mg twice a day. It is said to be effective in mild or moderate depression, but it should not be administered in conjunction with other antidepressants. It has anticholinergic properties.

L-Tryptophan (Optimax, Pacitron) is an essential aminoacid which is a precursor of serotonin. It is marketed in tablet and powder form. The daily dosage is 6 g/day for 4 weeks then 4 g/day. L-Tryptophan preparations usually contain pyridoxine in order to avoid pyridoxine deficiency. Pyridoxine is, however, a coenzyme of dopa decarboxylase and when given to patients on L-dopa it increases the breakdown of this drug with loss of control of Parkinson's disease. Preparations without pyridoxine are available on the market for this situation. Side-effects are few, but nausea and drowsiness may occur. The value of L-tryptophan in the treatment of depression is still controversial.

Lithium is not strictly speaking an antidepressant, but is used for the treatment and prophylaxis of manic depressive disease. Plasma levels should be monitored, as overtreatment may cause tremor, diarrhoea, vomiting, polyuria and polydipsia, confusion, fits, or coma. The therapeutic range is 0·8–1·2 mmol/l. Lithium calms manic patients, and maintains mood at a normal level for as long as it is taken. Its mechanism of action is only partly understood, but it appears to act through interfering with neurotransmitter metabolism. Diuretics can decrease renal clearance of lithium; it can cause nephrogenic diabetes insipidus. Hypothyroidism with goitre is a well-known complication.

Management of depression in the elderly
There are several causes of depression in old age. The most common form encountered is reactive, resulting from a reaction to environmental adversities to which elderly people living alone are particularly prone. The problems which may gradually sap the old person's self-confidence and capacity to enjoy life, include loss of social status following retirement, loss of social contacts, isolation, loneliness, chronic incapacitating diseases, bereavement, or a new severe disease. Endogenous depression which occurs with little relationship to external factors is much less common. Depression may also be a manifestation of an organic disease, such as myxoedema, thyrotoxicosis, hypercalcaemia, or a viral infection, especially influenza. It may also be iatrogenic, caused by the prolonged administration of some drugs such as tranquillizers, methyldopa, some β-blockers, reserpine and corticosteroids.

All depressed patients should receive a full medical examination after a careful medical and social history has been taken. This may reveal an organic cause which usually responds to treatment of the precipitating disease or discontinuation of the drug responsible. If the patient suffers from a reactive depression, the first step should be to try to manipulate the patient's environment in order to make it less hostile by providing adequate moral support and those supporting services that may help the patient to lead an independent and meaningful life. Social contacts should be stimulated by encouraging the patient to attend social day centres and luncheon clubs.

If depression persists despite these measures and endangers the patient's life, or if he suffers from endogenous depression, it is reasonable to try antidepressant drugs. Imipramine, desipramine, amitriptyline, nortriptyline are the drugs most commonly used in these circumstances, and do indeed bring relief to a great number of these patients. Anxious, depressed patients may require the addition of a tranquillizer especially if they are agitated and have hallucinations and delusions. Some, however, do not respond while others develop drug reactions requiring discontinuation of therapy. Bereaved patients respond worse than the others; one is often left to wonder whether the loss of a spouse can be satisfactorily replaced by an antidepressant tablet.

Minor forms of depression can be treated at home, but drug compliance is particularly unreliable in these patients, and there is also a higher than average risk of self-poisoning. These patients require frequent visits and close monitoring by doctors and nurses. No more than 1 week's supply should be issued at a time.

Severe depression is better treated in hospital in a psychiatric ward. If the history of depression goes back only a few months the chances of a good recovery without relapses are good. In these patients treatment should continue for 3–6 months, and then be tapered off over a period of 2–3 months. If depression goes back a year or more the prognosis is less good and the chances of relapses are higher; it is probably advisable to continue the antidepressant drugs indefinitely. If depression does not respond to treatment within 1–2 months, or the number and severity of side-effects are intolerable, electroconvulsive therapy (ECT) should be considered. This is usually given twice a week up to a total of between four and eight sessions. Electroconvulsive therapy is the most effective form of treatment for depression with often dramatic improvements of mood even in very old patients. Some memory loss for recent events may follow ECT, but this usually clears within 1–3 months.

ANTIEPILEPTIC DRUGS

Idiopathic epilepsy is decidedly rare in old age, and mainly occurs in patients whose disease started earlier in life, and have carried it into their old age. Epilepsy due to a clearly definable pathology is a relatively common occurrence. Cerebrovascular accidents are the commonest cause, followed by other intracranial diseases such as cerebral tumours, subdural haematomas, and posthead trauma cerebral scars. Epilepsy is also a recognized feature of senile dementia, while generalized convulsions may occur in severe myxoedema as well as in hypocalcaemia, hyponatraemia, hypoglycaemia, and

Stokes–Adams crisis. Epileptic fits may be precipitated by stress, alcohol, and a variety of drugs such as phenothiazines, tricyclic antidepressants, or corticosteroids. The most common form in old age is Jacksonian or focal epilepsy, which may spread to a generalized tonic–clonic fit. Generalized convulsions not preceded by focal phenomena, such as an aura or localized tonic–clonic contractions, occur less commonly in old age. The two forms of epilepsy may be difficult to differentiate because of the retrograde amnesia that these patients suffer, and the absence of witnesses to the fit.

Until recently, epilepsy was generally treated with a cocktail of drugs, in the belief that their therapeutic effects were additive, but their toxic effects were not. The reverse has been shown to be true, the number of side-effects increasing with the number of drugs used. It has been shown that when a single drug is correctly used, by monitoring its plasma level and keeping it within the therapeutic range, 95% of patients do not need the addition of a second drug[28]. A good correlation has been found between plasma and brain concentrations of phenobarbitone and phenytoin in patients undergoing temporal lobectomy for Temporal lobe epilepsy. The aim of antiepileptic therapy is to achieve and maintain a steady, adequate brain level of the drug being used. This is achieved by maintaining an adequate plasma level of the drug, administering it at intervals of at least one plasma half-life. After the initial dose, the daily dose should be slowly adjusted on clinical grounds, until cessation of fits or onset of side-effects. Once steady state is achieved the plasma level should be measured and the dose adjusted accordingly. It is more important to become familiar with the therapeutic plasma range and the plasma half-life than with a fixed recommended dosage of antiepileptic drugs, as the dose required will greatly vary from patient to patient. The therapeutic plasma range should be considered in a fairly elastic manner, balancing maximal antiepileptic effect with tolerable side-effects. Patients with mild forms of epilepsy may, however, be controlled with serum levels below the therapeutic range.

Phenobarbitone is the oldest of all antiepileptic drugs, having been used to treat epilepsy since 1912, and is still the most widely prescribed. Phenobarbitone has a plasma half-life of 3–6 days in the elderly; it is slowly metabolized in the liver, but some 30% is excreted unchanged by the kidney. It may take up to 30 days to achieve constant plasma levels. It should be given in a single dose at night-time, starting with 60 mg; seldom more than 90 mg/day are required. The therapeutic plasma concentration is 40–100 μmol/l (10–25 μg/ml).

Its mode of action is unknown although it is probably through its generally depressant effect on nerve cell membranes. It is effective in the treatment of grand mal epilepsy and also in suppressing the focus itself in focal epilepsy. It has also been claimed that phenobarbitone increases the brain level of serotonin and of catecholamines, and inhibits the uptake of calcium in the neurones, all facts which may contribute in stabilizing the cell membrane of the affected neurones. The main drawback is that phenobarbitone has a strong sedative action and may at times cause confusion in old age. Its dose should be reduced in liver and renal failure. It is a strong liver enzyme-inducer, and may increase the rate of its own metabolism, as well as that of other drugs and chemicals. Folate and vitamin D deficiency may occur, as during phenytoin treatment.

Primidone (Mysoline) is not widely used nowadays because it is partly metabolized in the body into phenobarbitone which makes the establishment and monitoring of therapeutic plasma ranges very difficult.

Diphenylhydantoin (Epanutin) was introduced in the treatment of epilepsy in 1938, and is still one of the most popular antiepileptic drugs. It is considered by some as the drug of choice in grand mal epilepsy. It cannot, however, suppress the focus itself in focal epilepsy, although it stops the spread of a focal fit to other areas of the brain. It probably works through its membrane stabilizing properties on the neurones, an effect seen on other tissues as well, such as the heart, hence its use to treat some cardiac dysrhythmias. Its antiepileptic effect has also been attributed to its capacity to elevate serotonin and catecholamine brain levels, and to decrease the metabolism of gamma-aminobutyric acid (GABA).

Half the administered dose is hydroxylated in the liver to an inert form. Its plasma half-life is about 30 hours, and administration should be once daily. The plasma half-life is much longer in a small proportion of people who have a genetically determined enzyme defect. The plasma therapeutic range is 40–80 μmol/l (10–20 μg/ml). The initial dose is 150–200 mg/day; the daily dose is slowly increased until seizure control, or the appearance of signs of toxicity. Plasma concentrations should be measured 2–4 weeks after beginning treatment, and the dose adjusted accordingly. The signs of toxicity most commonly encountered are cerebellar and lethargy. As a rough guideline, nystagmus is said to occur with serum levels of over 100 μmol/l, ataxia and dysarthria over 120 μmol/l, lethargy at serum levels over 160 μmol/l[24]. The dose of phenytoin should be reduced in liver failure. In renal failure phenytoin is less protein-bound and should be given in smaller amounts. Phenytoin is a powerful enzyme-inducer.

Folate deficiency is found in up to 50% of patients on phenytoin, but megaloblastic anaemia seldom occurs. This deficiency may be due to malabsorption of folic acid, or induction of enzymes that metabolize folic acid, or increased consumption of folate-containing coenzymes, necessary for the hydroxylation of phenytoin. The administration of folic acid may cause loss of control of epilepsy as more phenytoin will be metabolized. Osteomalacia may occur through the increased breakdown of vitamin D caused by phenytoin enzyme induction. Gum hypertrophy is rare in the elderly, as it does not occur in the edentulous. Systemic lupus erythematosus (SLE), and a Hodgkin type of lymphoma may occur, but are extremely rare.

Other hydantoins seldom used are methoin (Mesontoin) which is more toxic than phenytoin, and ethotoin (Peganone) which is less effective.

Carbamazepine (Tegretol) is considered by some to be as powerful as phenobarbitone and phenytoin in grand mal epilepsy, and more powerful in focal epilepsy, and to have fewer side-effects than any other antiepileptic drug. It has a structure that three-dimensionally resembles phenytoin, although two-dimensionally is more similar to the tricyclic antidepressants. Its mode of action is unknown. It has a short half-life and requires a twice daily administration. The initial dose is 100 mg b.d. which can be slowly increased up to 800–1200 mg/day. The therapeutic plasma concentration is 15–50 μmol/l (4–12 μg/ml). It is a powerful enzyme-inducer. It is also effective in the treatment of tabetic pains, as well as in trigeminal neuralgia. Side-effects encountered in the elderly are sedation and hyponatraemia, and less commonly diplopia; an erythematous skin rash may also occur. Bone marrow depression and agranulocytosis are rare complications. Carbamazepine may become the drug of first choice in the treatment of epilepsy in old age. It has also been claimed to improve mood and behaviour, but this is likely to be a consequence of changing from barbiturates or other drugs with more sedative effect.

Sodium valproate (Epilim) has been recently introduced from France. It is a two-chain fatty acid. Its mode of action is thought to be inhibition of GABA metabolism, thus increasing the concentration of this inhibitory neurotransmitter in the brain. Its half-life is short, requiring a twice-daily administration. Initial dose is 200 mg b.d., increasing the daily dose by 200 mg/day every 3 days up to a maximum dose of 2400 mg/day. Plasma levels should not exceed 200 μg/ml. It has few side-effects, but reversible hair loss and thrombocytopenia have been described. Tremor may occur at high dosage but is usually controlled by dose reduction. Abnormalities of liver function have been reported in some patients on this drug. It is a liver microsomal enzyme-inducer. It is effective in grand mal and focal epilepsy, but probably not as powerful as the previously described drugs.

A number of benzodiazepine drugs have anticonvulsant properties, and are used for the treatment of several types of epilepsy. They are not generally used in the elderly, for they commonly cause adverse drug reactions in this age group. Intravenous diazepam (Valium) is the only exception as it is the drug of choice in status epilepticus.

Sulthiame (Ospolot), a sulphonamide derivative, is said to work mainly through inhibition of the metabolism of other antiepileptic drugs concurrently administered. It is not much used nowadays as it is generally deemed preferable to increase the dose of just the one antiepileptic drug the patient is taking if fits persist, instead of adding an extra drug.

Phenacemide, now obsolete, and pheneturide (Benuride) are seldom used as intolerance is common. Pheneturide inhibits phenytoin metabolism.

Succinimides are not effective in major and focal epilepsies although useful in petit mal and myoclonic epilepsies.

General principles in the management of epilepsy
The onset of epilepsy in old age requires full investigation to exclude curable pathology. An adequate history, clinical examination, including a detailed inspection of the fundi, blood tests including blood urea, electrolytes, plasma calcium, phosphorus, alkaline phosphatase, blood glucose, thyroid function tests and skull x-ray, EEG, brain scan, CAT scan; ECG to exclude heart pathology are all necessary.

Although some patients can be successfully treated by neurosurgical procedures, control of metabolic disorders or withdrawal of certain drugs, a large proportion of patients require long-term antiepileptic drugs. The majority suffer from cerebrovascular disease. The patient should be closely followed and a careful record made of the occurrence and number of fits. Precipitating factors such as stress, alcohol, or drugs should be identified and avoided. The aim of treatment is to fully control attacks with the smallest dose of any one drug. The daily dose should be increased every 3–4 days for the rapidly acting drugs, and every week for the slow acting ones, as maximum effect may take time to develop. When fits occur infrequently, dose adjustments are clearly difficult. After steady state of plasma concentration is reached, plasma levels should be checked and the dose adjusted accordingly. It may take up to 3 months to evaluate the value of a drug and if after this time the convulsive fits are not controlled, a new drug should only then be tried. An adequate dose of a new drug must be given before discontinuing the previous drug as there is a real risk of precipitating status epilepticus on sudden discontinuation of any antiepileptic drugs. The patient's drug compliance must be carefully assessed; this is a common problem in epileptic patients, as at least 40% of outpatients fail to take all the tablets recommended[29]. If the patient is confused, suffers from dementia, or is forgetful, a younger person, either a relative or a district nurse, should be put in charge of the medication. Evaluation of plasma levels will also give some guide to the patient's drug compliance. Therapy should be continued for at least 2 years after the last recorded fit. During this time periodical checks are carried out, usually every 3–4 months, to assess the drug plasma level, haematological status, to detect folate deficiency and vitamin D status. At the end of the 2 years, the drug should be gradually tapered off over a period of weeks.

For patients suffering from depression as well as epilepsy, one should ensure that both antidepressant and antiepileptic drugs are given in adequate doses, checking their plasma levels at regular intervals. Problems may occur when phenytoin is used, as some tricyclic drugs can elevate phenytoin plasma levels through enzyme inhibition. Maprotyline should be avoided as it is the most epileptogenic of all antidepressant drugs. Viloxazine may be of use in this situation, as it possesses antiepileptic activity.

Status epilepticus
Status epilepticus is a medical emergency, and should be terminated as quickly as possible. The risk of permanent brain damage through hypoxia, or even death, is very high. There are many drugs which are highly effective in such a situation. In the elderly, intravenous diazepam is the drug of first choice, usually given as a slow i/v injection of 10 mg. Larger doses may be necessary at times, and can be given by intravenous drip up to several hundred mg in 24 hours, but this is seldom necessary. Intravenous diazepam carries the risk of respiratory depression and hypotension; this seems to occur mainly when other drugs such as phenobarbitone had been given previously. Phenobarbitone 200 mg intramuscularly used to be very commonly given but its onset of action is too slow, and in the

elderly it may cause respiratory depression. Phenytoin 100–200 mg by intravenous injection is rapidly effective in arresting status epilepticus. Phenytoin given intramuscularly is not well absorbed and is too irritant. Paraldehyde 2–8 ml intramuscularly used to be very popular in this situation; it has, however, the disadvantages already described, and is more safely given as an intravenous injection after dilution.

If all else fails, chlormethiazole should be tried, 30–50 ml of chlormethiazole 0·8% aqueous solution (8 mg/ml) should be set up as an infusion and administered at a rate of 4 ml/min (60 drops), until the fits are terminated. It should then be decreased to 10–15 drops/min, the drip rate and the amount given depending on the patient's response. During this period the patient should be kept under close observation, as temporary hypotension and respiratory depression may occur, especially if the patient has previously received phenobarbitone. In this situation, an oral airway tube may be necessary, or more rarely assisted respiration. Mild thrombophlebitis at the site of injection is very common. Some authorities use chlormethiazole as the drug of first choice in status epilepticus. In the very rare patient who does not respond to any of the above procedures, it may be necessary to give intravenous anaesthetics and curare to terminate the episode. The cooperation of the anaesthetist is necessary as artificial respiration must be instituted. Once the acute episode is controlled, phenytoin 200 mg or phenobarbitone 90 mg should be administered parenterally to prevent recurrences.

NARCOTIC ANALGESICS AND RELATED DRUGS

Dependence-producing analgesic drugs have been used for medical purposes longer than any other. Some occur naturally, some are synthetic. Their use is regulated in the United Kingdom by a number of Acts, the last of which is the Misuse of Drugs Act 1971.

Physiology of pain
Pain is perceived by specific receptors which are free nerve endings found in most but not all tissues of the body. They originate from nerve cells in the sensory ganglia; these cells send nerve fibres that relay with other nerve cells in the substantia gelatinosa and posterior grey horn of the spinal chord. From these neurones ascending fibres reach the ventroposterior and intralaminar nuclei of the contralateral thalamus, via the lateral spinothalamic tract. Painful stimuli reach the brainstem reticular formation via side branches of

the spinothalamic tract and via the spinoreticular tract. The intrala-minar nuclei send their axons to various areas of the cortex, which relay information to the limbic system. Descending pathways from these higher centres reach the posterior horn and substantia gelatin-osa in the spinal chord.

Pain sensation is carried in the posterior or sensory root by two types of fibres: A delta, relatively large, fast conducting, and C fibres, much thinner, slow conducting. Painful stimuli carried in the A delta fibres can inhibit further transmission of pain sensation carried in the C fibres; stimuli carried in the C fibres enhance fur-ther transmission of pain sensation carried both in the A and C fibres. Diseases of the peripheral nervous system affect large fibres more than small ones with loss of moderation of C fibres pain. This is thought to be the mechanism of the severe pain often encountered in herpes zoster and other peripheral neuropathies.

It is now considered that the sensation of pain is perceived at a subcortical level, probably in the thalamus. The intensity of the sensation of pain perceived is thought to be regulated by the physio-logical state of the substantia gelatinosa which is considered to act· as a 'gate' to painful stimuli. This gate can be opened or shut by stimuli coming from higher centres in the central nervous system, or from peripheral nerves.

Recent research has shown that specific neurotransmitters and synaptic receptor sites exist in the pain pathways in the central nervous system. These neurotransmitters are peptides of which at least three have been identified, leucine and methionine enkephalins, which contain five aminoacids, and beta-endorphin, which is a 31 amino acid peptide, and is probably a precursor of methionine enke-phalin. These substances are inhibitory neurotransmitters which are thought to dampen pain sensation by binding to specific receptor sites in physiological conditions. Narcotic analgesics are now thought to act by binding to the same receptors.

From the practical point of view there are two types of pain: that arising from somatic structures, skin, muscles, bone and joints, which is sharp, well localized and usually controllable with non-narcotic drugs, and visceral pain, poorly localized, dull, seldom adequately controlled by non-narcotic drugs. Pain is only a symp-tom of an underlying disease, at times the only symptom. To relieve it before a diagnosis is made and an adequate plan of treatment is established may endanger the patient's life. Analgesic drugs are not necessarily the best treatment for pain; thus anginal pain is better treated with vasodilators, psychogenic pain with tranquillizers or antidepressants, gout with colchicine (Colbenemid). Analgesics are indicated either for temporary relief as the underlying disease is being treated, or for the long-term relief of pain in incurable diseases such as inoperable cancer. Pain sensation, like most other sensations, is decreased in normal old age; the mechanism is not well understood. About three-quarters of elderly patients with acute myocardial infarctions present without pain. Burns, skeletal fractures, perforations of hollow viscera, peritonitis may not give rise to pain in old age which can cause serious diagnostic difficulties. Some people, however, do retain normal pain sensation into their old age.

Pharmacology of narcotic analgesics
These drugs (Table 4) have a number of effects in various tissues of the body. They both depress and excite the central nervous system.

Table 4 Narcotic analgesics

(1) Naturally occuring		Morphine
(2) Synthetic	(a)	With a 5-ring structure: diamorphine (heroin)
	(b)	Morphinans: have a 4-ring structure, one of the morphine rings having been opened: levorphanol (Dromoran)
	(c)	Benzmorphans, which possess a 3-ring molecule, a further morphine ring having been opened: phenazocine (Narphen), pentazocine (Fortral)
	(d)	Pethidine group: 2-ring drugs: pethidine (Meperidine), phenoperidine (Operidine), fentanyl (Sublimaze)
	(e)	Methadone group: methadone (Amidone, Physeptone) dextromoramide (Palfium), dextropropoxyphene (Depronol SA)

They produce analgesia in the ways already described, but also alter the patient's emotional response to pain by inducing relaxation, sleepiness and a sense of euphoria. In some patients, however, they may produce a sensation of malaise and dysphoria. Depression of the respiratory centre and the cough reflex may occur; the capacity to do so parallels the analgesic effect. They may stimulate the third nerve nucleus causing miosis, and the vagal nuclei causing sweating and bradycardia. They may cause nausea and vomiting through stimulation of the chemoreceptor trigger zone. Spinal reflexes become brisker and convulsions may be precipitated. They may cause an increase in intracranial pressure. Hypotension may be produced by depression of ganglionic function. They increase smooth muscle tone and may cause spasm of the sphincter of Oddi, constipation, and retention of urine. They may release histamine, cause pruritus and urticaria. Physical dependence may occur after only 48 hours of regular administration leading to a withdrawal syndrome of tremor, confusion and agitation if the drug is suddenly stopped. These drugs are generally metabolized by the liver, and therefore contraindicated in liver failure. They are contraindicated in hypothyroidism where they may precipitate coma. Their action is potentiated by alcohol, sedative drugs especially phenothiazines and barbiturates, monoamine oxidase inhibitors. When given to elderly people narcotic analgesics may cause drowsiness, confusion, hallucinations. The reasons are not fully understood, but Chan in 1975[30] showed that giving the same dose of pethidine to young and old people the latter developed higher blood levels which lasted longer. Confusion and drowsiness are less likely to occur if smaller doses are used to begin with and these are increased more slowly.

Naturally occuring opium derivatives
Opium is a powder obtained from the seed head of the opium poppy. It contains a number of alkaloids, the most important being morphine, codeine, and papaverine, the latter having no analgesic properties.

Morphine has a five-ring phenanthrene structure. It possesses all the actions already described. It is slowly absorbed when given by mouth but acts within 15 min when given intramuscularly or subcutaneously. Its analgesic effect lasts 4–6 hours. This drug is also used in elixirs with cocaine, and sometimes chlorpromazine (Brompton cocktails). Initial dose: 10–15 mg 4 hourly.

Papaveretum (Omnopon) is a mixture of purified soluble opium alkaloids in the same proportions in which they occur in opium (50% morphine). It is available in tablets and injections. It has no advantages over morphine.

Codeine (methylmorphine) has an analgesic potency one-fourth to one-fifth that of morphine. It is non narcotic, dependence seldom occuring. It causes too much constipation in analgesic doses to be useful in clinical practice on its own. Small doses of codeine, however, greatly potentiate the analgesic effect of other drugs. It is mainly used in the treatment of somatic pain in combination with aspirin: codis which contains aspirin 500 mg and codeine phosphate 8 mg per tablet and compound codeine tablets BP containing phenacetin 250 mg, aspirin 250 mg, codeine phosphate 8 mg. Codeine is also used for the treatment of diarrhoea, and for suppression of cough.

Synthetic narcotic analgesics

Diamorphine or heroin is chemically diacetylmorphine. This drug causes more analgesia and euphoria than morphine, and less hypotension, nausea, vomiting and constipation. It is more addictive than morphine, and for this reason its use is illegal in the United States of America. It is better absorbed by mouth than morphine. Dose is 5–10 mg orally or parenterally, and its duration of action is 4–6 hours. Heroin is also used in elixirs containing cocaine, and at times chlorpromazine (Brompton cocktails).

Dihydrocodeine (DF118) has an analgesic power halfway between codeine and morphine. It causes less respiratory depression and sedation, but more constipation than morphine. It is a cough depressant. Dose is 30 mg 4–6 hourly by mouth or parenterally. Although it is not a narcotic drug, the injection is a controlled drug.

Levorphanol (Dromoran) causes less drowsiness, nausea and constipation than morphine, but the advantage is minimal. It is well absorbed by mouth; the dose is 1·5–2 mg either orally or parenterally given 6–8 hourly.

Phenazocine (Narphen) is weight for weight more powerful than morphine. Its principal advantage is that it does not contract the sphincter of Oddi. The dose is 5 mg 4–6 hourly by mouth; 500 μg – 3 mg intramuscularly 4–6 hourly up to a maximum of 12 mg/day.

Pentazocine (Fortral) originally developed as a narcotic antagonist, can cause a withdrawal syndrome when given to narcotic addicts. It is not a controlled drug. It is unreliably absorbed when given by mouth. A 50 mg dose of oral pentazocine is less powerful than two tablets of Codis[31]. It can cause hallucinations and vivid unpleasant dreams[32]. It increases pulmonary and systemic arterial pressure, and therefore is not recommendable for use in myocardial infarction. The dose is 30–60 mg intramuscularly or intravenously 4–6 hourly.

The pethidine group of drugs generally have fewer side-effects than morphine. Their duration of action is short. Pethidine (Meperidine, Demerol) causes less sedation, euphoria, respiratory depression, nausea and vomiting than morphine, but is also less powerful. It is a very useful analgesic, once claimed to have spasmolytic effects which have never been substantiated. It does not cause miosis. Absorption is unreliable by mouth, and the recommended dose is 1 mg/kg body weight 6 hourly either intramuscularly or intravenously.

Phenoperidine (Operidine) and fentanyl (Sublimaze) are two powerful analgesics that belong to this group. They are short-acting, and mainly used together with a butyrophenone for the induction of neuroleptanalgesia, a kind of 'twilight state' used for short minor surgical procedures. Respiratory depression may however occur. This usually responds to nalorphine intravenously.

The methadone group of drugs only remotely resemble morphine chemically. Methadone (Amidone, Physeptone) is well absorbed when given by mouth; it is less sedative than morphine and causes less respiratory depression and euphoria. It has a longer half-life than morphine. The dose is 5–10 mg orally or subcutaneously 8 hourly. Dextromoramide (Palfium) has a shorter half-life and is a milder analgesic. The dose is 5–10 mg 4 hourly orally or parenterally. Dextropropoxyphene is a non-narcotic analgesic chemically related to methadone, but with less analgesic effect. Preparations containing dextropropoxyphene alone (Depronal SA, Doloxene) are not as popular as those in which this drug is combined with other analgesic drugs such as distalgesic (dextropropoxyphene and paracetamol). Side-effects are rare but do occur. Dependence and overdosage have been described.

Narcotic antagonists
Nalorphine (Lethidrone), levallorphan (Lorfan), naloxone (Narcan) are structurally similar to morphine, and possess mild analgesic properties. They specifically counteract the respiratory depressant effect of most narcotic drugs, but the first two drugs have a respiratory depressant effect of their own. They should not be used as analeptics in respiratory depression due to non-narcotic drugs, which would be made worse. They can cause thought and mood disorders and hallucinations. Naloxone is the drug of first choice as it is a pure antagonist. It is the only one effective against pentazocine as well. The dose is 0·4–1·2 mg intramuscularly or intravenously, repeated every few hours if necessary. The dose of nalorphine is 5–10 mg intramuscularly or intravenously repeated after 10–15 min if the response is not satisfactory. The dose of levallorphan is 0·2–1·0 mg intravenously or intramuscularly.

Indications for narcotic analgesic drugs
The management of acute pain in the elderly varies little from that of younger patients. Narcotic analgesics are likely to be required for the short-term management of some patients suffering from fractures or other injuries, and of most patients following major surgery. They should be given for as short a period as possible, as the main objective of treatment is early mobilization in order to prevent the

catastrophic complications of bed rest and excessive sedation. Morphine 10 mg intramuscularly 4–6 hourly, or diamorphine 5 mg generally prove adequate in these circumstances.

In myocardial infarction the drug of choice is diamorphine 5 mg intravenously, as this drug is less likely to cause hypotension, nausea and vomiting than morphine. It effectively relieves the anxiety which so often complicates painful myocardial infarction, and greatly reduces dyspnoea which may occur if the patient develops pulmonary oedema.

Patients with chronic pain due to advanced and inoperable cancer should be given the benefit and comfort of the powerful analgesia obtainable with narcotic drugs. Dependence and addiction are not a problem in these patients, but tolerance may develop and may require the administration of increasingly larger doses of such drugs.

Pain due to bone metastasis may respond to radiotherapy. Severe headache due to intracranial secondaries may respond to large doses of corticosteroids, such as dexamethasone 4 mg 6 hourly. Pain in terminal illness may produce depression but this is seldom seen if the euphoriant Brompton cocktail is used.

The dose of analgesic drugs should be adjusted to each individual patient, and should provide complete relief of pain for at least 4 hours. This is obtained by gradually increasing the dose until the patient is free from pain. The frequency of administration should be at such intervals that the next dose is given before the pain recurs, preventing it not just suppressing it. The anxiety due to anticipating the pain may be relieved using this simple technique.

Oral preparations are used for as long as possible, usually until the last few days of life, when parenteral preparations may be needed. Methadone may be quite satisfactory, but morphine and diamorphine are more widely used because of their euphoriant effect. They can be given in the form of elixirs which contain cocaine and alcohol as well (the Brompton cocktails). Heroin and cocaine mixtures seem to be the most effective preparations; the starting dose contains diamorphine 5 mg and cocaine 5 mg, and is given 4–6 hourly, according to the patient's needs. The dose is adjusted up as necessary and antiemetic drugs such as chlorpromazine may be added. Constipation often occurs in terminal illness and should be treated with bulk purgatives, stool softeners and bowel stimulants.

Adequate control of pain in terminal illness is one of the most important services a doctor can provide for his patients, and requires a combination of skills, commonsense and humanity. Every human being should be allowed to conclude his life free from pain and preserving his dignity. His needs, though, are greater than just adequate medication: companionship, affection, sensitive under-standing, adequate supporting care either in hospital or at home are equally if not more important than drugs.

ANTIEMETIC DRUGS

Vomiting is produced by the activity of the emetic centre in the brain stem. This can be stimulated by the cerebral cortex when this is activated by the perception of unpleasant smells, or by unpleasant sights, or thoughts, by the vestibular nuclei as in motion sickness and Ménière's disease, by increased intracranial pressure, or by sti-muli from intrathoracic or abdominal viscera. It can also be ac-tivated by the chemoreceptor trigger zone (CTZ) which lies nearby in the floor of the fourth ventricle. This trigger zone may be stimulated by drugs, such as morphine, oestrogens, or by endogenous chemicals such as in uraemia, terminal cancer, diabetic ketoacidosis, after irradiation. Phenothiazines are effective in CTZ-mediated vomiting. Anticholinergic and some antihistamine drugs suppress vomiting from any cause as they depress the activity of the emetic centre. Antihistamine drugs include dimenhydrate (Dramamine), given in a dose of 50–100 mg three times daily or promethazine hydrochloride (Phenergan) in a dose of 25 mg two to three times a day. Both drugs may cause sleepiness. Phenothiazines used as antiemetics include chlorpromazine (Largactil) 25 mg up to three times a day, cyclizine (Marzine) 50 mg t.d.s., prochlorperazine (Stemetil) 5–10 mg b.d., thiethylperazine (Torecan) 10 mg b.d.

Metoclopramide (Maxolon, Primperan), chemically similar to procainamide, has both central and peripheral actions. It depresses the chemoreceptor trigger zone, and accelerates gastric emptying by increasing peristalsis and relaxing pyloric and duodenal smooth muscle. It has extrapyramidal side-effects similar to the phenothiazines[33]. It can be given orally, intramuscularly or in-travenously at a dose of 10 mg up to three times a day. It is con-traindicated in carcinoma of the breast as it produces a release of prolactin from the pituitary gland.

MUSCLE-RELAXANT DRUGS

Muscle spasticity due to lesions of the upper motor neurone, or pyramidal tract, is a frequent problem in elderly patients, mainly in those suffering from the consequences of cerebrovascular disease.

When present it prolongs and hinders the rehabilitation of the patient.

Many drugs are advertised as effective in controlling this type of increased muscle tone. Mephenesin (Myanesin) is considered to act by depressing polysynaptic reflexes in the spinal chord. Diazepam (Valium) has been claimed to decrease muscle tone by increasing presynaptic inhibition in the spinal chord. Dantrolene (Dantrium), a hydantoin drug, is thought to have a direct effect on voluntary muscles, while baclophen (Lioresal), a derivative of GABA, has a general depressant action on spinal chord neurones. However, many geriatricians consider that muscle-relaxant drugs have not proved as beneficial as these claims might have suggested. Doses that decrease muscle tone generally cause too many side-effects, especially sedation and confusion. Unfortunately we do not have at present any muscle-relaxant drugs of real clinical value for the treatment of spasticity in the elderly.

References

1 Gibson, I. I. J. M. and O'Hare, M. M. (1968). Prescription of drugs for old people at home. *Gerontol. Clin.*, **10**, 271
2 Shaw, S. M. and Opit, L. J. (1976). Need for supervision in the elderly receiving long-term prescribed medication. *Br. Med. J.*, **1**, 505
3 Law, R. and Chalmers, C. (1976). Medicines and elderly people: a general practice survey. *Br. Med. J.*, **1**, 565
4 Williamson, J., (1978). Principles of drug action and usage. *Recent Advances in Geriatric Medicine, 110.* (Edinburgh: Churchill, Livingstone)
5 Learoyd, B. M. (1972). Psychotropic drugs and the elderly patient. *Med. J. Aust.*, **1**, 1131
6 Corsellis, J. A. N. (1976). Ageing and the dementias. In W. Blackwood and J. A. N. Corsellis. *Greenfield's Neuropathology*, 796–848. (London: Arnold)
7 Davison, A. N. (1978). Biochemical aspects of the ageing brain. *Age Ageing*, 7, Supplement, 4
8 Davies, P. and Maloney, A. J. F., (1976). Selective loss of central cholinergic neurons in Alzheimer's disease. *Lancet*, **ii**, 1403
9 Perry, E. K., Perry, R. H., Blessed, G. and Tomlinson, B. E. (1977). Necropsy evidence of central cholinergic deficits in senile dementia. *Lancet*, **i**, 189
10 White, P., Hiley, C. R., Goodbardt, M. J., Carrasco, L. H., Keet, J. P., William, I. E. I. and Bowen, D. M. (1977). Neocortical cholinergic neurones in elderly people. *Lancet*, **i**, 668
11 Perry, E. K., Tomlinson, B. E., Blessed, G., Bergman, K., Gibson, P. H. and Perry, R. H. (1978). Correlation of cholinergic abnormalities with senile plaques and mental test scores in senile dementia. *Br. Med. J.*, **2**, 1457
12 Exton-Smith, A. N. (1965). Tranquillizers and sedatives in old age. *Prescribers' J.*, **5**, 49
13 Irvine, R. E., Grove, J., Toseland, P. A. and Trounce, J. R. (1974). The effect of age on the hydroxylation of amylobarbitone sodium in man. *Br. J. Clin. Pharmacol.*, **1**, 41

14 Boston collaborative drug surveillance program (1973). Clinical depression of the central nervous system due to diazepam and chlordiazepoxide in relation to cigarette smoking and age. *N. Engl. J. Med.*, **288,** 277

15 Klotz, U., Avant, G. R., Hoyumpa, A., Schenker, S. and Wilkinson, G. R. (1975). The effects of age and liver disease on the disposition and elimination of diazepam in adult man. *J. Clin. Invest.*, **55,** 347

16 Castleden, C. M., George, C. F., Marcer, D. and Hallett, C. (1977). Increased sensitivity to nitrazepam in old age. *Br. Med. J.*, **1,** 10

17 Grimley-Evans, J. and Jarvis, E. H. (1972). Nitrazepam and the elderly. *Br. Med. J.*, **4,** 487

18 Majundar, S. K., Shaw, G. K. and Thomson, A. D. (1978). Effect of chlormethiazole on serum prolactin. *Br. Med. J.*, **2,** 1266

19 Herbert, M. (1978). Studies of sleep in the elderly. *Age Ageing,* **7,** Supplement, 41

20 Gerard., P., Collins, K. J., Dore, C. and Exton-Smith, A. N. (1978). Subjective characteristics of sleep in the elderly. *Age Ageing,* **7,** Supplement, 55

21 Davison, W. (1978). Neurological and mental disturbances due to drugs. *Age Ageing,* **7,** Supplement, 119

22 Silverman, G. (1977). Management of the elderly agitated demented patient. *Br. Med. J.*, **2,** 318

23 Williamson, J. (1978). Depression in the elderly. *Age Ageing,* **7,** Supplement, 35

24 Stockley, I. (1977). Drug Interactions and Their Mechanisms. (London: Pharmaceutical Press) 55–63

25 Carr, A. C. and Hobson, R. P. (1977). High serum concentrations of antidepressants in elderly patients. *Br. Med. J.*, **2,** 1151

26 Montgomery, S. A., Braithwaite, R. A. and Crammer, J. L. (1977). Routine nortriptyline levels in the treatment of depression. *Br. Med. J.*, **2,** 166

27 Montgomery, S. A., McAuley, R., Rani, S. J., Montgomery, D. B., Braithwaite, R. and Dawling, S. (1979). Amitriptyline plasma concentration and clinical response. *Br. Med. J.*, **1,** 230

28 Reynold, E. H. (1978). How do anticonvulsants work? *Br. J. Hosp. Med.*, **19,** 505

29 Richens, A. (1978). Choice of drugs in epilepsy. *Prescribers' J.*, **18,** 125

30 Chan, M. J., Kendall, M. J., Mitchard, M., Wells, W. D. E. and Vickers, M. D. (1975). The effect of ageing on plasma pethidine concentrations. *Br. J. Clin. Pharmacol.*, **2,** 297

31 Twycross, R. G. (1978). Relief of pain in advanced cancer. *Prescribers' J.*, **18,** 117

32 Taylor, M., Galloway, D. B., Petrie, J. C., Davidson, J. F., Gallon, S. C. and Moir, D. C. (1978). Psychomimetic effects of pentazocine and dihydrocodeine tartrate. *Br. Med. J.*, **2,** 1198

33 Nimmo, W. S. (1977). Metoclopramide. *Prescribers' J.*, **17,** 90

8

Cerebral activating drugs

D. E. Hyams

INTRODUCTION

The term 'cerebral activating drugs' is used for the title of this chapter as a convenient way to embrace a wide variety of drugs which have been used in attempts to improve cerebral function in old age. Such drugs include vasodilators, drugs influencing cerebral metabolism, stimulants and drugs which are claimed to improve the flow of blood in the cerebral microcirculation by virtue of actions on blood viscosity, red cell deformability, or one or more biochemical effects at the cellular level.

Many of these drugs are collectively known as 'vasoactive drugs'. Some also have more general metabolic effects – such as on blood lipids or fibrinolysis and/or effects on platelet function.

Many drugs formerly advocated as vasodilators have been shown to have one or more of these other properties in addition to their vasodilating capabilities, as the emphasis has shifted away from the feasibility or safety of cerebral vasodilatation and towards metabolic effects in brain and blood, including those which may alter the physical properties of the blood itself.

CEREBRAL BLOOD FLOW (CBF)

General considerations
Blood flow depends on perfusion pressure and vascular resistance, but in normal circumstances the cerebral circulation is protected from reflecting systemic arterial pressure changes; this phenomenon of *autoregulation* depends on an intrinsic mechanism within the vascular smooth muscle, influenced to some extent by autonomic

295

neurogenic influences. Although that might suggest a role for drugs which influence autonomic nervous function, it appears that the threshold for such drug effects on the cerebral circulation is much higher than that for the peripheral circulation[1]; thus, peripheral vasodilators are unlikely to have much influence on intracerebral circulation unless they drop the systemic aterial pressure to undesirably low levels, when autoregulation is overcome but hypotension is then a clinical problem.

Vascular resistance
(a) *Structural changes in cerebral blood vessels with ageing* The blood vessels of the cerebral circulation (intracerebral and extracerebral, including the microcirculation) show structural changes in old age which increase with each decade from 55 years onwards[2].
(b) *Cerebral vascular tone* This is controlled by interacting metabolic influences, mainly CO_2 tension of arterial blood (PCO_2); but PO_2 and concentrations of hydrogen, potassium, magnesium and calcium ions and adenosine levels may also play important roles.

Physical properties of the blood
Blood viscosity in disease states has attracted much interest recently[3]. Patients with raised haematocrit may have low mean CBF[4] and decreased cortical CBF[5]; in each of these studies the CBF increased after the haematocrit was reduced by venesection. In the microcirculation, blood viscosity depends mainly on plasma viscosity (largely influenced by fibrinogen levels) and erythrocyte flexibility[3,6].

Red cell membrane flexibility depends largely on the concentration of adenosine triphosphate (ATP) in the erythrocytes[7]: ATP-depleted erythrocytes are more rigid than normal[8] and their passage through the microcirculation may be markedly impaired[9]. ATP modulates calcium-ion concentrations, but other influences include pH, PO_2 and PCO_2[6,10]. The viscosity of the intracellular contents is mainly determined by the state of the haemoglobin[6]. An exciting therapeutic possibility is to find drugs which increase erythrocyte flexibility. Some of the drugs discussed below may be able to achieve this, but the evidence is still equivocal.

Cerebral blood flow in old age

Normal old age
In normal old age CBF and autoregulation show no significant change from younger ages[11], and there is evidence to suggest that cerebral functional reserve is normal during ageing[12].

Disease states in old age

(a) *Diseases associated with raised haematocrit* Older patients are less able to maintain CBF when blood viscosity is raised due to increased haematocrit[4].

(b) *Dementia* It is increasingly important to recognize two main types of dementia – that due to cerebrovascular disease (multi-infarct dementia, MID)[13] and that due to primary neuronal degeneration (PND, 'senile dementia') often, though not invariably, of Alzheimer-type (SDAT)[14]. The evidence suggests that cerebrovascular disease may lead to reduced CBF, whereas the lesser decrease of CBF found in PND or SDAT is compensatory to reduced metabolic need[15,16]. However, in both types of dementia autoregulation is normal[15].

The concept of 'cerebral arteriosclerosis' as a diagnosis to explain mental deterioration in old age has been severely criticized[13], but the same group subsequently conceded that attempts to increase blood supply to underperfused but viable areas of brain are worth exploring[16]. Restoration of function has been demonstrated in ischaemic neurons in cats[17] and an optimistic view appears justified[18].

(c) *Transient ischaemic attacks (TIAs)* These attacks are common in old age[19]. Transient changes in rCBF and autoregulation occur[20]. Following carotid endarterectomy, CBF may not change[21] or may increase independently of improvement in cerebral function[22]. Management is based on the likelihood of a subsequent cerebral infarction: about one-third of patients with TIAs will have a stroke within 5 years[23], the risk increasing with age. In patients unsuitable for surgery, the mainstay of treatment has hitherto been anticoagulant therapy[24]. Treatment with vasoactive drugs has occasionally been advocated[25,26], but today interest is focused largely on drugs influencing platelet function, notably aspirin[27,28].

(d) *Focal neurological disease* It is difficult to forecast the effects of vasoactive drugs on rCBF in patients with focal cerebrovascular disease; deleterious effects may occur[29], although local increases in perfusion were seen after injection of a xanthine derivative, papaverine-like drugs and low molecular weight dextran[29].

(e) *Acute strokes* An ischaemic lesion causes widespread reduction in CBF but an area of hyperaemia develops around the ischaemic zone ('luxury perfusion'[30]) and autoregulation is lost. Vasoactive drugs may be harmful in this situation: if a fall in systemic blood pressure occurs, a dangerous reduction in CBF could follow, possibly involving areas far removed from the original lesion; or an 'intracerebral steal' phenomenon[31] may occur. However, a more aggressive approach has been advocated with selective use of such drugs, provided that rCBF measurements are available for monitoring and conditions are carefully controlled[32].

CEREBRAL METABOLISM IN OLD AGE

Normal old age

There is little or no fall in the cerebral metabolic rate for oxygen ($CMRO_2$) in old age, but cerebral glucose consumption may be significantly reduced[11]. Some vasoactive drugs are claimed to increase $CMRO_2$ and cerebral glucose uptake, as well as increasing CBF.

A decreased supply of oxygen or glucose to the brain may lead to depletion of ATP and other energy-rich compounds which have multiple essential roles in cerebral functioning. Both ATP and cyclic adenosine monophosphate (cAMP) may influence the calibre of cerebral arteries[33,34], and cyclic nucleotides may be involved in memory processes[35]. There is evidence in rats that cAMP levels decrease in the cerebral cortex with ageing[36], although the activities of those enzymes which determine cAMP levels are apparently unchanged[37]. Other enzymes do show changed activities; these, and changes in neurotransmitter metabolism, have been the subject of much recent attention[38-41]. Further details will be considered later in this chapter.

Dementia

There is good evidence of reduced cerebral oxygen uptake in dementia and $CMRO_2$ is inversely related to the degree of dementia. In arteriosclerotic elderly subjects, reduced cerebral glucose consumption and a fall in CBF have been reported[11]. Tight coupling between CBF, cerebral energy metabolism and neuronal function is well-recognized[42], and interrelationships between metabolic and morphological changes in neuronal and glial cells, on the one hand, and the cerebral microcirculation, on the other, have also been stressed[43].

Neurotransmitters of the cholinergic, adrenergic, dopaminergic and other neuronal systems have been related to human cognitive function at various times but the evidence has been mainly qualitative and anecdotal[44] until the last few years. There is now impressive evidence to suggest that acetylcholine (ACh) is the neurotransmitter particularly involved in memory processes: anticholinergic agents such as scopolamine impair memory[44], whilst anticholinesterases may enhance it[45]; enzymes that synthesize and degrade ACh – that is, choline acetyltransferase (CAT) and acetylcholinesterase (AChE) – are significantly decreased in necropsy specimens and cortical biopsies from brains of patients with dementia of Alzheimer-type (senile or presenile) as compared to normal brain or the brain in MID[46,47], and the regional loss of CAT correlates with the distribution of the characteristic histopathological abnormalities[46]. In addition, there are reductions in glycolytic enzymes[47], and it has been shown that reduced ACh synthesis occurs when glucose oxidation is impaired by mild hypoxia[48]. However, neurotransmitter synthesis generally is susceptible to hypoxia[49].

REVIEW OF MAJOR CEREBRAL ACTIVATING DRUGS

Vasoactive drugs

Drugs acting via the autonomic nervous system
(a) *Alpha-adrenergic blocking drugs* These drugs can oppose cerebral vasospasm during or after neurosurgery, but evidence of cerebral vasodilatation and increased CBF in other patients (such as with dementia) is conflicting.
(i) Co-dergocrine mesylate (Hydergine, UK, USA; Deapril-ST, Circanol, USA) This mixture of hydrogenated alkaloids of ergotoxine – dihydroergocornine, dihydroergocristine and dihydroergokryptine – has been used for over a quarter of a century. Evidence for increase of CBF is conflicting[1,50,51]. More recent work has shifted the emphasis from gross changes in CBF to the effects of Hydergine on cerebral metabolism and the cerebral microcirculation[38,43]. It is claimed that the drug improves neuronal and glial metabolism in several ways, involving enzymes, ATP metabolism and protein synthesis, resulting in improved aerobic metabolism and increased electrical activity of the brain[38]. These metabolic changes are said to reduce the size of brain cells and their pseudopodial extensions and thus to improve microcirculatory flow. Hydergine may also react with neurotransmitters at the synapses[52].

There are many clinical reports of the use of Hydergine in elderly patients with mental deterioration, including several double-blind controlled studies of up to 16 weeks duration. Significant improvements were found mainly in mild to moderate cases, and usually took 3 weeks to appear. A wide range of mental and physical functions were included, with many differences in points of detail and frequent apparent contradictions between authors. This problem is common to most studies with cerebral activating drugs.

In a critical review of 12 clinical trials of Hydergine in dementia[53], it was noted that despite the statistically significant ($p < 0.05$) improvement in 13 clinical features of dementia demonstrated in these studies, the degree of improvement was small and there was no evidence of long-term benefit. The only long-term study[54] showed maximum improvement after 12 weeks of therapy, with subsequent loss of that improvement over a 1 year period. The reviewers[53] concluded that Hydergine was of little value in the treatment of dementia; but it must be remembered that in individual patients even a little improvement (or the prevention of further deterioration) may make a disproportionately large difference to the quality of life. Clearly, improved methodology and trial design, with more long-term studies, are needed. Another review[55] included 17 double-blind studies and illustrated the difficulty in evaluating the literature due to the diversity of methods and findings. It is worth noting that in double-blind comparative studies against papaverine[56-58], Hydergine has been considered significantly superior after 12 weeks of therapy in improving mental alertness, confusion, irritability, hostility, emotional lability, depressive mood and lack of motivation.

A recent placebo-controlled double-blind study[59] of Deapril-ST (1 mg sublingually thrice daily) showed significant efficacy in 34 mentally deteriorated elderly patients in a psychiatric hospital, often within 4 weeks, but more notably after 16 weeks of treatment.

Intravenous injection of 0.3 mg of Hydergine improved EEG patterns in a pilot study in 12 elderly female demented patients[60]; EEG changes correlated with improvements in several psychometric tests. It is well known that Hydergine produces changes in the EEG of experimental animals[38,43], and previous reports have appeared correlating such changes with clinical improvement in mentally deteriorated elderly patients treated with 1.5 mg Hydergine orally thrice daily for 6[61] or 12[62] weeks.

A double-blind controlled study of intramuscular dihydroergocristine was reported to show the value of this therapy in patients with cerebral and peripheral vascular disorders[63]. This drug has also been evaluated by studying the conjunctival microcirculation in elderly patients with 'cerebrovascular insufficiency'[64]: Treatment periods varied from 30–90 days, 0.6 mg/day being given intravenously for the first 3 days and 1.5 mg orally thrice daily thereafter. Of the 48 subjects 36 (75%) showed improved conjunctival microcirculation and reduced erythrocyte sludging, as compared with only eight (17%) of 47 control subjects given placebo.

Dosage: The usual dose is one 1·5 mg tablet thrice daily. A sublingual tablet is available in the United States. At least 6 weeks of therapy should be given before assessing the potential value of this drug. Improvement may continue for at least 12 weeks from the start of treatment. Side-effects are very rare; the only remarkable one in over 25 years of extensive use of the drug has been a marked sinus bradycardia[65].

(ii) Other α-blockers These are not recommended for cerebral problems. Phenoxybenzamine (Dibenyline, UK, Dibenzyline, USA) and thymoxamine (Opilon, UK) may oppose cerebral arterial spasm; phentolamine (Rogitine, UK, Regitine, USA, Australia, South Africa) and tolazoline (Priscol, UK, Priscoline, Canada, USA, Zoline, Australia) do not appear to influence CBF.

(b) *β-Adrenergic stimulants*
(i) Isoxsuprine (Duvadilan, Defencin, Vasotran, UK; Vasodilan, Canada, USA) This drug (which in large doses also has alpha-blocking properties) has had variable effects on CBF, but it has been reported that 10 mg intramuscularly can reverse the EEG changes caused by hyperventilation-induced cerebral vasoconstriction, both in young women and in older women with cerebral arteriosclerosis[66]. However, in normal men a similar intramuscular dose did not increase internal carotid artery flow over the 13 minute period studied[67]. It is claimed that isoxsuprine lowers blood viscosity[68] and inhibits red-cell clumping[69].

Clinical benefit has been reported in patients with TIAs and also in cerebral arteriosclerosis. The incidence of TIAs was halved in isoxsuprine-treated patients during a 1 year double-blind placebo-controlled crossover study in 32 elderly patients[25]; no change in mental status or behaviour was observed. An uncontrolled study claimed that isoxsuprine not only reduced the incidence of TIAs but also improved the patients' mental status[70]. Double-blind controlled studies of isoxsuprine in elderly patients have shown significant improvements in some intellectual activities; one study[71] used 80 mg/day isoxsuprine by mouth for 14 weeks; another study[72] used a graded-release preparation (40 mg twice daily for 16 weeks) and assessed performance by a teaching machine[73]. In a large-scale open general practice study of isoxsuprine resinate, 40 mg twice daily for 12 weeks, it was reported[74] that one-third of the 3050 patients on the drug improved in all functions tested (mood, intellect, locomotion, and daily living activities) with a statistical significance of $p < 0.001$

for all functions. A remarkable result in an uncontrolled study!

Dosage: Oral dosages have been mentioned; parenteral administration is also possible, but usually limited to patients with peripheral vascular disease – ampoules contain 5 mg/ml isoxsuprine hydrochloride. Side-effects (flushing, palpitation) are rare and transient after oral administration.

(ii) Nylidrin (Buphenine, Arlidin, USA; not available in the United Kingdom.) It resembles isoxsuprine in structure and effects, and there is conflicting evidence over its effects on CBF. It has been reported to be of some benefit in cerebrovascular insufficiency[75], and further clinical evaluation in the elderly is continuing in the United States.

Drugs with direct effect on vascular smooth muscle

(a) *Papaverine* (many trade names in the United States) Papaverine acts directly on smooth muscle; this effect may be partly mediated by inhibition of cAMP PDE and, in the brain, by increased output of adenosine. Intravenous papaverine increases CBF and decreases cerebrovascular resistance in patients with strokes or cerebrovascular spasm[76–79]. Intravenous and intracarotid arterial injection of papaverine has increased rCBF in some focal ischaemic areas of the brain in stroke patients[32,79], but there were no neurological improvements clinically, and the dangers of this approach may outweigh the possible advantages. Nevertheless, in a controlled study of papaverine in 70 patients with cerebral infarction, neurological improvements have been reported[80].

Intravenous papaverine has improved cerebral oxygen availability in stroke patients[81]. Improved glucose metabolism was reported in perfused cat brain[38], though to a lesser extent than with Hydergine, but there was no change in capillary morphometry after papaverine. Oral papaverine (300 mg twice daily for 1 week) produced small increases in CBF in healthy young adults, at rest and on hyperventilation[82]. However, in elderly patients with mental deterioration, the results of double-blind controlled studies with oral papaverine show the variability of response so characteristic of trials of cerebral activating drugs[55–58,83–87]. More consistent improvements are seen in the EEG[85–87]; it was previously shown that papaverine prevents slowing of the EEG on hyperventilation[88]. Nevertheless, papaverine seems to be less effective than Hydergine in elderly demented patients[56–58] and some authorities do not recommend it for the improvement of intellectual function[89].

Dosage: Papaverine hydrochloride is available as soft gelatin capsules (150 mg) but the short half-life of the drug (90–120 minutes) demands frequent administration – one capsule 6 hourly is usually recommended but 4 hourly administration would seem more appropriate, though not very practical. A total dose of 900 mg/day is acceptable.

Sustained-release preparations of papaverine (150 mg) are popular in the United States but may provide less effective vasodilatation than the gelatin capsules[90]. A new controlled-release tablet containing 300 mg papaverine hydrochloride (Papacontin) appears to hold more promise as a sustained-action preparation; a bioavailability study[91] showed a rise in plasma papaverine levels to a therapeutic range within 1 hour and maintenance of these levels for 10–12 hours, with no accumulation on repeated 12 hourly dosage. Side-effects are those of vasodilators in general; a fall in systemic blood pressure may occur, and intravenous papaverine has given rise to cardiac arrhythmias[92]. An important side-effect is hepatotoxicity[93,94], which is probably allergic in nature[95]; though said to be rare, mild degrees of hepatic disturbance may be commoner than formerly thought, since 12 of 40 patients on papaverine showed elevated levels of serum transaminases and alkaline phosphatase[95].

(b) *Cyclandelate* (Cyclospasmol, UK) This drug is three times as potent as papaverine (to which it bears a structural resemblance) in producing vasodilatation by direct action on vascular smooth muscle[96]; it is also claimed to improve cerebral metabolism and increase resistance to cerebral hypoxia.

Cyclandelate has been shown to increase CBF in patients with cerebral arteriosclerosis[97–99]; but clinical correlations were few or absent in these studies. There are several double-blind controlled clinical studies of cyclandelate in such patients[97,99–105]; the results are inconsistent and the usual problems of interpretation arise. Improvement is seen most often, perhaps not surprisingly, in patients below 75 years.

In some marginally successful cases, the drug may have been acting as an antidepressant[103]; depression may mimic dementia if retardation is marked, and effective antidepressant treatment may improve psychomotor test performance[106]. However, in a double-blind study, demented or depressed psychogeriatric patients showed no mental improvement, intellectual or affective, despite treatment with 1200 mg/day cyclospasmol for 6 weeks[107].

In a double-blind crossover study of cyclandelate (1200 mg/day for 2 months) in 'normal' old people living at home[108], the women showed significant improvement in intellectual tests, but the men showed steady intellectual and behavioural deterioration despite the therapy. The prophylactic effect claimed for cyclandelate in patients with TIAs[25,26] was not confirmed[100]. Large doses (1600–2400 mg/day) significantly improved sensorimotor recovery after strokes[109].

(c) *Betahistine* (Serc, UK)   This histamine analogue has most of the H_1-receptor effects of histamine, but only a minimal effect on gastric secretion. Its value in Ménière's disease is attributed to vasodilatation in the microcirculation of the labyrinth. Betahistine can increase CBF[110–112], and it has been suggested that the drug is particularly effective in increasing rCBF in the vertebrobasilar arterial system[110,113].

Three double-blind controlled studies[114–116] in cerebral arteriosclerosis showed a degree of improvement in psychological test performance, especially in relation to intellectual function, after betahistine treatment. A fourth study[117], in patients with vertebrobasilar artery insufficiency and TIAs, was reported as showing subjective improvements but no change in frequency of TIAs. Oral betahistine has been considered to be more effective than oral papaverine or hexobendine in cerebral ischaemia[110,118].

(d) *Nicotinic acid and its derivatives*   Nicotinic acid is a well-known vasodilator, but despite the ability of large doses to cause facial flushing, there is no convincing evidence that nicotinic acid can increase CBF. The use of smaller doses with other cerebral activating drugs is considered below; an alternative approach is to use a derivative or preparation with less side-effects.

(i) Inositol hexanicotinate (Hexopal, UK, Hexanicit, South Africa, Germany, Sweden; Linodil, Canada; Vasodil, Australia)   Each molecule contains six nicotinic acid moieties. The drug produces increased blood levels of nicotinic acid. Direct evidence of increased CBF is lacking but metabolic effects (improved lipid metabolism, stimulation of fibrinolysis, and decreased blood viscosity) are documented and claimed to improve blood circulation in ischaemic areas of cerebrum. It appears that no satisfactory double-blind clinical trials of adequate doses of Hexopal in brain failure have been published.

(ii) Tetranicotinoylfructose (Nicofuranose, Bradilan, UK)   There is little or no evidence that this drug (a slow-release preparation) is of value in cerebral disorders. It has been used together with meclofenoxate in psychiatric disorders, but the results do not assist in evaluating the use of Bradilan alone in cerebrovascular insufficiency or in dementia.

(iii) Nicotinyl alcohol tartrate (β-pyridylcarbinol, Ronicol, UK; Roniacol, Canada, USA)   This is the alcohol corresponding to nicotinic acid, with similar properties. There is conflicting evidence concerning its effect on CBF and on cerebral carbohydrate metabolism, but the drug has found some favour in Europe, where benefit was reported in cerebral impairment[119,120]. However, an American double-blind study in nine atherosclerotic patients with chronic brain syndrome showed no benefit from the drug in doses of 150 mg twice daily for 6 weeks[121].

Dosage: The dosage usually recommended for peripheral vascular disease is 25–50 mg nicotinyl alcohol four times daily. Each tablet of Ronicol contains 59·4 mg of the tartrate, equivalent to 25 mg of the alcohol. A slow-release tablet, containing six times this amount, is available; dosage is one or two tablets night and morning. There is no recommended dosage given for cerebrovascular indications in the United Kingdom. The side-effects are transient facial flushing on moderate doses; large doses may lower systemic blood pressure.

(iv) Xanthinol nicotinate (Complamex, UK; Complamin, Europe, Canada, South Africa) Each molecule consists of a xanthine base linked to nicotinic acid; the drug is claimed to have effects superior to those of concomitant therapy with theophylline and nicotinic acid. It has undoubted efficacy as a peripheral vasodilator, and is claimed to increase CBF[122] and to encourage development of collaterals in the microcirculation[123]. In addition, a wide range of metabolic effects has been described, including increase of nucleotides in the brain[124], erythrocytes[125], and liver[126], and lowering of blood viscosity and lipids[123]. In healthy adults made hypoxic, xanthinol nicotinate improved mental concentration[127] and prevented a fall in erythrocyte ATP concentrations[128].

The manufacturers state that the drug is a 'haemokinator' rather than a vasodilator – in other words it promotes blood flow (by opening up microcirculatory channels, by improving flow properties of blood and by improving haemodynamics). Most of the evidence suggesting benefit from this drug in patients with 'cerebrovascular insufficiency' comes from uncontrolled studies. A double-blind crossover study, using a teaching machine for assessing 28 elderly demented patients after 22 weeks of treatment[129], showed mental improvement in 18 patients, persisting after the drug was stopped.

Dosage: Tablets of 150 and 300 mg are available; the recommended dose is 300 mg thrice daily, with meals. A retard preparation (500 mg) is available in Europe. Parenteral administration has been effective in peripheral vascular disease. Side-effects are the same as those of nicotinic acid.

(e) *Methylxanthines*

(i) Caffeine (1,3,7-trimethylxanthine) and theophylline (1,3-

dimethylxanthine) are cerebral stimulants and have diuretic as well as peripheral vasodilator properties.

(ii) Aminophylline is theophylline ethylenediamine. It is a respiratory stimulant, useful in management of Cheyne – Stokes respiration. Aminophylline was once thought to increase CBF[130] but it is now known that the drug actually constricts cerebral vessels in man[1,131]; a fall in CBF has been demonstrated in normal volunteers[1], and an even greater fall in patients with cerebrovascular disease, following intravenous aminophylline[1,132]. Hopes that aminophylline-induced cerebral vasoconstriction might produce an 'inverse steal' effect[133], of benefit in acute cerebrovascular disorders, were not borne out in animal experiments[134].

(iii) Pentifylline with nicotinic acid (Cosaldon, UK) Pentifylline (1-hexyl,3,7-dimethylxanthine) is said to dilate cerebral blood vessels as much as CO_2 inhalation doses[135]; the addition of small doses of nicotinic acid is said to potentiate this. Metabolic and EEG effects have been reported[136].

Two double-blind crossover studies – one in elderly patients with cerebral sclerosis[137] and one in healthy volunteers aged from the third to the ninth decade[138] – reported improved mental function, but the design of both studies has been criticized[139].
Dosage: One tablet (pentifylline 200 mg + nicotinic acid 50 mg) four times daily with food. Side-effects (flushing, gastrointestinal disturbances), if they occur, are usually transient.

(f) *Hexobendine* (Ustimon, South Africa, France; Reoxyl, Germany) This is a synthetic agent with a prolonged vasodilator effect shown in animal experiments. Parenteral injection has produced increased CBF in animals and man. The drug has been widely used in Austria and Germany but has not been approved for general use in the United States and is unavailable in the United Kingdom.

(g) *Suloctidil* (Sulocton, Europe) This synthetic drug has a direct vasorelaxant effect on peripheral and cerebral circulations which is greater than that of papaverine[140]. In addition, suloctidil reduces plasma fibrinogen levels, blood viscosity and blood cholesterol and has antiplatelet aggregation and antithrombotic properties[140]; there is also evidence of improved cerebral metabolism[140]. In psychogeriatric patients, significant improvements in performance of psychometric tests[141] and in behavioural and functional patterns[142] have been reported in double-blind controlled studies.

Drugs with combined effects
(a) *Oxpentifylline* (Pentoxifylline, Trental, UK and Europe) This drug [3,7-dimethyl-1-(5-oxohexyl)xanthine] is a more recent intro-

duction from the makers of Cosaldon. Vasodilatation may result from several mechanisms[143] – direct action, antagonism of vasoconstrictor effects of catecholamines, potentiation of beta-sympathomimetic agents and PDE inhibition (leading in turn to increased cAMP levels and relaxation of vascular smooth muscle). Blood pressure does not fall. Blood viscosity is reduced, due largely to increase in erythrocyte flexibility consequent upon elevation of erythrocyte ATP levels[143,144].

CBF may increase[145]. Several published open and blinded studies of oxpentifylline in cerebrovascular disorders have been reviewed[146] and a further study reported[147]. Most of the recent studies lack precision in patient definition, study design and evaluation techniques; but some double-blind controlled studies seem to give satisfactory evidence of improvement in symptoms, mood and performance. Beneficial results have also been reported in patients recovering from stroke[146].

Dosage: 100–400 mg thrice daily, taken with food. Side-effects are usually mild and transient. Parenteral therapy is available for peripheral vascular disease.

(b) *Naftidrofuryl* (Nafronyl oxalate, Praxilene, UK) This synthetic compound has several actions[148]: vasodilator properties (papaverine-like and sympatheticolytic), local anaesthetic properties, antagonism to serotonin and bradykinin, and analgesic and antidepressant effects. In addition, various metabolic effects have been demonstrated: improved cerebral glucose metabolism[149], with activation of succinate dehydrogenase, and increased cerebral PO_2 and oxygen availability[150]. These metabolic enhancements may lead to increase of energy-rich substrates in the brain, as found in mice[149].

Naftidrofuryl has been used in Europe as a peripheral vasodilator since 1968; however, there is little convincing evidence that it increases CBF. Several double-blind controlled studies of its use in cerebral arteriosclerosis and dementia have been reported[151–157]. The overall picture is of improved mental function, but with much individual variability. One striking observation was the significant improvement in intellect and coping behaviour in severely demented patients[152]; such dramatic results have not been reproduced but many worthwhile gains have been reported. Further evidence of intellectual improvement has come from a controlled study in which global performance was measured by an 'Impairment Index' which the authors claimed to be more reliable and accurate than psychiatric global impressions[158].

A recent publication described beneficial results from the use of naftidrofuryl in recent acute stroke[159]; the design of the study has been criticized[160] and the caution advocated earlier, page 297, regarding the use of vasoactive drugs in acute stroke should be borne in mind.

Dosage: The usual recommended dose is one 100 mg capsule thrice daily. Parenteral administration is useful in some instances of peripheral vascular disease. Side-effects are rare and transient on oral therapy: headache, gastrointestinal disturbances, paraesthesiae and agitation have been reported. Intravenous infusion has led to severe local thrombophlebitis in elderly patients[161] but this is contrary to general experience with this preparation[162] and has been attributed to contamination rather than to the drug or the pH of the parenteral solution[163].

Antagonists of vasoconstriction: vasorelaxants
These drugs block calcium influx into depolarized smooth muscle cells in arterial walls[164]. Since free intracellular calcium ions are required for muscular contraction, relaxation of muscle is promoted – hence the term 'vasorelaxants' which is intended to differentiate this class of drugs from 'vasodilators'[165]. Vasorelaxants inhibit vasoconstriction caused by various agents or physiological states – *cf.* the protective effect of cromoglycate against bronchoconstriction, as distinct from the effect of bronchodilators in brochial asthma[165].

The drugs in this category include cinnarizine, flunarizine and nifedipine.

(a) *Cinnarizine* (Stugeron, UK; Stutgeron, Germany; Midronal, France) This piperazine derivative has antihistamine properties and is used against vertigo and travel sickness. Cinnarizine inhibits vasoconstriction induced by KCl-depolarization more markedly than do several other vasoactive agents[166]. It prolonged the reactive hyperaemia after a period of peripheral arterial occlusion in normal volunteers[167,168] and in patients with peripheral vascular disease[168–170]. The use of cinnarizine in clinical and pharmacological studies in peripheral vascular disease has been well documented[165,171].

Blood viscosity is reduced, probably by an effect of the drug on erythrocyte flexibility[172] (which is in turn related to calcium-ion flux[19]). There is some evidence of increased CBF in man[173,174].

Double-blind studies in patients with cerebrovascular insufficiency have been favourable in Europe[175–178] but not in the United Kingdom[179–181]. Of the UK studies, two[179,180] were in severely affected patients who were not always matched for type of disease; the third study[181] was a multicentre general practice study of less severely affected patients.

Dosage: 15 mg tablets and 75 mg capsules (cinnarizine forte) are available. For circulatory disorders, 75 mg thrice daily may be given. Side-effects include fullness in the head, dizziness or somnolence; occasional mild and transient nausea and vomiting have been reported.

(b) *Flunarizine* (Sibelium, Germany)   This is the difluoro-derivative of cinnarizine, but is more potent than cinnarizine[167,168]. There are as yet no published studies showing an effect on CBF or blood flow in man.

(c) *Nifedipine* (Adalat, UK and Europe)   This pyridine derivative has been studied mainly as a coronary artery vasodilator.

Drugs acting on microcirculation
Many of the drugs already considered are claimed to improve microcirculation. Another is low molecular weight dextran.

(a) *Low molecular weight dextran* (Dextran 40, Rheomacrodex, UK, USA; Lomodex 40, Gentran 40, UK)   Infusion of this agent lowers blood viscosity by haemodilution, and blood flow may thus be facilitated. Increased CBF and rCBF have been noted in patients with cerebrovascular problems treated with low molecular weight dextran[1,29,132] and beneficial effects have been reported in acute strokes[182].

For management of brain failure (chronic brain syndrome) this type of therapy with repeated infusions is clearly of little practical value, and oral agents which may reduce blood viscosity are of more interest. Hypersensitivity reactions may occur; they are rare but most likely in subjects with an allergic history.

Cerebral 'metabolic improvers'
Several of the drugs previously discussed are claimed to improve cerebral metabolism. Certain other agents are of importance in this category.

(a) *Agents enhancing acetylcholine levels in the brain*   The rationale for this approach has been discussed earlier in this chapter (see pages 298–299). (i) Anticholinesterases – physostigmine is the only such agent to cross the blood-brain barrier effectively. When used to antagonize the anticholinergic effects of overdoses of tricyclic antidepressants or antiparkinsonian drugs, it has improved defects in recent memory caused by such intoxications[183]; disease-induced amnesia has been improved[145] and long-term memory has been enhanced even in normal subjects[184]. It has also been helpful in reducing postoperative mental aberrations and somnolence after narcotic drugs in patients up to 94 years of age[185].

Side-effects may be central (vomiting) or peripheral (parasympathetic) and these, together with the need for parenteral administration and the short duration of action, limit the usefulness of this drug for the treatment of SDAT. A search for a more selective cholinesterase inhibitor with predominantly central effects – the cholinergic equivalent of carbidopa – has been advocated[186].

(ii) Choline is the precursor of ACh and increases brain ACh levels in animals; in man direct measurements of brain ACh have not been made, but increased serum and cerebrospinal fluid levels of choline result from taking choline orally[187].

Lecithin, a natural source of choline, is more potent than choline itself in increasing blood choline levels[188]. Choline has improved memory in normal volunteers[189,190], but not in the majority of elderly demented patients studied in the small trials reported so far[191–193]. More promising are the early results from a small uncontrolled study in early cases of Alzheimer's disease[194], but clearly an adequate evaluation in SDAT will only be obtained by a full-scale clinical trial in early cases, carefully assessed over 6–12 months; the trial design will need to include the recognition of an arrest or slowing down of progressive deterioration as well as a more obvious reversal of an established condition[195]. The therapeutic agent need not necessarily be choline, but might be lecithin or deanol (see below, with or without an anticholinesterase; such a study, though expensive, would be justified since even a moderate therapeutic success would have large-scale social consequences. The question of possible adverse effects must be considered; choline therapy has been associated with urinary incontinence[192,193] and depression[193,196].

(iii) Deanol (2-dimethylaminoethanol, DMAE; Deaner, USA, Australia)   DMAE is a precursor of choline and can increase ACh levels in animal brains. DMAE is converted to choline in the liver, where it is incorporated into phosphatidylcholine; blood choline levels rise and choline enters the brain in both free and lipid-bound forms. Deaner is the *p*-acetamidobenzoic acid salt of DMAE; it has been used mainly for learning and behaviour disorders in children and more recently (with variable results) in tardive dyskinesia. Healthy volunteers have shown increased mental concentration on this drug[197]. An uncontrolled study of Deaner in chronic brain syndrome[198] used doses of up to 500 mg/day by mouth in severe cases, without improvement.

Dosage: Tablets of Deaner are in 25 mg, 100 mg and 250 mg strengths; it has been suggested that up to 1 g/day may be needed in adults[199]. In tardive dyskinesia doses up to 2 g/day have been used.

Side-effects are cholinergic; they may be severe with large doses.

(iv) Dopaminergic drugs   Drugs may stimulate dopamine receptors directly (for example, bromocriptine) or indirectly (such as levodopa, a precursor of dopamine; and d-amphetamine, which releases dopamine). All these drugs increase ACh levels in brains of experimental animals.

Ageing of the extrapyramidal system is associated with notable losses of striatal tyrosine hydroxylase and dopa decarboxylase activities, leading to reduced synthesis of dopamine and other catecholamines[39,40]. Striatal dopamine loss is not infrequently associated with intellectual impairment which may show improvement after levodopa treatment[200,201]; and it is possible that derangement of mesocortical dopaminergic neurons may occur in SDAT[202].

Histological evidence of Alzheimer's disease occurs more frequently in brains of patients with Parkinson's disease than in age-matched controls, which supports the concept of a link between the dopaminergic and the cholinergic systems[203]. Results of levodopa treatment in senile dementia without extrapyramidal features have been encouraging[204,205] but the improvement may not be sustained[206]. In presenile dementia neither levodopa[207] nor bromocriptine[202] has improved cognitive function. Piribedil (Trivastal, France) is a dopamine agonist which is used in Europe as a treatment for failing mental functions in old age.

(b) *Cholinomimetic agents*

Arecoline   This natural alkaloid from the betel nut has cholinomimetic effects. Although not in clinical use, it has been injected into normal volunteers before and after scopolamine (a drug which is known to impair memory function[44]); in both circumstances learning was enhanced[189].

(c) *Agents related to neurotransmitters*

(i) Piracetam (Nootropil, South Africa; Nootropyl, France; Normabrain, Germany)   This is a cyclic derivative of gamma-aminobutyric acid (GABA), which is the major inhibitory neurotransmitter throughout the brain. It has several effects on the brain[208]; of interest here is its reported ability to protect the brain from hypoxia and to facilitate learning and memory – although this latter effect may be seen clearly only in very mildly demented subjects. The mechanism of action is uncertain; it may relate to increase in ATP/ADP ratio and in glucose consumption in cerebral cells.

In studies on psychogeriatric patients, evidence of improvement was dose-dependent; significant results were reported in a double-blind study when the dose was 4·8 g/day[209,210] but not in studies in which only 2·4 g/day was given[209,211,212].

Dosage: 4·8 g/day in divided doses. Side-effects are uncommon, but fatigue, nausea, diarrhoea and nightmares have been reported.

(d) *Neuropeptide hormones and drugs affecting them*   Animal experiments implicate neuropeptides of hypothalamo-hypophyseal origin in learning and memory processes[213,214]. In man, ACTH injections have improved the attention/arousal process in elderly subjects[215] and vasopressin has improved various aspects of memory processes[215,216], especially in Korsakoff's syndrome[217]. However, in senile dementia, the effect has been much less[217].

The possible mechanisms of these effects have been reviewed[215,216] and include regulation of rapid eye movement (REM) sleep (of importance in memory consolidation) and hippocampal theta rhythm (reflecting a functional state of the brain which facilitates learning and memory formation)[218]. Other drugs which enhance learning and memory in animals produce changes in REM sleep similar to those induced by vasopressin[219].

Vasopressin release is stimulated by carbamazepine (which improves mental function in epileptics[220]) and inhibited by ethanol (which impairs various aspects of memory[221]). Lithium carbonate depresses vasopressin function and may impair memory[222].

Dosage: Lysine-8-vasopressin may be given as a nasal spray, one puff to each nostril three times daily (16–22 international units). It has a short half-life.

DDAVP (1-deamino-8-d-vasopressin) is a potent vasopressin analogue free of vasoactive properties. It can also be given as a nasal spray, and its half-life is considerably longer than that of lysine-8-vasopressin. Trials in SDAT would be of great interest.

(e) *Agents enhancing levels of ribonucleic acid in the brain*   A fall in ribonucleic acid (RNA) in the brain occurs with ageing[223]. RNA increases in the brain during learning and training[224] and RNA synthesis has been linked to the storage process of memory[225]. The transfer of learned behaviour by injection of brain RNA from trained rats to naive rats has been reported[226].

RNA from yeast has improved memory in the elderly[227]. However, RNA does not itself enter cerebral neurons and the effect may be via a breakdown product[228].

(f) *Drugs enhancing synthesis of brain RNA*   TCAP (tricyanoaminopropene) was of no value in elderly patients with severe dementia[229].

Pemoline (5-phenyl-2-imino-4-oxo-oxazolidine, Ronyl, Kethamed, UK; Volital, Cylert, UK and USA) This has been used in Europe as a cerebral stimulant since 1956[230,231]. Its level of stimulation is between that of amphetamine and that of caffeine[230].

It is said to increase the rate of synthesis of dopamine in the brain[232]. Magnesium pemoline is said to be more active than pemoline itself[233].

Improved performance in psychological tests was reported in healthy adults given pemoline[234] and magnesium pemoline[235]. However, a double-blind crossover study in 22 elderly women in a residential home showed no effect of pemoline on psychological test results or on EEG patterns[236]. Psychogeriatric patients were said to show improved memory[233] but subsequent investigators have been unable to confirm this[237-239].

Dosage: Recommended dose of pemoline is 20–120 mg/day depending on age and condition. In the elderly with memory impairment, 10 mg (half a tablet) morning and midday is usually stimulant enough. Side-effects include agitation, confusion and insomnia.

Meclofenoxate (centrophenoxine, Europe; Lucidril, UK) This synthetic agent is the dimethylaminoethyl ester of *para*-chlorophenoxyacetic acid; it was formerly known as ANP[235]. It is a cerebral stimulant[240] and various metabolic effects have been reported in animal brains – enhanced cerebral glucose uptake and resistance to cerebral anoxia and, most notably, protection against cyanide poisoning. In addition, the drug markedly reduces lipofuscin pigment formation in animals although this effect has not been recorded in man. Lipofuscin increases in ageing neurons, probably formed from lysosomes (intracellular autophagocytic vesicles containing enzymes); the amount of lipofuscin is inversely related to the amount of Nissl substance, which contains ribosomal RNA as its major nucleic acid component – and RNA is related to memory (see above, page 312). In old mice treated with meclofenoxate, learning and memory improvements were associated with reduction in neuronal lipofuscin in both cerebral cortex and hippocampus[241]; conversely, rats on a vitamin E-deficient diet showed significant impairments of learning and memory, and an increased deposition of neuronal lipofuscin[241]. Possible improvement in intellectual function in old age by the use of meclofenoxate has been discussed[242]. Normal old people living in the community treated with meclofenoxate for 6 months in a double-blind study, then followed up for 3 more months, showed a highly significant ($p < 0.001$) improvement in the delayed free-recall test[243]. This suggested that new information could be processed more efficiently – an area where the elderly are most vulnerable. These subjects also had a greater sense of wellbeing. The authors suggested that old people who appear depressed because everyday life is becoming harder to cope with may benefit more from meclofenoxate than from antidepressants or tranquillisers.

A small double-blind study[244] evaluated the effect of meclofenoxate in six matched pairs of elderly women patients in two short-stay geriatric units, using a teaching machine. The treated patients all improved relative to the controls ($p < 0.05$).

A 1 year multicentre hospital trial in 62 patients with dementia did not give conclusive results[245]. However, after 3 months on meclofenoxate patients showed improved performance in the delayed free-recall test, and over the 12 month period the meclofenoxate-treated group showed a trend towards improvement of memory and sense of wellbeing, as compared to the placebo group.

Dosage: One 300 mg tablet three to five times daily. The drug has been used parenterally in Europe. Overstimulation may result in confusion and insomnia.

Cerebral stimulants

Although cerebral stimulants act by one metabolic pathway or another so that many of the drugs described earlier in this chapter could also be classified as stimulants (such as pemoline, deanol) certain drugs will be considered here because they are usually regarded as stimulants *per se*: these drugs are related to amphetamine and camphor.

Amphetamine and its derivatives

(a) *Amphetamine* First synthesized in 1887, the stimulant effects of amphetamines were not noted until 1930. The *d*-isomer is more potent in this regard than the *l*-isomer. The drug has many pharmacological, biochemical and physiological effects: apart from being a potent central stimulant, inhibiting uptake and promoting release of catecholamines at the neuronal level, amphetamine is an anorexigenic agent and vasoconstrictor. In animals, it enhances learning and memory, thus implicating catecholamines in these processes[246]. Amphetamine has been used for treatment of obesity, nasal congestion, fatigue states, hyperkinesis and mild depression. It has also had some use in Parkinsonism[247,248].

The use of amphetamine has largely fallen away because of the risk of habituation and the development of psychoses. It may still be useful in the elderly patient with physical disability in whom poor motivation is impairing or preventing successful rehabilitation[248,249], but if a limited trial proves unsuccessful, it should be discontinued.

Dosage: Five to 15 mg twice daily, preferably in gradually increasing doses over 3 weeks, with the second dose each day no later than 4 p.m.

Amphetamine has been the starting-point of many derivatives which are more in current use than amphetamine itself. Of particular concern to us here are pemoline (discussed earlier in this chapter, page 312) and methylphenidate.

(b) *Methylphenidate* (Ritalin, UK, USA, Methidate, Canada) This cyclized amphetamine derivative contains a piperidine ring. It may act on a number of central nervous pathways – enhancement of hypothalamic sympathetic centres, stimulation of the brain-stem reticular formation, and depression of inhibitory pathways in the thalamic region.

Benefit has been claimed in elderly patients with various degrees of psychomotor retardation and depression, in mainly uncontrolled studies. The drug has reduced apathy and increased motivation[248,250,251].

In one study oxprenolol, a beta-adrenergic-blocking drug, was used to counter undesirable sympathomimetic side-effects; the authors considered that 50% of the patients so treated were prevented from becoming long-stay hospital patients[251]. The use of a beta-blocker is of interest for another reason: it has been suggested that beta-blockers may improve learning, by reducing autonomic end-organ arousal[252]. Double-blind studies have given conflicting results[250,253,254], but the overall impression has been favourable, one well-conducted study being particularly so[250].

Dosage: Initially, 5 mg (half a tablet) morning and midday. This may be increased gradually, up to a maximum dose of 30 mg/day in two divided doses. Overstimulation may occur; the value of adding a beta-blocker has been mentioned above.

Fencamfamin (Reactivan, UK and Europe)
Fencamfamin is a camphor derivative with a stimulant action on the reticular formation and cerebral cortex equivalent to that of amphetamine, but apparently with no peripheral effects or dangerous synergism with other drugs. It is combined with vitamins B_1, B_6, B_{12} and C in Reactivan, which has been widely used in Europe since 1960 for debility and fatigue states. In the United Kingdom, general practice studies have confirmed its value in these indications[255,256].

In double-blind studies in dementia, it has shown significant effects in mild to moderate cases[257] but not in severely demented psychogeriatric patients[258].

Dosage: Two tablets at breakfast and one at midday. Side-effects include agitation and restlessness.

A more detailed review of thè use of the use of cerebral stimulants in the elderly is available[259].

OXYGEN

The idea that oxygen-enrichment of inspired air might improve cognitive function in the aged is attractive[260]; this approach has improved function in stroke patients[261]. Hyperbaric oxygen therapy has been used with success in the management of senile dementia by some investigators[262,263] but not by others[264,265]. This treatment has been critically reviewed[266]. Recent studies have used both hyperbaric and normobaric oxygen therapy in dementia, either in parallel groups of patients[267] or sequentially in the same individuals[258]. In neither study did the oxygen therapy lead to any improvement.

On the other hand, a double-blind controlled study of continuous normobaric portable oxygen therapy in healthy elderly men with some degree of failing memory showed statistically significant improvements in IQ and memory tests[269]. The report on this well-designed and conducted study includes an analysis of differences from previously published studies which is valuable. But in regard to hyperbaric oxygen, it is difficult to argue with the view that such therapy is not recommended for elderly demented patients, as it is 'impractical, expensive and not without danger'[118].

MISCELLANEOUS OTHER DRUGS

Space precludes consideration of many other relevant agents which, however, seem less important than those already discussed. Of course, time may prove this wrong. Such agents include other stimulants, metabolic improvers (pyritinol, vincamine), enzymes, carbonic anhydrase inhibitors, hormones, phospholipids, nucleosides, ornithine alpha-glutarate, and various vitamins. Last but not least, the controversial but disappointing Gerovital-H_3 has been reviewed several times in recent years[270-272].

CONCLUSIONS

Attempts to improve brain failure are justified, since even marginal improvements could make the difference between coping and non-coping, or between being manageable or non-manageable by an existing support system, at home or in an institution. In early cases, the improvement may be seen at a more sophisticated level of organization, with disproportionate improvement in the quality of life.

Furthermore, there are grounds for believing that improvements are indeed possible in the integrity of brain cells in hypoxic or ischaemic or degenerating brain. Brain tissue has only small stores of oxygen and substrate and only a limited capacity for anaerobic respiration; even small changes may improve the situation or at least prevent deterioration.

Even though some drugs may increase CBF, there may be no correlation with cerebral function as measured by formal psychometric tests. It is important to adopt a global functional emphasis in evaluation; this is less precise ('scientific') but far more meaningful in terms of the happiness and self-sufficiency of ageing populations.

The variability of the design and results of the many published studies ('double-blind does not mean 'valid'!) makes it difficult to compare different drugs, or even to evaluate whether such therapy is of any value at all; yet properly conducted multicentre studies, with meticulous attention to entry criteria, diagnosis, grading of patients, treatment regimens and their duration, and standardized assessment procedures along the lines outlined above are clearly essential if the medical profession is ever to do more than dabble with the massive and growing problem of brain failure in the elderly.

It must be understood that the aims of such therapy may be to prevent deterioration rather than to reverse pathological and functional changes which have already occurred. This may be achieved by a variety of mechanisms – vasodilatation in macrocirculations or microcirculations, improved flow properties of blood, resistance to cerebral hypoxia, enhancement of glucose metabolism in brain cells (including the facilitation of anaerobic routes of metabolism), increase in energy-rich compounds in the brain, and so on.

Another aspect worth considering is the extent to which 'activator' therapy really acts as antidepressant therapy in patients who adapt poorly to the functional impairments (or even to the very concept) of ageing. Cerebral stimulants may be doing this rather than (or as well as) having more specific effects on cognitive function.

It is perhaps self-evident that the author is a therapeutic optimist; but he is also a realist. In the light of present knowledge, it is impossible to know with a reasonable degree of certainty precisely which patients will benefit from the use of cerebral activating drugs.

Continued uncritical prescribing of such drugs will not help to define the issue any more clearly. Pending the much-needed adequate trials, it is suggested that such drugs might find a limited use in clinical practice according to criteria such as: mild to moderate brain failure, certain cases of mild reactive depression and retardation, poor motivation towards physical rehabilitation yet likelihood of compliance, practicable functional assessments, adequate duration of therapy. In this way a sufficient harvest of improvement or arrest of decline may be achieved to warrant the therapeutic endeavours.

References

1 Gottstein, U. (1969). The effect of drugs on cerebral blood flow especially in patients of older age. *Pharmakopsychiatr. Neuro-Psychopharmakol.*, **2**, 100

2 Fang, H. C. H. (1976). Observations on aging characteristics of cerebral blood vessels, macroscopic and microscopic features. In R. D. Terry and S. Gershon (eds.). *Neurobiology of Aging* (*Aging*, Vol. 3), pp. 155–166. (New York: Raven Press)

3 Leading article (1977). Hyperviscosity in disease. *Lancet*, **ii**, 961

4 Thomas, D. J., Marshall, J. and Russell, R. W. R. (1978). Haematocrit and cerebral blood flow. *Lancet*, **i**, 41

5 York, E. L. and Sproule, B. J. (1978). Cerebral blood flow and polycythaemia. *Lancet*, **i**, 152

6 Leading article (1978). Red-cell deformability. *Lancet*, **ii**, 1348

7 Nakao, M., Nakao, T. and Yamazoe, S. (1960). Adenosine triphosphate and maintainance of shape of the human red cells. *Nature*, **187**, 945

8 Nakao, M., Wada, T. and Kamiyama, T. (1962). A direct relationship between adenosine triphosphate level and *in vivo* viability of erythrocytes. *Nature*, **194**, 877

9 La Celle, P. L., Kirkpatrick, F. H., Udkow, M. P. and Arkin, B. (1973). Membrane fragmentation and Ca^{++}-membrane interaction: potential mechanisms of shape change in the senescent red cell. In M. Bessis, R. I. Weed and P. F. Leblond (eds.). *Red Cell Shape*, pp. 69–78. (Berlin: Springer Verlag).

10 Weed, R. I., La Celle, P. L. and Merrill, E. W. (1969). Metabolic dependence of red cell deformability. *J. Clin. Invest.*, **48**, 795

11 Sokoloff, L. (1975). Cerebral circulation and metabolism in the aged. In S. Gershon and A. Raskin (eds.). *Genesis and Treatment of Psychologic Disorders in the Elderly* (*Aging*, Vol. 2), pp. 45–54. (New York: Raven Press)

12 Meyer, J. S. (1978). Improved method for noninvasive measurement of regional cerebral blood flow by [133]xenon inhalation. Part II: Measurements in health and disease. *Stroke*, **9**, 205

13 Hachinski, V. C., Lassen, N. A. and Marshall, J. (1974). Multi-infarct dementia. A cause of mental deterioration in the elderly. *Lancet*, **ii**, 207

14 Tomlinson, B. E. (1977). The pathology of dementia. In C. E. Wells (ed.). *Dementia* (Edition 2), pp. 113–153. (Philadelphia: F. A. Davis Co.)

15 O'Brien, M. D. and Mallett, B. L. (1970). Cerebral cortex perfusion rates in dementia. *J. Neurol. Neurosurg. Psychiatr.*, **33**, 497

16 Hachinski, V. C., Iliff, L. D., Zilkha, E., Du Boulay, G. H., McAllister, V. L., Marshall, J., Ross Russell, R. W. and Symon, L. (1975). Cerebral blood flow in dementia. *Arch. Neurol.*, **32**, 632

17 Heiss, W.-D., Hayakawa, T. and Waltz, A. G. (1976). Cortical neuronal function during ischemia. Effects of occlusion of one middle cerebral artery on single-unit activity in cats. *Arch. Neurol.,* **33,** 813

18 Millikan, C. H. (1978). Cerebral circulation. *J. Am. Med. Assoc.,* **239,** 1313

19 Ross Russell, R. W. (1976). Transient cerebral ischaemia. In R. W. Ross Russell (ed.). *Cerebral Arterial Disease,* pp. 125–145. (Edinburgh and London: Churchill Livingstone)

20 Skinhøj, E., Høedt-Rasmussen, K., Paulson, O. B. and Lassen, N. A. (1970). Regional cerebral blood flow and its autoregulation in patients with transient focal cerebral ischemic attacks. *Neurology (Minneap.),* **20,** 485

21 Boysen, G., Ladegaard-Pedersen, J. H., Valentin, N. and Engell, H. C. (1970). Cerebral blood flow and internal carotid artery flow during carotid surgery. *Stroke,* **1,** 253

22 Perry, P. M., Drinkwater, J. E. and Taylor, G. W. (1975). Cerebral function before and after carotid endarterectomy. *Br. Med. J.,* **4,** 215

23 Toole, J. F., Janeway, R., Choi, K., Cordell, R., Davis, C., Johnston, F. and Miller, H. S. (1975). Transient ischemic attacks due to atherosclerosis. *Arch. Neurol.,* **32,** 5

24 Whisnant, J. P. (1977). Indications for medical and surgical therapy for ischemic stroke. In R. A. Thompson and J. R. Green (eds.). *Stroke (Advances in Neurology,* Vol. 16), pp. 133–144. (New York: Raven Press)

25 Dhrymiotis, A. D. and Whittier, J. R. (1962). Effect of a vasodilator (isoxsuprine) on cerebral ischemic episodes. *Curr. Ther. Res.,* **4,** 124

26 Van der Drift, J. H. A. and Kok, N. K. D. (1971). Transient ischaemic attacks. In G. Stöcker, P. A. Kuhn, P. Hall, G. Becker and E. van der Veen (eds.). *Assessment in Cerebrovascular Insufficiency,* pp. 132–135. (Stuttgart: Georg Thieme)

27 Leading article (1978). Aspirin and stroke prevention. *Lancet,* **ii,** 245

28 Leading article (1978). Transient ischemic attacks and the prevention of strokes. *N. Engl. J. Med.,* **299,** 93

29 Heiss, W.-D. (1973). Drug effects on regional cerebral blood flow in focal cerebrovascular disease. *J. Neurol. Sci.,* **19,** 461

30 Lassen, N. A. (1966). The luxury perfusion syndrome. *Lancet,* **ii,** 1113

31 Lassen, N. A. and Pálvölgyi, R. (1968). Cerebral steal during hypercapnia and the inverse reaction during hypocapnia observed by the 133-xenon technique in man. *Scand. J. Clin. Lab. Invest.,* **22** (Suppl. 102), XIII: D

32 McHenry, L. C. (1972). Cerebral vasodilator therapy in stroke. *Stroke,* **3,** 686

33 Forrester, T., Harper, A. M., MacKenzie, E. T. and Thomson, E. M. (1975). Vascular and metabolic effects of systemic ATP on the cerebral circulation. In A. M. Harper, W. B. Jennett, J. D. Miller and J. O. Rowan (eds.). *Blood Flow and Metabolism in the Brain.* (Edinburgh and London: Churchill Livingstone)

34 Flamm, E. S., Kim, J., Lin, J. and Ransohoff, J. (1975). Phosphodiesterase inhibitors and cerebral vasospasm. *Arch. Neurol.,* **32,** 569

35 McIlwain, H. (1977). Extended roles in the brain for second messenger systems. *Neuroscience,* **2,** 357

36 Zimmerman, I. and Berg, A. (1974). Levels of adenosine 3′, 5′, cyclic monophosphate in the cerebral cortex of aging rats. *Mech. Ageing Dev.,* **3,** 33

37 Zimmerman, I. D. and Berg, A. P. (1975). Phosphodiesterase and adenyl-cyclase activities in the cerebral cortex of the aging rat. *Mech. Ageing Dev.,* **4,** 89

38 Meier-Ruge, W., Enz, A., Gygax, P., Hunziker, O., Iwangoff, P. and Reichlmeier, K. (1975). Experimental pathology in basic research of the aging brain.

In S. Gershon and A. Raskin (eds.). *Genesis and Treatment of Psychologic Disorders in the Elderly (Aging,* Vol. 2), pp. 55–126. (New York: Raven Press)

39 McGeer, E. and McGeer, P. L. (1976). Neurotransmitter metabolism in the aging brain. In R. D. Terry and S. Gershon (eds.). *Neurobiology of Aging (Aging,* Vol. 3), pp. 389–403. (New York: Raven Press)

40 Davison, A. N. (1978). Biochemical aspects of the ageing brain. *Age Ageing,* **7** (Suppl.), 4

41 Perry, E. K., Perry, R. H., Blessed, G. and Tomlinson, B. E. (1978). Changes in brain cholinesterases in senile dementia of Alzheimer type. *Neuropathol. Appl. Neurobiol.,* **4,** 273

42 Sokoloff, L. (1978). Local cerebral energy metabolism: its relationships to local functional activity and blood flow. In *Cerebral Vascular Smooth Muscle and its Control.* Ciba Foundation Symposium 56 (new series), pp. 171–191; and subsequent Discussion, pp. 191–197

43 Emmenegger, H. and Meier-Ruge, W. (1968). The actions of Hydergine on the brain: A histochemical, circulatory and neurophysiological study. *Pharmacology,* **1,** 65

44 Drachman, D. A. and Leavitt, J. (1974). Human memory and the cholinergic system. A relationship to aging? *Arch. Neurol.,* **30,** 113

45 Peters, B. H. and Levin, H. S. (1977). Memory enhancement after physostigmine treatment in the amnesic syndrome. *Arch. Neurol.,* **34,** 215

46 Perry, E. K., Tomlinson, B. E., Blessed, G., Bergmann, K., Gibson, P. H. and Perry, R. H. (1978). Correlation of cholinergic abnormalities with senile plaques and mental test scores in senile dementia. *Br. Med. J.,* **2,** 1457

47 Bowen, D. M., White, P., Spillane, J. A., Goodhardt, M. J., Curzon, G., Iwangoff, P., Meier-Ruge, W. and Davison, A. N. (1979). Accelerated ageing or selective neuronal loss as an important cause of dementia? *Lancet,* **i,** 11

48 Gibson, G. and Blass, J. P. (1976). A relation between [NAD$^+$]/[NADH] potentials and glucose utilization in rat brain slices. *J. Biol. Chem.,* **251,** 4127

49 Siesjö, B. K. (1978). *Brain Energy Metabolism.* (New York: John Wiley and Sons)

50 Heyck, H. (1961). Der Einfluss der Ausgangslage auf Sympathikolytische Effekte am Hirnkreislauf bei Cerebrovascularen Erkrankungen. *Artzl. Forsch.,* **15,** 243. (English abstract)

51 McHenry, L. C., Jaffe, M. E., Kawamura, J. and Goldberg, H. I. (1971). Hydergine effect on cerebral circulation in cerebrovascular disease. *J. Neurol. Sci.,* **13,** 475

52 Loew, D. M., Vigouret, J. M. and Jaton, A. L. (1976). Neuropharmacological investigations with two ergot alkaloids, hydergine and bromocriptine. *Postgrad. Med. J.,* **52** (Suppl. 1), 40

53 Hughes, J. R., Williams, J. G. and Currier, R. D. (1976). An ergot alkaloid preparation (hydergine) in the treatment of dementia: critical review of the clinical literature. *J. Am. Geriatr. Soc.,* **24,** 490

54 Soni, S. D. and Soni, S. S. (1975). Dihydrogenated alkaloids of ergotoxine in nonhospitalized elderly patients. *Curr. Med. Res. Opin.,* **3,** 464

55 Hyams, D. E. (1978). Cerebral function and drug therapy. In J. C. Brocklehurst (ed.). *Textbook of Geriatric Medicine and Gerontology,* 2nd Ed., pp. 670–711. (Edinburgh and London: Churchill Livingstone)

56 Bazo, A. J. (1973). An ergot alkaloid preparation (Hydergine) versus papaverine in treating common complaints of the aged: double-blind study. *J. Am. Geriatr. Soc.,* **21,** 63

57 Nelson, J. J. (1975). Relieving select symptoms of the elderly. *Geriatrics,* **30,** 133 (March)

58 Rosen, H. J. (1975). Mental decline in the elderly: pharmacotherapy (ergot alkaloids versus papaverine). *J. Am. Geriatr. Soc.*, **23**, 169

59 Novo, F. P., Ryan, R. P. and Frazier, E. L. (1978). Dihydroergotoxine mesylate in treatment of symptoms of idiopathic cerebral dysfunction in geriatric patients. *Clin. Ther.*, **1**, 359

60 Buchan, T., Styles, I. M. and Newton, J. (1978). The EEG response to intravenous dihydroergotoxine mesylate. *Pharmatherapeutica*, **2**, 59

61 Herzfeld, U., Christian, W., Ronge, J. and Wittgen, M. (1972). Richtgrossen fur die Beurteilung der Hirnfunktion nach Langzeittherapie mit Hydergin. *Ärztl. Forsch.*, **26**, 215

62 Arrigo, A., Braun, P., Kauchtschischwili, G. M., Moglia, A. and Tartara, A. (1973). Influence of treatment on symptomatology and correlated electroencephalographic (EEG) changes in the aged. *Curr. Ther. Res.*, **15**, 417

63 Calisti, G., Biscarini, L. and Miseo, A. (1977). Studio clinico controllato sull' impiego della diidroergocristina nelle vasculopatie cerebrali e periferiche. *Clin. Terap.*, **83**, 371

64 Massoni, G. and Falciola, N. (1978). Studio 'controllato' della microcircolazione congiuntivale nel soggetto anziano dopo impiego di diidroergocristina. *G. Gerontol.*, **26**, 117

65 Cayley, A. C. D., MacPherson, A. and Wedgwood, J. (1975). Sinus bradycardia following treatment with hydergine for cerebrovascular insufficiency. *Br. Med. J.*, **4**, 384

66 Whittier, J. R. and Dhrymiotis, A. D. (1962). Prevention of slow wave response to hyperventilation in the human electroencephalogram by a vasodilator. *Angiology*, **13**, 324

67 Miyazaki, M. (1971/2). Effect of cerebral circulatory drugs on cerebral and peripheral circulation, with special reference to aminophylline, papaverine, cyclandelate and isoxsuprine. *Eur. Neurol.*, **6**, 162

68 Schlichting, K. and Heidrich, H. (1976). Influence of isoxsuprine on blood viscosity. *Vasa*, **5**, 51

69 Di Perri, T., Forconi, S., Guerrini, M. and Agnusdei, D. (1977). *In vitro* activity of isoxsuprine on blood plasma and serum viscosity. *Pharmatherapeutica*, **1**, 447

70 Elliott, C. G., Brown, A. L. and Smith, T. C. G. (1973). Multicentre general practitioner trial of isoxsuprine in cerebrovascular disease: a pilot study. *Curr. Med. Res. Opin.*, **1**, 554

71 Affleck, D.C., Treptow, K. R. and Herrick, H. D. (1961). The effects of isoxsuprine hydrochloride (Vasodilan) on chronic cerebral arteriosclerosis. *J. Nerv. Ment. Dis.*, **132**, 335

72 Hussain, S. M. A., Gedye, J. L., Naylor, R. and Brown, A. L. (1976). The objective measurement of mental performance in cerebrovascular disease. A double-blind controlled study, using a graded-release preparation of isoxsuprine. *Practitioner*, **216**, 222

73 Gedye, J. L. and Wedgwood, J. (1966). Experience in the use of a teaching machine for the assessment of senile mental changes. *Proc. 7th Int. Congr. Gerontol., Vienna*, **8**, 205

74 Guyer, B. M. (1978). Cerebrovascular disease in the elderly: Response to isoxsuprine resinate (Defencin CP) therapy. *Clin. Trials J.*, **15**, 49

75 Winsor, T., Hyman, C. and Knapp, F. M. (1960). The cerebral peripheral circulatory action of nylidrin hydrochloride. *Am. J. Med. Sci.*, **239**, 594

76 Jayne, H. W., Scheinberg, P., Rich, M. and Belle, M. S. (1952). The effect of intravenous papaverine hydrochloride on the cerebral circulation. *J. Clin. Invest.*, **31**, 111

77 Karlsberg, P., Elliott, H. W. and Adams, J. E. (1963). Effect of various pharmacologic agents on cerebral arteries. *Neurology (Minneapolis)*, **13**, 772

78 Gottstein, U. (1965). Pharmacological studies of total cerebral blood flow in man with comments on the possibility of improving regional cerebral blood flow by drugs. *Acta Neurol. Scand.*, **41**, Suppl. 14, 136

79 McHenry, L. C., Jaffe, M. E., Kawamura, J. and Goldberg, H. I. (1970). Effect of papaverine on regional blood flow in focal vascular disease of the brain. *N. Engl. J. Med.*, **282**, 1167

80 Gilroy, J. and Meyer, J. S. (1966). Controlled evaluation of cerebral vasodilator drugs in the progressive stroke. In R. G. Sickert and J. P. Whisnant (eds.). *Cerebral Vascular Diseases. Trans. 5th Princeton Conf.*, pp. 197–202. (New York: Grune and Stratton)

81 Meyer, J. S., Gotoh, F., Gilroy, J. and Nara, N. (1965). Improvement in brain oxygenation and clinical improvement in patients with strokes treated with papaverine hydrochloride. *J. Am. Med. Assoc.*, **194**, 957

82 Wang, H. S. and Obrist, W. D. (1976). Effects of oral papaverine on cerebral blood flow in normals: evaluation by the xenon-133 inhalation method. *Biol. Psychiatr.*, **11**, 217

83 Stern, F. H. (1970). Management of chronic brain syndrome secondary to cerebral arteriosclerosis, with special reference to papaverine hydrochloride. *J. Am. Geriatr. Soc.*, **18**, 507

84 Ritter, R. M., Nail, H. R., Tatum, P. and Blazi, M. (1971). The effect of papaverine on patients with cerebral arteriosclerosis. *Clin. Med.*, **78**, 18

85 McQuillan, L. M., Lopec, C. A. and Vibal, J. R. (1974). Evaluation of EEG and clinical changes associated with Pavabid therapy in chronic brain syndrome. *Curr. Ther. Res.*, **16**, 49

86 Cole, J. O., Branconnier, R. J. and Martin, G. F. (1975). Electroencephalographic and behavioral changes associated with papaverine administration in healthy geriatric subjects. *J. Am. Geriatr. Soc.*, **23**, 295

87 Culebras, A. (1976). Effect of papaverine on cerebral electrogenesis. *Neurology (Minneapolis)*, **26**, 673

88 Korenyi, C. and Whittier, J. R. (1969). Prevention of brain vasospasm: effect of sustained release form of papaverine (Pavabid) on blocking of hyperventilation electroencephalogram in the human. *Physicians' Drug Manual*, **1**, 81

89 Prien, R. F. and Cole, J. O. (1978). The use of psychopharmacological drugs in the aged. In W. G. Clark and J. del Giudice (eds.). *Principles of Psychopharmacology*, pp. 593–605. (New York and London: Academic Press)

90 Lee, B. Y., Sakamoto, H., Trainor, F., Brody, G. and Cho, Y. W. (1978). Comparison of soft gelatin capsule vs. sustained release formulation of papaverine HCl: vasodilation and plasma levels. *Int. J. Clin. Pharmacol.*, **16**, 32

91 Miller, R. B., Leslie, S. T., Black, F. M. and Boroda, C. (1978). A controlled release papaverine tablet (Papacontin): a study in normal volunteers. *Br. J. Clin. Pharmacol.*, **5**, 51

92 Elek, S. R. and Katz, L. N. (1942). Some clinical uses of papaverine in heart disease. *J. Am. Med. Assoc.*, **120**, 434

93 Rønnov-Jessen, V. and Tjernlund, A. (1969). Hepatotoxicity due to treatment with papaverine. *N. Engl. J. Med.*, **281**, 1333

94 Zimmerman, H. J. (1969). Papaverine revisited as a hepatotoxin. *N. Engl. J. Med.*, **281**, 1364

95 Kiaer, H. W., Olsen, S. and Rønnov-Jessen, F. (1974). Hepatotoxicity of papaverine. *Arch. Pathol.*, **98**, 292

96 Bijlsma, U. G., Funcke, A. B. H., Tersteege, H. M., Rekker, R. F., Ernsting, M. J. E. and Nauta, W. Th. (1956). The pharmacology of Cyclospasmol. *Arch. Int. Pharmacodyn.*, **105**, 145

97 Eichhorn, O. (1965). The effect of cyclandelate on cerebral circulation. A double-blind trial with clinical and radiocirculographic investigations. *Vasc. Dis.*, **2**, 305

98 O'Brien, M. D. and Veall, N. (1966). Effects of cyclandelate on cerebral cortex perfusion rates in cerebrovascular disease. *Lancet*, **ii**, 729

99 Ball, J. A. C. and Taylor, A. R. (1967). Effect of cyclandelate on mental function and cerebral blood flow in elderly patients. *Br. Med. J.*, **3**, 525

100 Rogers, W. F., Shaikh, V. A. R. and Clark, A. N. G. (1970). Cyclandelate in long-standing cerebral arteriosclerosis. *Gerontol. Clin.*, **12**, 88

101 Fine, E. W., Lewis, D., Villa-Landa, I. and Blakemore, C. B. (1970). The effect of cyclandelate on mental function in patients with arteriosclerotic brain disease. *Br. J. Psychiatr.*, **117**, 157

102 Aderman, M., Giardina, W. J. and Koreniowski, S. (1972). Effect of cyclandelate on perception, memory and cognition in a group of geriatric subjects. *J. Am. Geriatr. Soc.*, **20**, 268

103 Young, J., Hall, P. and Blakemore, C. (1974). Treatment of the cerebral manifestations of arteriosclerosis with cyclandelate. *Br. J. Psychiatr.*, **124**, 1977

104 Westreich, G., Alter, M. and Lundgren, S. (1975). Effect of cyclandelate on dementia. *Stroke*, **6**, 535

105 Capote, B. and Parikh, N. (1978). Cyclandelate in the treatment of senility: a controlled study. *J. Am. Geriatr. Soc.*, **26**, 360

106 Brasseur, R. (1978). Clinical value of a combined antiischemic and anticholinergic substance with antidepressant properties. *Angiology*, **29**, 121

107 Davies, G., Hamilton, S., Hendrickson, E., Levy, R. and Post, F. (1977). The effect of cyclandelate in depressed and demented patients: a controlled study in psychogeriatric patients. *Age Ageing*, **6**, 156

108 Judge, T. G., Urquhart, A. and Blakemore, C. B. (1973). Cyclandelate and mental functions: a double-blind crossover trial in normal elderly subjects. *Age Ageing*, **2**, 121

109 Sourander, L. and Blakemore, C. B. (1978). Effects of cyclospasmol upon sensory parameters in patients recovering from cerebrovascular accidents. *Angiology*, **29**, 133

110 Meyer, J. S., Mathew, N. T., Hartmann, A. and Rivera, V. M. (1974). Orally administered betahistine and regional blood flow in cerebrovascular disease. *J. Clin. Pharmacol.*, **14**, 280

111 Seipel, J. H. and Floam, J. E. (1975). Rheoencephalographic and other studies of betahistine in humans. I. The cerebral and peripheral circulatory effects of single doses in normal subjects. *J. Clin. Pharmacol.*, **15**, 144

112 Seipel, J. H., Fisher, R., Floam, J. E. and Bohm, M. (1975). Rheoencephalographic and other studies of betahistine in humans. II. The cerebral and peripheral microcirculatory effects of single doses in geriatric patients with 'pure' arteriosclerotic dementia. *J. Clin. Pharmacol.*, **15**, 155

113 Anderson, W. D. and Kubicek, W. G. (1971). Effects of betahistine-HCl, nicotinic acid and histamine on basilar blood flow in anesthetized dogs. *Stroke*, **2**, 409

114 Esser, A. H. and Reis, J. (1968). Preliminary study of betahistine in chronic psychiatric patients with symptoms of arteriosclerosis cerebri. *Curr. Ther. Res.*, **10**, 122

324   *The Treatment of Medical Problems in the Elderly*

115 Rivera, V. M., Meyer, J. S., Baer, P. E., Faibish, G. M., Mathew, N. T. and Hartmann, A. (1974). Vertebrobasilar arterial insufficiency with dementia. Controlled trials of treatment with betahistine. *J. Am. Geriatr. Soc.*, **22**, 397
116 Pathy, J., Menon, G., Reynolds, A. and Van Strik, R. (1977). Betahistine hydrochloride (Serc) in cerebrovascular disease: a placebo-controlled study. *Age Ageing*, **6**, 179
117 Spruill, J. H., Jr., Toole, J. F., Kitto, W. and Miller, H. E. (1975). A comparison of betahistine hydrochloride with placebo for vertebral-basilar insufficiency: a double-blind study. *Stroke*, **6**, 116
118 Meyer, J. S., Mathew, N. T. and Hartmann, A. (1976). Cerebral blood flow and metabolism changes in the epilepsies and during cerebral anoxia, ischemia and edema. In H. E. Himwich (ed.). *Brain Metabolism and Cerebral Disorders*, 2nd ed., pp. 207-229. (New York: Spectrum Publications, Inc.)
119 Cornu, F. (1969). Zur Kreislaufphysiologie und Biochemie zerebraler Abbauprozesse und der Verhaltensbeeinflussung von Kranken durch Phamakotherapie. *Wien. Klin. Wochenschr.*, **81**, 426
120 Boudouresques, J., Papy, J. J. and Daniel, F. (1970). Une thérapeutique retard dans les insuffisances circulatoires cérébrales chroniques. *Sem. Thér.*, **46**, 789
121 Stuart, S. E. (1967). Long-acting form of the peripheral vasodilator, nicotinyl alcohol: double-blind evaluation. *J. Am. Geriatr. Soc.*, **15**, 780
122 Schreiber, H. (1970). Untersuchungen über die Änderung der Durchblutungsgröße des Gehirns unter 3-(Methyl-oxyäthylamino)-2-oxopropyl-theophyllin nikotinat mit Hilfe der Schädelrheographie. *Med. Klin.*, **55**, 509
123 Davis, E. and Rozov, H. (1973). The effects of xanthinol nicotinate on the small blood vessels. In J. Ditzel and D. H. Lewis (eds.). *7th Europ. Conf. Microcirculation, Aberdeen, 1972, Part I*, Bibl. Anat. No. 11, pp. 334-339. (Basel: Karger)
124 Brenner, G. and Brenner, H. (1972). The effect of xantinol nicotinate on the metabolism of the brain. *Arzneim. Forsch.*, **22**, 754
125 Brenner, G. (1973). Beeinflussbarkeit des ATP-Gehaltes menschlicher und tierischer Erythrozyten in vivo und in vitro durch xantinol-nicotinat. *Arzneim. Forsch.*, **23**, 562
126 Brenner, G. (1968). Über den Einfluss von Xantinol-nicotinat auf die Biosynthese der oxydierten Pyridinnucleotide in der Rattenleber. *Arzneim. Forsch.*, **18**, 1153
127 Held, K., Wünsche, O. and Reuter, N. (1973). The effect of xantinol nicotinate on man in altitude oxygen deficiency. *Ärtzl. Praxis*, **26**, 91
128 Held, K. (1973). Experiments on effect and mechanism of xantinol nicotinate in man during oxygen deficiency. *Therapiewoche*, **37**, 3270
129 Braverman, A. M. and Naylor, R. (1975). Vasoactive substances in the management of elderly patients suffering from dementia. *Mod. Geriatr.*, **5**, 20
130 Mainzer, F. (1949). Frühbehandlung des Schlaganfalls mit Aminophyllin. *Schweiz. Med. Wochenschr.*, **79**, 108
131 Gottstein, U. and Paulson, O. B. (1972). The effect of intracarotid aminophylline infusion on the cerebral circulation. *Stroke*, **3**, 560
132 Herrschaft, H. (1975). The efficacy and course of action of vaso- and metabolic-active substances on regional cerebral blood flow in patients with cerebrovascular insufficiency. In A. M. Harper, W. B. Jennett, J. D. Miller and J. O. Rowan (eds.). *Blood Flow & Metabolism in the Brain*, pp. 11.24-11.28. (Edinburgh and London: Churchill Livingstone)
133 Skinhøj, E. and Poulson, O. B. (1970). The mechanism of action of aminophylline upon cerebral vascular disorders. *Acta Neurol. Scand.*, **46**, 129

134 McGraw, C. P., Crowell, G. F. and Howard, G. (1978). Effect of aminophylline on cerebral infarction in the Mongolian gerbil. *Stroke*, **9**, 477

135 Cugurra, F. and Echinard-Garin, P. (1960). Alcuni aspetti dell' attivita farmacologica di un nuovo teofillinico; 1'1-exil-3,7-dimetilxantine (SK-7). *Arch. Int. Pharmacodyn.*, **123**, 481

136 Quadbeck, G. and Tarragó-Humet, P. (1972). Ricerche sperimentali sull' influenza dei derivati xantinici sul metabolismo cerebrale. *Clin. Ter.*, **60**, 125

137 Kirchberger, F., Kehl, R. and Gutmann, W. (1969). Zur Behandlung zerebraler Ernährungsstörungen. Eine Doppelblind-Studie. *Med. Welt*, **20**, 1542

138 Amthauer, R. (1971). Veränderung psychischer Leistungen durch ein Pharmakon, das den Stoffwechsel im Gehirn beeinflusst. *Wien Klin. Wochenschr.*, **83**, 659

139 *Drug Ther. Bull.* (1972). Cosaldon for vascular disorders? *Drug Ther. Bull.*, **10**, 66

140 Roba, J., Roncucci, and Lambelin, G. (1977). Pharmacological properties of Suloctidil. *Acta Clin. Belg.*, **32**, 3

141 Jacquy, J. and Noel, G. (1977). Double-blind trial with Suloctidil, a new vasoactive agent, in elderly patients with psycho-organic brain syndrome. *Acta Clin. Belg.*, **32**, 22

142 Bargheon, J. (1977). Evaluation de l'activité thérapeutique du Suloctidil chez le vieillard atteint d'insuffisance cerebrovasculaire. Étude en double insu par comparaison à un placebo. *Acta Clin. Belg.*, **32**, 15

143 Stefanovich, V. (1978). The biochemical mechanism of action of pentoxifylline. *Pharmatherapeutica*, **2**, Suppl. 1, 5

144 Müller, R. (1978). The haemorheological profile of pentoxifylline: a review. *Pharmatherapeutica*, **2**, Suppl. 1, 27

145 Koppenhagen, K., Wenig, H. G. and Muller, K. (1977). Measurement of cerebral blood flow following intravenous administration of pentoxifylline (Trental). *Curr. Med. Res. Opin.*, **4**, 521

146 Theis, H., Lehrach, F. and Muller, R. (1978). A 5-year review of clinico-experimental and therapeutic experience with pentoxifylline. *Pharmatherapeutica*, **2**, Suppl. 1, 150

147 Dominguez, D., De Cayaffa, C. L., Gomensoro, J. and Aparicio, N. J. (1977). Modification of psychometric, practical and intellectual parameters in patients with diffuse cerebrovascular insufficiency during prolonged treatment with pentoxifylline: a double-blind, placebo-controlled trial. *Pharmatherapeutica*, **1**, 498

148 Fontaine, L, Grand, M., Chabert, J., Szarvasi, E. and Bayssat, M. (1968). Pharmacologie générale d'une substance nouvelle, vasodilatatrice du naftidrofuryl. *Bull. Chim. Thér.*, **6**, 463

149 Meynaud, A., Grand, M., Belleville, M. and Fontaine, L. (1975). Effet du naphtidrofuryl sur le métabolisme énergétique cérébral chez la souris. *Thérapie*, **30**, 777

150 Plotkine, M., Paultre, C. Z., Boulu, R. and Rossignol, P. (1975). Intérêt pharmacologique d'une technique d'enregistrement de la PO_2 tissulaire du cortex cérébral chez le lapin. Réponse à la papaverine et au naftidrofuryl. *Thérapie*, **30**, 713

151 Robinson, K. (1972). A double-blind clinical trial of naftidrofuryl in cerebral vascular disorders. *Med. Dig.*, **17** (12), 50

152 Judge, T. G. and Urquhart, A. (1972). Naftidrofuryl—a double-blind crossover study in the elderly. *Curr. Med. Res. Opin.*, **1**, 166

153 Gerin, J. (1974). Double-blind trial of naftidrofuryl in the treatment of cerebral arteriosclerosis. *Br. J. Clin. Pract.*, **28**, 177

154 Bouvier, J. B., Passeron, O. and Chupin, M. P. (1974). Psychometric study of Praxilene. *J. Int. Med. Res.*, **2**, 59

155 Bargheon, J. (1975). Essai en double aveugle du Praxilene en gériatrie. *Gaz. Méd. Fr.*, **82**, 4755.

156 Cox, J. R. (1975). Double-blind evaluation of naftidrofuryl in treating elderly confused hospitalized patients. *Gerontol. Clin.*, **17**, 160

157 Brodie, N. H. (1977). A double-blind trial of naftidrofuryl in treating confused elderly patients in general practice. *Practitioner*, **218**, 274

158 Branconnier, R. J. and Cole, J. O. (1978). The Impairment Index as a symptom-independent parameter of drug efficacy in geriatric psychopharmacology. *J. Gerontol.*, **33**, 217

159 Admani, A. K. (1978). New approach to treatment of recent stroke. *Br. Med. J.*, **2**, 1678

160 Steiner, T., Capildeo, R. and Rose, F. C. (1979). New approach to treatment of recent stroke. (Letter). *Br. Med. J.*, **1**, 412

161 Woodhouse, C. R. J. and Eadie, D. G. A. (1977). Severe thrombophlebitis with Praxilene. *Br. Med. J.*, **1**, 1320

162 Heidrich, H. (1978). Incidence of thrombophlebitis with naftidrofuryl. *Br. Med. J.*, **1**, 618

163 Standing, V. F., Wiggins, P. A., Pratt, D. and Kester, R. C. (1977). Thrombophlebitis with intravenous naftidrofuryl oxalate. *Br. Med. J.*, **2**, 895

164 Emanuel, M. B. and Will, J. A. (1977). Cinnarizine in the treatment of peripheral vascular disease: mechanisms related to its clinical action. *Proc. R. Soc. Med.*, **70** (Suppl. 8), 7

165 Godfraind, T. and Kaba, A. (1972). The role of calcium in the action of drugs on vascular smooth muscle. *Arch. Int. Pharmacodyn.*, **196**, Suppl., 35

166 Van Neuten, J. M. (1969). Comparative bioassay of vasoactive drugs using isolated perfused rabbit arteries. *Eur. J. Pharmacol.*, **6**, 286

167 Jageneau, A., Loots W. and Brugmans, J. (1974). Prolongation of anoxia-induced hyperemia in healthy middle-aged men treated with cinnarizine and flunarizine. *Arzneim. Forsch.*, **24**, 1839

168 Verhaegen, H., Roels, V., Adriaensen, H., Brugmans, J., De Cock, W., Dony, J., Jageneau, A. and Schuermans, V. (1974). The arteriolar effects of cinnarizine and flunarizine. Multitechnical investigations in normal volunteers and in patients with occlusive disease of the extremities secondary to arteriosclerosis. *Angiology*, **25**, 261

169 Ellis, F. and Hyams, D. E. (1977). Vascular responses with cinnarizine to standard exercise in patients with intermittent claudication. *Proc. R. Soc. Med.*, **70** (Suppl. 8), 13

170 De Cree, J., Jageneau, A. H. M., Geukens, H. and Loots, W. (1977). Use of the ECG-triggered venous occlusion plethysmograph to study hyperaemic response patterns in patients with intermittent claudication treated with cinnarizine. *Proc. R. Soc. Med.*, **70** (Suppl. 8), 21

171 Staessen, A. J. (1977). Treatment of peripheral circulatory disturbances with cinnarizine. A multi-centre double-blind, placebo-controlled evaluation. *Proc. R. Soc. Med.*, **70** (Suppl. 8), 17

172 Di Perri, Forconi, S., Guerrini, M., Pasini, F. L., Del Cipolla, R., Rossi, C. and Agnusdei, D. (1977). Action of cinnarizine on the hyperviscosity of blood in patients with peripheral obliterative arterial disease. *Proc. R. Soc. Med.*, **70** (Suppl. 8), 25

173 Wilcke, O. (1966). Ergebnisse der Behandlung zerebraler Durchblutungsstörungen mit Cinnarizin. *Med. Welt.*, **17**, 1472

174 Weigelin, E. and Sayegh, F. (1968). Zur Objectivierung der zerebralen durch-blutungsfordernden Effektes vasoaktiver Substanzen unter besonderer Beruck-sichtigung von Cinnarizin. In K. Heinrich (ed.). *Aktuelle Probleme der psychiatrischen Pharmakotherapie in Klinik und Praxis*, pp. 3–12. (Stuttgart: Schattauer)

175 Behrens, E. (1966). Medikamentose Beeinflussung der Hirndurchblutung durch Stugeron. *Med. Welt.*, **38**, 2029

176 Van der Meer-Van Manen, A. H. E. (1967). Klinische evaluatie can cinnarizine bij geriatrische patienten. *Ned. T. Geneesk.*, **111**, 256

177 Bernard, A. and Goffart, J. M. (1968). A double-blind crossover clinical evalua-tion of cinnarizine. *Clin. Trials J.*, **5**, 945

178 Toledo, J. B., Pisa, H. and Marchese, M. (1972). Clinical evaluation of cinnari-zine in patients with cerebral circulatory deficiency. *Arzneim. Forsch.*, **22**, 448

179 Irvine, R. E., Greenfield, P. R., Griffith, D. G. C., Paget, S. C., Strouthidis, T. M. and Vaughan, V. St. G. (1970). Cinnarizine in cerebrovascular disease. *Gerontol. Clin.*, **12**, 297

180 Droller, H., Jayaram, V. K., Bevans, H. G. and Bentinck, S. J. (1971). A re-evaluation of cinnarizine with geriatric inpatients. *Gerontol. Clin.*, **13**, 89

181 General Practitioner Research Group (1969). Manifestations of cerebral arter-iosclerosis unaffected by a vasodilator. *Practitioner*, **203**, 695

182 Gilroy, J., Barnhart, M. I. and Meyer, J. S. (1969). Treatment of acute stroke with dextran 40. *J. Am. Med. Assoc.*, **210**, 293

183 Granacher, R. P. and Baldessarini, R. J. (1975). Physostigmine: Its use in acute anticholinergic syndrome with antidepressant and anti-Parkinson drugs. *Arch. Gen. Psychiatr.*, **32**, 375

184 Davis, K. L., Mohs, R. C., Tinkleberg, J. R., Pfefferbaum, A., Hollister, L. E. and Kopell, B. S. (1978). Physostigmine: improvement of long-term memory processes in normal humans. *Science*, **201**, 272

185 El-Naggar, M., El-Ganzouri, A.-R., Heller, F. and Sadove, M. S. (1978). Physostigmine: its use in the management of postoperative mental aberrations. *Anesthesiol. Rev.*, **6**, 49

186 Comfort, A. (1978). Cholinesterase inhibition in the treatment of Alzheimer's dementia. *Lancet*, **i**, 659

187 Growdon, J. H., Cohen, E. L. and Wurtman, R. J. (1977). Effects of oral choline administration on serum and CSF choline levels in patients with Huntington's disease. *J. Neurochem.*, **28**, 229

188 Wurtman, R. J., Hirsch, M. J. and Growdon, J. H. (1977). Lecithin consump-tion elevates serum free choline levels. *Lancet*, **ii**, 68

189 Sitaram, N., Weingartner, H. and Gillin, J. C. (1978). Human serial learning: enhancement with arecholine and choline and impairment with scopolamine. *Science*, **201**, 274

190 Sitaram, N., Weingartner, H., Caine, E. D. and Gillin, J. C. (1978). Choline: selective enhancement of serial learning and encoding of low imagery words in man. *Life Sci.*, **22**, 1555

191 Boyd, W. D., Graham-White, J., Blackwood, G., Glen, I. and McQueen, J. (1977). Clinical effects of choline in Alzheimer senile dementia. *Lancet*, **ii**, 71

192 Etienne, P., Gauthier, S., Johnson, G., Collier, B., Mendis, T., Dastoor, D., Cole, M. and Muller, H. F. (1978). Clinical effects of choline in Alzheimer's disease. *Lancet*, **i**, 508

193 Smith, C. M., Swash, M., Exton-Smith, A. N., Phillips, M. J., Overstall, P. W., Piper, M. E. and Bailey, M. R. (1978). Choline therapy in Alzheimer's disease. *Lancet*, **ii**, 318

194 Signoret, J. L., Whiteley, A. and Lhermitte, F. (1978). Influence of choline on amnesia in early Alzheimer's disease. *Lancet*, **ii**, 837
195 Levy, R. (1978). Choline in Alzheimer's disease. *Lancet*, **ii**, 944
196 Tamminga, C. A., Smith, R. C., Ericksen, S. E., Chang, S. and Davis, J. M. (1977). Cholinergic influences in tardive dyskinesia. *Am. J. Psychiatr.*, **134**, 769
197 Pfeiffer, C. C. and Murphree, H. B., Jr. (1958). Stimulant effect of 2-dimethylaminoethanol in human subjects. *J. Pharmacol. Exp. Ther.*, **112**, 60A
198 Lawrence, R. M. and Leichman, N. S. (1965). Comparison of the effects of heparin sodium, xanthinol nicotinate (Complamin) and 2-dimethylamino-ethanol (Deaner) in institutionalized geriatric groups. *J. Am. Geriatr. Soc.*, **13**, 325
199 Ré, O. (1974). 2-dimethylaminoethanol (deanol): a brief review of its clinical efficacy and postulated mechanism of action. *Curr. Ther. Res.*, **16**, 1238
200 Murphy, D. L. (1973). Mental effects of L-dopa. *Ann. Rev. Med.*, **24**, 209
201 Drachman, D. A. and Stahl, S. (1975). Extrapyramidal dementia and levodopa. *Lancet*, **i**, 809
202 Phuapradit, P., Phillips, M., Lees, A. M. and Stern, G. M. (1978). Bromocriptine in presenile dementia. *Br. Med. J.*, **1**, 1052
203 Hakim, A. M. and Mathieson, G. (1978). Basis of dementia in Parkinson's disease. *Lancet*, **ii**, 729
204 Lewis, C., Ballinger, B. R. and Presly, A. S. (1978). Trial of levodopa in senile dementia. *Br. Med. J.*, **1**, 550
205 Renvoize, E. B., Jerram, T. and Clough, G. (1978). Levodopa in senile dementia. *Br. Med. J.*, **2**, 504
206 Johnson, K., Presly, A. S. and Ballinger, B. R. (1978). Levodopa in senile dementia. *Br. Med. J.*, **1**, 1625
207 Kristensen, V., Olsen, M. and Theilgaard, A. (1977). Levodopa treatment of presenile dementia. *Acta Psychiatr. Scand.*, **55**, 41
208 Richardson, A. E. and Bereen, F. J. (1977). Effect of piracetam on level of consciousness after neurosurgery. *Lancet*, **ii**, 1110
209 Kretschmar, J. H. and Kretschmar, C. (1976). Zur Dosis-Wirkungs-Relation bei der Behandlung mit Piracetam. *Arzneim. Forsch.*, **26**, 1158
210 Dorn, M. (1978). Piracetam bei vorzeitiger biologischer Alterung. *Fortschr. Med.*, **96**, 1
211 Abuzzahab, F. S., SR., Merwin, G. E. Sherman, M. C. (1973). A controlled investigation of piracetam versus placebo on the memory of geriatric patients. *Pharmacologist*, **15**, 456
212 Gedye, J. L., Ibrahimi, G. S. and McDonald, C. (1978). Double-blind controlled trial of piracetam (2-pyrrolidone acetamide) on two groups of psychogeriatric patients. *IRCS Med. Sci.* **6**, 202
213 De Wied, D. (1977). Peptides and behavior. *Life Sci.*, **20**, 195
214 Gold, P. W., Goodwin, F. K. and Reus, V. I. (1978). Vasopressin in affective illness. *Lancet*, **i**, 1233
215 Legros, J. J., Gilot, P., Seron, X., Claessens, J., Adam, A., Moeglen, J. M., Audibert, A. and Berchier, P. (1978). Influence of vasopressin on learning and memory. *Lancet*, **i**, 41
216 Oliveros, J. C., Jandali, M. K., Timsit-Berthier, M., Remy, R., Benghezal, A., Audibert, A. and Moeglen, J. M. (1978). Vasopressin in amnesia. *Lancet*, **i**, 42
217 Leboeuf, A., Lodge, J. and Eames, P. G. (1978). Vasopressin and memory in Korsakoff syndrome. *Lancet*, **ii**, 1370
218 Urban, I. and De Wied, D. (1978). Neuropeptides: effects on paradoxical sleep and theta-rhythm in rats. *Pharmacol. Biochem. Behav.*, **8**, 51

219 Longo, V. G. and Loizzo, A. (1973). Effects of drugs on the hippocampal θ-rhythm. In F. E. Bloom and J. H. Acheson (eds.). *Pharmacology and the Nature of Man. Proc. 5th Int. Congr. Pharmacology, San Francisco, 1972.*, Vol. 4, p. 46. (Basel: Karger)

220 Dadrill, C. B. and Troupin, A. S. (1977). Psychotropic effects of carbamazepine in epilepsy: a double-blind comparison with phenytoin. *Neurology*, **27**, 1023

221 Ryback, R. S. (1971). The continuum and specificity of the effects of alcohol on memory: a review. *Q. J. Stud. Alc.*, **32**, 995

222 Kusumo, K. S. and Vaughan, M. (1977). Effects of lithium salts on memory. *Br. J. Psychiatr.*, **131**, 453

223 Samorajski, T. and Rolsten, C. (1973). Age and regional differences in the chemical composition of brains of mice, monkeys, and humans. In D. H. Ford (ed.). *Neurological Aspects of Maturation and Aging. Progr. Brain Res.*, **40**, 251. (Amsterdam: Elsevier)

224 Glassman, E. (1969). The biochemistry of learning: an evaluation of the role of RNA and protein. *Ann. Rev. Biochem.*, **38**, 605

225 Cameron, D. E. (1966). Evolving concepts of memory. In J. Wortis (ed.). *Recent Advances in Biological Psychiatry, IX*, pp. 1–12. (New York: Plenum Press)

226 Babich, F. R., Jacobson, A. L., Bubash, S. and Jacobson, A. (1965). Transfer of a response to naive rats by injection of ribonucleic acid extracted from trained rats. *Science*, **149**, 656

227 Cameron, D. E., Sved, S., Solyom, L. and Wainrib, B. (1963). Effects of ribonucleic acid on memory defect in the aged. *Am. J. Psychiat.*, **120**, 320

228 Kral, V. A., Solyom, L., Enesco, H. and Ledwidge, B. (1970). Relationship of vitamin B_{12} and folic acid to memory function. *Biol. Psychiatr.*, **2**, 19

229 Talland, G. A., Mendelson, J. H., Koz, G. and Aaron, R. (1965). Experimental studies of the effects of tricyanoaminopropene on the memory and learning capacities of geriatric patients. *J. Psychiatr. Res.*, **3**, 171

230 Schmidt, L. (1956). 5-phenyl-2-imino-4-oxo-oxazolidine-ein zentral erregender Stoff. *Arzheim. Forsch.*, **6**, 423

231 Plotnikoff, N. (1971). Pemoline: review of performance. *Tex. Rep. Biol. Med.*, **29**, 467

232 Valle-Jones, J. C. (1978). Pemoline in the treatment of psychogenic fatigue in general practice. *Practitioner*, **221**, 425

233 Cameron, D. E. and Brand, M. I. (1966). Magnesium pemoline and memory. *Proc. IV World Congr. Psychiatr.*, **4**, 2558. (Amsterdam: Excerpta Medica Foundation)

234 Dureman, I. (1962). Behavioral patterns of antibarbituric action after 5-phenyl-2-imino-4-oxo-oxazolidine, amphetamine and caffeine. *Clin. Pharmacol. Ther.*, **3**, 163

235 East, M. O'N. and Mann, R. D. (1966). A clinical trial of magnesium and pemoline: a central nervous system stimulant. *J. Ther.*, **1**, 22

236 Droller, H., Bevans, H. G. and Jayaram, V. K. (1971). Problems of a drug trial (pemoline) on geriatric patients. *Gerontol. Clin.*, **13**, 269

237 Smart, R. G. (1967). Magnesium pemoline. *Science*, **155**, 603

238 Talland, G. A., Hogen, D. Q. and James, M. (1967). Performance tests of amnesic patients with Cylert. *J. Nerv. Ment. Dis.*, **144**, 421

239 Eisdorfer, C., Conner, J. F. and Wilkie, F. A. (1968). Effect of magnesium pemoline on cognition and behavior. *J. Gerontol.*, **23**, 283

240 Coirault, R., Jarret, T. Ramel, P., Cadour, E., Crocq, L. and Vincent, A. (1962). Dimethyl-amino-ethyl ester of *parachorophenoxy*-acetic acid – its psychopathological action. *J. Neuropsychiatr.*, **3**, 367

241 Nandy, K. (1978). Centrophenoxine: effects on aging mammalian brain. *J. Am. Geriatr. Soc.*, **26**, 74

242 Leading article (1970). A new line on age pigment. *Lancet*, **ii**, 451

243 Marcer, D. and Hopkins, S. M. (1977). The differential effects of meclofenoxate on memory loss in the elderly. *Age Ageing*, **6**, 123

244 Gedye, J. L., Exton-Smith, A. N. and Wedgwood, J. (1972). A method of measuring mental performance in the elderly and its use in a pilot clinical trial of meclofenoxate in organic dementia (preliminary communication). *Age Ageing*, **1**, 74

245 Morton, O. (1977). Personal communication.

246 McGaugh, J. L. (1973). Drug facilitation of learning and memory. *Ann. Rev. Pharmacol.*, **13**, 229

247 Parkes, J. D., Tarsy, D., Marsden, C. D., Bovill, K. T., Phipps, J. A., Rose, P. and Asselman, P. (1975). Amphetamine in the treatment of Parkinson's disease. *J. Neurol. Neurosurg. Psychiatr.*, **38**, 232

248 Miller, E. and Nieburg, H. A. (1973). Amphetamines. *NY State J. Med.*, **73**, 2657

249 Clark, A. N. G. (1978). Morale and motivation. *Practitioner*, **220**, 735

250 Kaplitz, S. E. (1975). Withdrawn, apathetic geriatric patients responsive to methylphenidate. *J. Am. Geriat. Soc.*, **23**, 271

251 Pritchard, J. G. and Mykyta, L. J. (1975). Use of a combination of methylphenidate and oxprenolol in the management of physically disabled, apathetic, elderly patients: a pilot study. *Curr. Med. Res. Opin.*, **3**, 26

252 Eisdorfer, C., Nowlin, J. and Wilkie, F. (1970). Improvement of learning in the aged by modification of autonomic nervous system activity. *Science*, **170**, 1327

253 Darvill, F. T. (1959). Double-blind evaluation of methylphenidate (Ritalin) hydrochloride. Its use in the management of institutionalized geriatric patients. *J. Am. Med. Assoc.*, **169**, 1739

254 Holliday, A. R. and Joffe, J. P. (1965). A controlled evaluation of protriptyline compared to a placebo and to methylphenidate hydrochloride. *J. New Drugs*, **5**, 257

255 General Practitioners Medical Research Unit (1972). Double-blind comparison trial of Reactivan and placebo in the treatment of debility. *Med. Dig.*, **17** (11), 64

256 General Practitioner Group (1974). Studies with Reactivan in general practice. *Med. Dig.*, **19** (4), 68

257 Magnus, R. V. and Cooper, A. J. (1974). A controlled study of Reactivan in geriatrics. *Mod. Geriatr.*, **4**, 270

258 Carney, M. W. P., Cashman, M. D., King, A., Rogan, P. A. and Sheffield, B. F. (1976). Severely demented patients beyond help of drugs. *Mod. Geriatr.*, **7**, 36

259 Lehmann, H. E. and Ban, T. A. (1975). Central nervous system stimulants and anabolic substances in geropsychiatric therapy. In S. Gershon and A. Raskin (eds,). *Genesis and Treatment of Psychologic Disorders in the Elderly* (*Aging*, Vol. 2), pp. 179–202. (New York: Raven Press)

260 Ben-Yishay, Y. and Diller, L. (1973). Changing of atmospheric environment to improve mental and behavioral function. Applications in treatment of senescence. *NY State J. Med.*, **73**, 2877

261 Ben-Yishay, Y., Haas, A. and Diller, L. (1967). The effects of oxygen inhalation on motor impersistence in brain-damaged individuals: a double-blind study. *Neurology*, **17**, 1003

262 Jacobs, E. A., Winter, P. M., Alvis, H. J. and Small, S. M. (1969). Hyperoxygenation effect on cognitive functioning in the elderly. *N. Engl. J. Med.*, **281**, 753

263 Edwards, A. E. and Hart, G. M. (1974). Hyperbaric oxygenation and the cognitive functioning of the aged. *J. Am. Geriatr. Soc.*, **22**, 376

264 Goldfarb, A. I., Hochstadt, N., Jacobson, J. H. and Weinstein, E. A. (1972). Hyperbaric oxygen treatment of organic mental syndrome in aged persons. *J. Gerontol.*, **27**, 212

265 Thompson, L. W., Davis, G. C., Obrist, W. D. and Heyman, A. (1976). Effects of hyperbaric oxygen on behavioral and physiological measures in elderly demented patients. *J. Gerontol.*, **31**, 23

266 Eisner, D. A. (1975). Can hyperbaric oxygenation improve cognitive functioning in the organically impaired elderly?: a critical view. *J. Geriatr. Psychiatr.*, **8**, 173

267 Raskin, A., Gershon, S., Crook, T. H., Sathananthan, G. and Ferris, S. (1978). The effects of hyperbaric and normobaric oxygen on cognitive impairment in the elderly. *Arch. Gen. Psychiatr.*, **35**, 50

268 Ben-Yishay, Y., Diller, L., Reich, T., Rosenblum, J. A. and Rusk, H. A. (1978). Can oxygen reverse symptoms of senility? *NY State J. Med.*, **78**, 914

269 Krop, H. D., Block, A. G., Cohen, E., Croucher, R. and Shuster, J. (1977). Neuropsychologic effects of continuous oxygen therapy in the aged. *Chest*, **72**, 737

270 Jarvik, L. F. and Milne, J. F. (1975). Gerovital-H_3: A review of the literature. In S. Gershon and A. Raskin (eds.). *Genesis and Treatment of Psychologic Disorders in the Elderly (Aging, Vol. 2)*, pp. 203–227. (New York: Raven Press)

271 Ostfeld, A., Smith, C. M. and Stotsky, B. A. (1977). The systemic use of procaine in the treatment of the elderly: A review. *J. Am. Geriatr. Soc.*, **25**, 1

272 Davison, W. (1978). The hazards of drug treatment in old age. In J. C. Brocklehurst (ed.). *Textbook of Geriatric Medicine and Gerontology* (2nd ed.), pp. 651–669. (Edinburgh and London: Churchill Livingstone)

9

Management of malignant disease in old age

A. E. Kark and D. F. Guéret Wardle

INTRODUCTION

Cancer presents with a vast array of symptoms and signs which produce classical disease patterns in every system and pose diagnostic and therapeutic challenges in the older age groups. Almost all malignant disease is more common in the older patient, particularly that of lung, skin, gut, breast and prostrate; it is also more common in men than women. In elderly patients, the standard indications for ablative treatment by surgery or radiotherapy have to be measured against the increased hazards of age and infirmity. This calls for fine judgement as to what constitutes the quality of the remaining years of life.

It is not easy to assess biological age. One man of 50 may be a livid bronchitic or obese with angina. Another of 80 may be spry, sharp-witted and physically well-preserved. While the latter is probably a good surgical risk, the former is decidedly not. There is no measure of tissue age or of the margin for safety that exists in ageing cardiovascular, pulmonary or renal systems. Such estimates must be made on the basis of clinical experience, an imprecise art at best. Most errors in therapeutic judgement in the elderly are made simply because of the increased number of unknown factors of organ deterioration.

Nevertheless the treatment of both early and advanced cancer in the elderly can be most satisfying because of the real possibilities of long-term alleviation and for the immense amount of relief which can be provided by palliative surgery or radiotherapy or judiciously used chemotherapy. Equally satisfying is an appreciation of the gains to be had by withholding radical or destructive treatment in slowly advancing disease and by treating each symptom as it arises.

This chapter will deal with: (a) the diagnosis and assessment of malignant disease, (b) the approach to the patient with cancer and to his family, particularly at the stage of terminal disease, (c) discussion of tumour growth and the application of treatment including chemotherapy, (d) the recognition and treatment of specific malignancies including the indications for purely symptomatic treatment, and (e) syndromes of advanced cancer including emergency situations that can arise.

DIAGNOSIS AND ASSESSMENT

A major dilemma occurs frequently in the management of elderly patients. There is a natural reluctance to use invasive techniques which are exhausting and by no means free from risk in those whose lifespan is limited. Yet the opportunity for many months, if not years, of palliation from unpleasant symptoms depends on accuracy in diagnosis and appropriate surgical, radiotherapeutic or chemotherapeutic measures. Therefore, as a general principle, one should investigate older patients as completely as possible unless there is good reason for omitting certain procedures, such as complex vascular radiological studies or lengthy pressure or motility studies which may be exhausting and which are unlikely to alter the course of treatment. When a patient presents with serious symptoms the routine investigations should be done expeditiously but spaced over a length of time which neither exhausts the patient nor causes unnecessary immobilization. An elderly patient with a lower abdominal mass may require sigmoidoscopy, barium enema and ultrasound. Careful co-ordination with the radiologist will make the studies tolerable. Venepunctures too should be kept to a minimum.

A particular problem concerns the 'occult primary'[1]. An elderly patient may present with a large node in the neck, axilla or groin or with backache and an isolated vertebral lesion on x-ray or a large liver which biopsy shows to be an adenocarcinoma. All these require further investigation to pinpoint the primary lesion. Even though the presentation of metastatic disease predominates, it is in the patient's interest that the primary site be known to determine whether subsequent radiotherapy or chemotherapy may be effective. Accordingly, the same principles for diagnostic tests and investigations obtain and these should be undertaken as thoroughly as possible.

Telling the patient the diagnosis

In our experience nothing is more worthwhile than a completely frank discussion at the outset. Apart from those few who are so dulled mentally as to be incapable of comprehension patients should be told the true nature of their condition. This is in the form, at the first interview, of a private discussion with a senior doctor usually with one or more family members present. Other staff and students should be excluded, with the exception of a house officer, so that the patient is not overwhelmed. The discussion should indicate the nature of the disease, the stage and likely prognosis. This is in many ways the hardest task and liable to be accompanied by distress and tears. However, from then on all interchange with the patient and family is on a firm basis of trust and acceptance that whatever is said by the doctor is honest.

In many years experience of facing this initial difficult interview there has not been a single instance of resistance, serious distress of a suicidal nature or later recrimination which would make us alter this approach. The widely practised, traditional approach of prevarication, guarded prognosis and sometimes outright deception may on occasion seem an acceptable attitude in the first instance; however, it leads inexorably to deception, distrust and disbelief. In the last analysis this will produce at best a resigned acceptance of the doctor's duplicity, the patient perhaps understanding the doctor to have done his best to be kind. In most instances, there will ensue antagonism and dislike for the betrayal of trust and worse still a frustrated feeling of being treated like a child with whispered decisions taken out of earshot. The inevitable end result of this approach is unease and the lack of any intelligent communication between doctor and patient in the terminal weeks and days. Instead of an adult and respectful interchange on ward visits, there occurs the quick, embarrassed, inarticulate mumblings and the rapid walking away from the bedside when a relaxed accepting discussion of real value could and should take place.

Obviously the initial discussion needs to be handled tactfully. The description should include the word cancer interchangeably with tumour, which is a more acceptable synonym, and should describe tumours as a broad range of diseases from cancers which are easily curable to more severe forms. The discussion must stress the positive optimistic view. There is no need to open up the medical dictionary with a definition of every complication and the worst prognostic features. However serious the phase of the disease there is always some comfort to be derived. This is what the patient wants to hear and is almost all that he will grasp during the first interview, usually a shattering experience for him. The discussion should be ended by the doctor saying that there is enough to think about, that there is a good deal to be thankful for and that subsequent meetings would be a good time for further questions. It is our practice to make a detailed note in the patient's case history chart of exactly what the patient was told and the prognosis given. It is essential that the general practitioner, the nursing staff and in particular the house staff know precisely what has been said. There is no more distressing occurrence than incomplete and confusing information being provided by ancillary, junior medical and nursing staff. It is to them that the patient invariably talks more freely and therefore they must be fully informed. Therefore one of the early interviews should take place with close family and a nursing staff member present so that all parties know what has been said and the optimistic view can later be reinforced when the myriad questions are put to non-medical individuals.

Inevitably, out of sight of the patient, the family will immediately bombard the doctor with questions about his truthfulness, the time-span of estimated survival and the likely need in the end phase for domiciliary and hospital nursing requirements. These, too, should be answered with an absolute assurance given of the complete truthfulness of the information. It is important at this time to establish the degree of religious feeling and the need for the involvement, at this or a later stage, of the appropriate minister.

From the patient's point of view the role the family play is as important as that of the medical team. The close family try all too often to protect the patient with cancer from painful truths in the mistaken belief that this is right and proper and most helpful. The commonest demand made by a spouse or devoted son or daughter is 'under no circumstances must Mum be told'. Except in the most unusual circumstances we do not agree with this and explain why the patient will be told, the most important reason being the fact that the patient has every right to be properly and responsibly informed. Deception within families divides them from the patient at the very time when he or she needs the comfort of being able to discuss the disease and its implications. For the patient such deceit is the beginning of isolation and establishes a pattern which in later stages plays a major part in entrenching bouts of depression, anxiety and loneliness. Most patients believe that cancer is uniformly fatal and will need to have this fallacy corrected. It will be apparent at subsequent meetings that in the majority of instances little of the detail described in the first meeting will have penetrated except the broad idea that he has a malignancy and that he will recover from the operation. It is the realization that the patient is seldom able to absorb more than these two basic facts which should limit the doctor's initial discussion to essential information without too much detail.

Even more difficult is the interview when the patient returns with secondary tumour spread. However optimistic the first interview and the promises inherent in them, the arrival of metastases is a doomladen sign for most patients as well as doctors. No amount of prevarication or dissembling will allay the patient's fear, and the seeds of trust planted with the frank approach of the initial interview will flourish only if the doctor persists with the same openness. Again a full description is necessary. The patient must be told that the tumour has spread but that there are a number of treatments which can further contain it. This is what the patient wishes to learn so it should be stressed with confidence. Emphasis should be placed on tumours as chronic diseases not unlike arthritis, diabetes, cardiac disease etc., and that the best way to come to terms with the disease is as people do with other diseases, that is taking one step at a time. It should be repeated to the patient that the present manifestation and all other subsequent signs and symptoms can be dealt with, that the patient will not be abandoned, and that pain, perhaps the most worrying unspoken fear, can be adequately controlled at all times.

Amongst elderly patients there is a greater proportion who are more resigned and who accept such news more stoically. This should not alter the doctor's frank and truthful approach.

MANAGEMENT OF THE TERMINALLY ILL

The final stages of the disease when the patient has multiple widespread cerebral, bony, serous, pulmonary or liver metastases are usually obvious to all. Most patients at this point are remarkably resilient and hopeful, some are resigned, some are very frightened and a few quite apathetic. It is at this time that maximum paramedical support is necessary[2-5]. It would be the kindest act for the original surgeon or physician to continue supervision but often this is impracticable in terms of hospital beds. In many cases the consultant is a busy man and cannot display the care or interest or time that he would like. Some turn away from the role of treatment of the incurable. This has its own professional psychological causes – doctors as well as patients are often frightened of and by the dying. The great majority of patients are therefore treated by general practitioners some of whom are skilled and sympathetic but many of whom lack the skill or the willingness to handle this prickly and demanding clinical problem which represents the antithesis of that which doctors are trained to achieve.

Therefore a large proportion of patients are pushed into hospitals where incarceration represents a mixture of antiseptic organized care, conscience soothing for family and doctor and a means of avoiding unpleasantness by busy medical and surgical units. There are very few hospitals equipped to take these patients who often occupy single lonely rooms at the end of a corridor with everyone waiting for the bed to be vacated and to be relieved of an uncomfortable chore.

There are features which can radically alter this dreary picture. One is the realization that the majority of patients can be nursed at home until they die, with perhaps a brief few days in hospital for drainage of ascites, help with infected areas or a colostomy, pain control etc., but with a rapid return home. This demands that essential facilities are available – a home nursing service, well integrated with the hospital, and a number of hospital beds set aside and staffed by doctors and nurses skilled in terminal care problems. In our unit, which handles 150 to 200 cases on chemotherapy, we have constant hospital access available for any of our patients yet there are never more than three to four beds occupied by the dying or those who are shortly to return home to die. Thus home and family care must be encouraged and this is far more acceptable to the family if they are fully briefed and supported. There are patients who are exceptions such as the very infirm, those who lack suitable home accommodation, or more rarely, those who have psychiatric disturbance or whose spouse is so afflicted.

The practicalities of the home – hospital – home sequences are considerable[4,6]. The general practitioner and social worker are essential partners with the hospital doctor. The general practitioner must be informed by telephone as well as in writing of the patient's return and the patient's state of mind and body, so that he and the social worker can help organize home help, district nursing and health visitor. In addition the social worker can very frequently assist in arranging financial help. Some practices have excellent home nursing attachments; others rely heavily on the hospital social worker. This cooperation helps to ensure that sensible decisions are made about the need for further active treatment.

The point will be quickly recognized that what is required is symptomatic treatment and improvement in day-to-day comfort rather than admission to hospital for parenteral feeding routines, etc. Voluntary help from neighbours with shopping or sitting with the patient to allow a spouse, son, or daughter to obtain a night's sleep is invaluable.

When dealing with clinical problems where the inevitable result is the early death of the patient, ethical and philosophical problems are bound to arise. The emotive question of euthanasia may eventually be posed. It is not defensible on any philosophical or moral basis. The only reason that the debate is kept alive is the prospect of needless suffering and the frightful helplessness and destruction of the body. Modern methods of pain control, allied to anti-anxiety regimens where necessary, largely eliminate the argument of those persuaded by the ease of administration of quick intravenous killing drugs. Intelligent and sympathetic use of increasing amounts of analgesics or narcotics is a daily occurrence among doctors and nurses, and helps the patient die more easily and in tranquillity. A small number remain who are afflicted by appalling disfigurement, incontinence and paralysis, and it is this group who stimulate the question of euthanasia. Unless there are excellent home facilities, such patients should usually be in hospital, in a unit with trained staff and with access to modern analgesic regimens. The failure of hospitals to provide both these facilities and the medical and nursing expertise is no argument in support of authorized killing of an indefinable group of patients.

TUMOUR CELL KINETICS

There are a number of popular misconceptions regarding the growth of tumours which are still current. One is that tumours grow exponentially. This may be true of the leukaemias for much of the time, and to a lesser extent with lung metastases but it presupposes that each generation of cells has exactly the same growth environment as the parent cell which gives rise to the tumour. With solid tumours the reality is very different. In normal tissues a cell which is lost is merely replaced by one more. In tumours where uncontrolled growth is taking place the tumour increases in size because more than the number of cells lost are replaced by new cells. Tumour cells in suspension can double their number and thus increase exponentially. This is also probably true of the smallest of solid tumours but, as it gets larger so the time it takes for a tumour to double its volume becomes longer[7,8].

A number of other factors need to be taken into account. All parts of the cell cycle except G_1 tend to be fairly constant in a particular

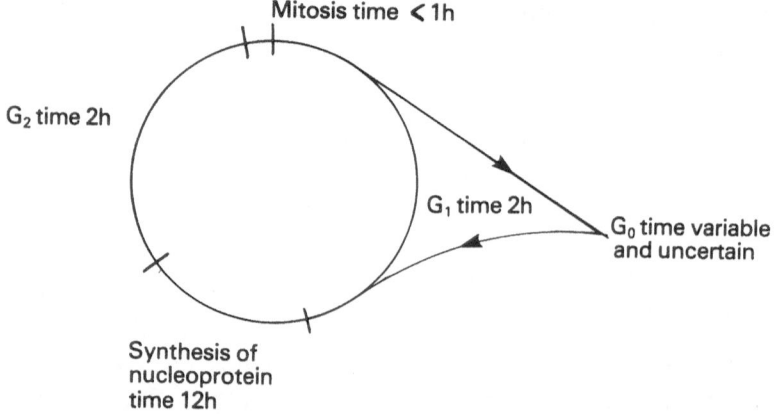

Figure 1   The phases through which a cell passes during cell division. G_1 = Gap between mitosis and synthesis phase. G_2 = Gap following synthesis phase before another mitosis. The times shown vary slightly from one tumour to another but G_0 represents a variably long time during which a cell is not actively in cycle and therefore not susceptible to most cytotoxic agents

tumour type (Figure 1). G_1 however, can be variably long. When a cell remains in G_1 for a long time it is sometimes said to be in 'G_0' or 'out of cell cycle'. Thus tumours are made up of actively dividing cells, cells out of cell cycle, cells which do not have the capacity to divide further or for only one or two further divisions (so called 'non-clonogenic cells'), plus areas of necrosis, together with blood vessels, fibroblasts, etc.

The way the tumour grows therefore depends on:

(1)   The cell cycle time, that is the time taken between the end of one mitosis in a cell to the end of mitosis in its progeny.

(2)   The growth fraction or that proportion of cells in the whole tumour which are actively in cell cycle and undergoing regular division.

(3)   The cell loss factor.

As a tumour grows larger so it appears that the cell loss factor becomes greater as the tumour outgrows its blood supply and nutrition, while the growth fraction may be smaller. Experimental tumours have given much of the data on which this is based but in human tumours, other than in the chest, growth rate information has been hard to gather since it is seldom possible ethically to inspect a tumour *in situ* more than once surgically. Ultrasound and CT scan may give more knowledge in this respect.

Steel and Lamerton[9] studied a variety of human primary and secondary tumour growth rates mostly in lung and found that tumour volume doubling times varied between 5 and 500 days, the great majority falling between 10 and 200 days. As with experimental tumour growth a further misconception is that cell cycle times or intermitotic times are shorter than in normal tissues. In fact cells from tumours tend to divide more slowly than those from the essential normal tissues such as bone marrow and gut mucosa and, as will be seen later, this provides an important therapeutic advantage when considering chemotherapy.

Thus the present concept of individual solid tumour enlargement is one of irregular growth, which may be rapid during early divisions of tumour cells but which slows as the tumour becomes larger and as the growth fraction becomes smaller, cell loss becomes greater. In addition it is possible that mutation and cell de-differentiation may continue so that the tumour may eventually be composed of more than one clone of malignant cells.

CHEMOTHERAPY

Antitumour chemotherapy[10-13] with cytotoxic drugs has gained an unnecessarily poor reputation among general physicians and surgeons. In unskilled hands and without knowledge of the limitations and principles underlying the use of such drugs unnecessary mortality and morbidity without therapeutic gain has been experienced.

In interfering with cell processes cytotoxic drugs affect normal tissues as well as tumour cells. Unfortunately there is little specificity with regard to a malignant cell line so that harmful effects to the whole patient can easily be brought about. It is generally true that such drugs exert greater effects on tissues with a large growth fraction where a large proportion of cells are actively in cell cycle. Thus normal tissue such as hair follicles, intestinal mucosa and bone marrow are particularly at risk. Exposure of these tissues to very large doses of cancer chemotherapeutic agents or to smaller doses given continuously for a prolonged period which span several cell cycle times, results in serious damage to them.

Until this was understood chemotherapy was given continuously at necessarily low dosage and without much benefit. It has become clear that greater therapeutic advantage can be gained by exploiting the knowledge that (a) tumour cell cycle times tend to be longer than those of the normal tissues at risk, and (b) tumour volume doubling times are usually longer than the time needed by damaged normal tissue such as bone marrow and intestinal mucosa to double its volume during regeneration.

Larger doses of chemotherapeutic agents given for short periods with appropriate intervals allow normal tissues to recover before the next dose is due. In this way cell loss in a tumour can be increased so that with intermittent treatment over a prolonged period it exceeds the number of new tumour cells that appear. Consequently a tumour will regress while normal tissues are damaged intermittently but temporarily. Therefore there may be only a small margin between severe toxicity to the patient and ineffective treatment at too low a dose and too long an interval between doses. This is particulary true in elderly patients where tissue reserve is less than in younger people.

Cell cycle specificity

Apart from their biochemical characteristics cytotoxic agents can be divided into three classes:

(1) Those which are believed to act in all phases of the cell cycle including 'G_0'. They are 'non-specific agents' such as irradiation.

(2) Those which act in a particular phase of the cell cycle, usually 'S' phase of DNA synthesis, and are termed 'phase specific agents'. Increasing dosage of these drugs over a short period causes increasing cell kill up to a plateau maximum after which further increase in dosage has no effect. Prolonged exposure, however, causes very definite increased effect both to tumour cells and the normal cell populations at risk with consequent greatly increased risk to the patient. Vincristine and methotrexate are such drugs.

(3) Cycle specific drugs damage cells in most phases of the cell cycle except those in resting or 'G_0' phase and include adriamycin and BCNU. Both increased dosage and exposure time cause steadily increasing tumour cell kill and host toxicity.

Bruce, Meeker and Valeriote[14] established these groups for lymphoma cells transplanted into mice. Although the work has not been repeated in human solid tumours these groups still form the basis of rationalizing the way in which chemotherapy drugs are combined. The classification of individual drugs can be seen in Table 1.

There is evidence that cytotoxic drugs given in high dosage over less than two haemopoietic stem cell cycle times have a higher therapeutic index (selective toxicity of an agent to tumour tissue compared to its effect on the most sensitive normal host tissue) than

Table 1　A classification of commonly used cytotoxic agents

Agent	Biochemical class	Kinetic group
Radiotherapy		non-specific
Prednisone	steroids	probably non-specific
Oestrogens	"	"
Androgens	"	"
Progesterone	"	"
Nitrogen mustard	alkylating agents	non-cycle-specific
Cyclophosphamide	"	"
Chlorambucil	"	"
Cytosine arabinside	antimetabolites	phase-specific
Methotrexate	"	"
6-Thioguanine	"	"
6-Mercaptopurine	"	"
5-Fluorouracil	"	"
Vincristine	plant alkaloids	phase-specific
Vinblastine	"	"
Actinomycin D	antibiotics	cycle-specific
Adriamycin	"	"
Daunorubicin	"	"
Bleomycin	"	"
Mitomycin	"	"
Mithramycin	"	"
BCNU	nitrosoureas	cycle-specific
CCNU	"	"
Streptozotocin	"	"
DTIC	miscellaneous	cycle-specific
Procarbazine	"	"
Hydroxyurea	"	"

the same drugs given in lower dosage over a longer period. This may be because over a longer period more haemopoietic stem cells are recruited from 'G$_0$' into active cell cycle and thereby become depleted being now sensitive to the agents employed[15].

Single drug versus multiple drug treatment
Tumour types are more or less sensitive to a variety of chemotherapeutic agents. There is a very large armamentarium from which to choose but it is still true that not all drugs have been evaluated in even the most common tumours. Providing that a drug used as a single agent has significant activity in making a specific type of tumour regress it is now often included in combination treatment with other drugs of similarly proven efficacy. It should be remembered, however, that the schedule and dosage in which a drug may have been evaluated for a particular malignancy may not be the optimum so that there may be some drugs which have been reported as inactive which may in fact have greater potential.

The principles governing combination chemotherapy are as follows:

(1)   Drugs should be combined so that they have an additive anti-tumour effect without increasing toxicity. This can be achieved by using drugs having different or minimal overlapping side-effects.

(2)   Drugs should be combined which cause multiple biochemical defects in malignant cells.

(3)   It is usual to include drugs from more than one of the classes of drugs described above with regard to the cell cycle.

(4)   It may be possible to combine drugs which have a synergistic rather than just an additive effect.

(5)   The combination of agents which produce antagonism with regard to the tumour effect should be avoided.

(6)   Some agents when combined together produce unexpectedly severe toxicity. These too should be avoided or at best used with great care. Examples are adriamycin with more severe cardiotoxicity after radiotherapy to the mediastinum[16], and cis-platinum, a nephrotoxic agent in combination with methotrexate, which is excreted predominantly unchanged by the kidneys[17,18]. Another example of where excretion may be affected is with allopurinol. This xanthine oxidase inhibitor is frequently used with cytotoxic chemotherapy, not for any cytotoxic effect but because it prevents the build up of urates, as a result of increased purine catabolism, which is potentially harmful to renal function. Allopurinol also slows the inactivation of 6-mercaptopurine by oxidation so that the dosage of 6-mercaptopurine in the presence of allopurinol should be greatly reduced to prevent serious toxicity without necessarily impairing the antineoplastic effect.

(7)   Small daily doses of both phase and cycle-specific agents are best avoided since greater therapeutic benefit with less toxicity is obtained when larger doses are given intermittently.

(8)   It may be possible to 'synchronize' tumour cells with one chemotherapeutic agent and then sequentially introduce other agents at the appropriate time when the synchronized cohort of cells is at that part of the cell cycle where the other agents may be expected to act. Cytosine arabinoside has been used in human acute leukaemia to 'synchronize' cells causing an in-

crease in the number of cells at the same stage of the cell cycle before administration of other drugs such as methotrexate and vincristine[19,20]. Price *et al.*[21] put together a kinetically based multiple drug regime for head and neck cancer, but in general synchronization remains largely a theoretical concept as yet of unproven practical use.

(9) A thorough knowledge of individual drug toxicities is essential and particularly important in the elderly. Drugs such as vincristine, which causes peripheral nerve damage, and adriamycin, which causes cardiomyopathy, have to be used with much greater care. This may also apply to bleomycin which causes pulmonary fibrosis. The specific side-effects of the last two drugs only appear after a threshold total dose has been administered, sometimes over several months. It is wise to lower this total permissible dose by 30–50% in the elderly since the effects once apparent are not reversible. Close supervision at home may be especially necessary in many patients to ensure correct dosage and correct timing.

Drug resistance
Drug resistance may already be present when chemotherapy is initiated so that the tumour does not respond at all. Experience has shown that, with notable exceptions, it is generally true that combinations of multiple drugs produce responses in a larger number of patients than with single agents, presumably overcoming drug resistance in these patients during early treatment.

Since the great majority of responses seen with solid tumours are partial, with eventual recrudescence of disease, drug resistance has appeared when this happens. Such resistance may be innate in a small proportion of cells from the onset in a drug-'sensitive' tumour or may be acquired as a result of further mutation. In either case such resistant clones will eventually be 'selected' and grow through as the sensitive cells are destroyed. There is evidence in solid tumours that more than one malignant cell line may be present in the same tumour[22].

Nutritional state
As adequate nutritional state is important to prevent undue toxicity from cancer chemotherapy, careful selection of drugs and dose schedules is necessary. Elderly patients with chronic disease, and living alone, may well be poor candidates for such treatment unless any existing nutritional deficiency can at least be partially corrected.

THE TREATMENT OF SYNDROMES
OF ADVANCED CANCER

A great deal can and should be done to relieve the patient of the symptoms of late disease. There are very few if any complications which cannot be helped and most of the accompanying anxiety can be removed. Much of the general complaint of pain and discomfort is bound up with fear and anxiety, fear of the next attack of pain and anxiety about the despair and helplessness induced by this. Commonly seen syndromes amongst those to be described are pain syndrome, bony metastases, recurrent ascites and effusions, oedema, recurrent and acute infections, acute renal failure, shortness of breath, nausea and vomiting, gastric and intestinal obstructions.

Pain

Whatever the source of the pain whether bony, soft tissue, visceral or neural, the chronicity and constant periodicity finally becomes intolerable for the patient. It can interfere with sleep, causes intense brooding anxiety and depression with increasing distress for both patient and family. It is this aspect which must be vigorously and sympathetically tackled by the medical attendant, before the patient becomes worn out or despondent.

There are many new and potent analgesics and much fascinating pharmacological work has been done to explain pain syndromes. The greatest single contribution and advance has been made by Cicely Saunders at St Christopher's Hospice, London[4]. The St Christopher's approach consists of the regular, carefully timed administration of an appropriate painkiller *before* the next pain cycle starts, even before the patient thinks it necessary. No other therapy plays so important a role in transforming a frightened and tense bedridden man or woman into a relaxed chairborne or ambulant personality, secure in the knowledge that the draining pain will not be allowed to happen. The 'p.r.n.' prescription must never be allowed and should be banned by any ward staff, both medical and nursing, who care for chronic pain syndromes – especially those due to cancer. Furthermore the outdated medical orthodoxy that preaches worry about addiction is in reality an unthinking cruelty. Addiction in the terminal stages of disease is of no consequence – what matter if the patient in the last weeks of life is receiving 20 or 40 or 60 ml of powerful narcotic formulas as long as he is comfortable, awake and aware for periods and able to talk to family and friends.

The basis of titration of a pain-killing drug against pain is to start with mild analgesics, to proceed to increasing doses, with appropriate anxiety-relieving drugs only if needed, and then to move on to more potent drugs and finally to morphine and its derivatives. The essence of successful therapy is regular timing based on individual assessment of each patient, and the willingness to move directly to stronger analgesics the moment that the patient's tolerance is exceeded. The correct dose is one which provides complete relief for periods of 3–4 hours. A useful guide is to prescribe a more potent drug when more than 3 tablets of a milder analgesic have become necessary. It is a repeated and disheartening experience to admit patients to hospital with severe pain which cannot be handled at home only to find that the patient is on a mixture of tablets and injections ranging from aspirin to morphine all given without relation to the patient's proper needs but usually taken at the height of the pain, at the peaks instead of in the valleys. The policy to be adopted in this situation should be the cessation of all drugs, followed by small doses of a mild analgesic on a regularly timed basis together with an anxiety-relieving drug such as diazepam or chlorpromazine, if required. The dosage may need to be increased or a more appropriate drug substituted. This will radically alter the whole picture. If pain is generalized it is often helpful to restart with an initial dose of diazepam (Valium) and diamorphine each of 10 mg. This will help allay extreme anxiety and allow more precise assessment. When the appropriate drugs have been properly titrated such patients can often be sent home for longer or shorter periods and the majority both prefer this and have less dread of further complication. Sedatives are too regularly added as a matter of routine to analgesic regimens. Adequate analgesia will usually obviate the need for such sedation, anxiety having been alleviated earlier. If sedation with drugs such as diazepam or chlorpromazine is required these should be titrated separately from analgesics so that again the correct maintenance dose can be achieved. An inert patient unable to communicate with those around him is too often seen. It is very rarely a therapeutic necessity. Additional medication is often valuable. For example, bony metastases may require aspirin as an anti-inflammatory agent. Nerve pain, especially where there is invasion of roots, may require chordotomy or nerve root blocks with phenol and an anaesthetist's opinion should be obtained. Table 2 outlines suitable regimes that may be used.

The clergyman or priest can play an important role at this stage but it is important that the doctor and cleric communicate so that both are aware of the stage of the patient's progress and the likely

Table 2 Drugs for the relief of pain

Degree of pain	Drug	Dose	Comments
MILD			
Oral	(a) Aspirin	600–1200 mg 4 hourly (up to 4 g/day)	Gastrointestinal bleeding problems, use soluble or enteric coated
	or		
	(b) Paracetamol	Two tabs 4 hourly	
	or		
	(c) Distalgesic (dextropropoxyphene + paracetemol)	Two tabs 4 hourly	
	or		
	(d) Benoral (Benorylate) (each 10 ml has 2.2 g aspirin and 1.8 g paracetemol)	10 ml twice a day or two tabs three times a day	Absorbed unaltered ∴ less likely to produce gastrointestinal irritation
	or		
	(e) Codeine	15, 30, 60 mg tabs	All constipating
	Codis (codeine 8 mg + 500 mg aspirin)	Two tabs 4 hourly	
	Panadeine (codeine 8 mg + paracetemol 1500 mg)	Two tabs four times a day	
	DF118 (dihydrocodeine)	One to two tabs 4 hourly	Weak narcotics
MODERATE			
(i) Oral	(a) Diconal (dipipanone hydrochloride 10 mg + Cyclyzine 30 mg)	One tab 4 hourly	Constipates; very useful for out-patients; nausea may be a problem
	or		
	(b) Omnopon (papervereetum 10 mg tab)	Two tabs 4 hourly	Moderate narcotic
	or		
	(c) Palfium (dextromoramide 5 mg, 10 mg tabs)	5–10 mg 2–4 hourly	Constipates; it is relatively shortlived but useful as a 'top-up' in addition to others
(ii) i.m.	(a) Pethidine	5–100 mg	
	or		
	(b) Paperveretum 20 mg amp.	20 mg 4 hourly	
	or		
	(c) Nepenthe (opium solution –	5–10 ml	

348

	Preparation	Dose	Comments
(i) Oral	(a) Diamorphine HCl in chloroform	5–10 mg up to 30 mg as a rule – even up to 100 mg	50% more potent than morphine due to better absorption
	or		
	(b) Brompton cocktail Diamorphine 5–10 mg Cocaine 5–10 mg Alcohol (50%) to 5 ml + Syrup + Chloroform water or syrup	5 ml, and increase either the diamorphine or both diamorphine and cocaine	Brompton does not need sedative. Add Largactil (chlorpromazine) or diazepam only if there is much anxiety. Chlorpromazine or diazepam should be given as a separate mixture and not as part of a Brompton. The required sedative effect can then be titrated separately from the analgesic effect. If too 'sickly' or 'alcoholic' to taste use diamorphine in chloroform water alone and patient adds own flavouring, such as blackcurrant
	or		
	(c) Narphen 5 mg (morphine analogue – phenazocine)	Two to three tabs 4 hourly	Five times more potent than morphine and longer action. Useful if patient prefers a tablet
	or		
	(d) Physeptone (Methadone) 5 mg tabs or 2 mg/5 ml lincture	5–30 mg	Has cumulated effect so not suitable in the elderly
(ii) Suppositories	Proladone (morphine supp.)	10–60 mg (15 mg = 10 mg morphine)	Extreme care in elderly (long plasma half-life)
(iii) i.m.	(a) Morphine sulph.	15–20 mg	This is preferable to morphine as it is more soluble (100 mg will dissolve in 0.2 ml)
	or		
	(b) Diamorphine HCl	5–10 mg	
	or		
	(c) Duromorph (morphine suspension)	1 vial = 64 mg/ml. Give $\frac{1}{3}$ oral dose two to three times a day	This is a long-acting preparation
(iv) i.v.	Same but smaller doses		

Note Dosages are given as a guide only. There is such a wide variation in each case and for each day that individual titration must be done.

problems that may occur. Above all sympathetic nursing and close family contacts should be fostered. Intellectual stimulation, diversion, the company of friends and home visits all play a very important role and make the last weeks and months at least tolerable and cheerful and at best may make it a meaningful and close family experience.

Painkilling regimes unfortunately have side-effects either by initiating symptoms such as nausea or exacerbating them if already present. Therefore an antiemetic, metoclopramide or cyclizine, should be prescribed or its need kept under regular review. They may be given in syrup form or as a tablet or i/m injection. Chlorpromazine may be used in suppository form. If one is ineffective it is preferable to add another antiemetic rather than to increase the dose.

Nausea and vomiting

These symptoms frequently accompany cancer, particularly of the gastrointestinal tract, but increasingly are side-effects of chemotherapeutic schedules. The need for control of them is 2-fold – firstly, for the patient's comfort, and secondly, in order to remove a serious bar to adequate food intake.

It is necessary first to distinguish whether the cause is local and obstructive or generalized. If local, and this is established primarily by x-ray, some form of surgical approach will be necessary. Any obstruction will be demonstrated by contrast studies and the commonest cause is a degree of pyloric obstruction, requiring a gastroenterostomy. This is a relatively minor surgical procedure and should seldom be withheld even in near-terminal patients. The alternative of having a permanent indwelling nasogastric tube is to be avoided if possible.

In an extensive clinical study Moertel[23] has shown, using patients on 5FU for advanced gastronintestinal cancer, that phenothiazine derivatives especially thiopropazate and prochlorperazine 5–10 mg (Stemetil, Compazine) have a significantly better antiemetic effect than placebos. Antihistamines effective for motion sickness are generally not of use for nausea and vomiting due to other causes.

While none of these drugs can be relied on to maintain control, they are effective in the majority of patients when given by injection. Metaclopramide (Maxolon) is particularly helpful in upper gastrointestinal tract lesions with nausea when increased gut motility is desirable. In non-specific cases of nausea and vomiting it is worth trying simple measures first. Sipping iced water or soda water combined with relief of pain may diminish nausea. If vomiting persists and no surgical relief is possible in the presence of obstruction then intermittent passage of a nasogastric tube either once daily before sleep or twice daily morning and evening is worthwhile. Alternatively an indwelling very fine (1 mm) plastic paediatric nasogastric tube may be tolerated for a week or more with rest periods of a few days.

Other malignant causes of nausea are leukaemia and lymphomatous infiltrations which cause meningitic symptoms and neck stiffness. Breast cancer can also occasionally cause meningitic symptoms but generally causes nausea and vomiting as do with other tumours through cerebral deposits and raised intracranial pressure.

Peripheral oedema, pleural effusions and ascites

Retention of fluid in malignant disease can be one of the most intractable and uncomfortable complications and one which is frequently treated inadequately. It should never be accepted that the cause of such fluid retention is the underlying malignant disease until proven, for example by demonstrating that pelvic masses are causing lymphatic and venous obstruction or that ascitic and pleural fluid contain malignant cells. Heart failure, hypoproteinaemia and portal hypertension are often present in the elderly and should be excluded since their effects can be more easily treated with appropriate diet and diuretics.

Peripheral oedema

Peripheral oedema[24] in the lower limbs, where this is due to malignant disease causing pelvic obstruction, can be treated with thigh-length elastic yarn stockings and intermittent but frequent elevation of the limbs often helps. If these measures work, then intermittent pressure using limb-encasing inflatable cuffs should be tried with pressure from an automatic pump being applied for 1 min every 2 min for periods of 20–30 min. This regimen two to four times daily may be very beneficial. Persistent limb swelling is considerably helped by compression stockings but this should be by a graduated stocking, that is, one specially measured for every contour. Those made by Jobst or Sigvaris are suitable. Diuretics may also be of benefit but if the tumour causing obstruction can be removed surgically or reduced in size with radiotherapy and/or chemotherapy, peripheral oedema will be more permanently relieved.

Malignant pleural effusion

This is a frequent complication of metastatic breast and bronchial carcinoma and less frequently of other metastatic disease. Although diuretics may be of some value such effusions inevitably require drainage. It has long been the practice to drain the effusion and then instill some agent such as nitrogen mustard, cyclophosphamide or thio-Tepa into the pleural cavity. It seems likely that these agents do not act by local effect on malignant cells in pleural deposits but by the following:

(1)   Systemic action after absorption.

(2)   Local inflammatory action causing the pleural surfaces to stick together with fibrosis and obliteration of the pleural space thus inhibiting fluid formation. This view is further strengthened by mepacrine and quinacrine also being of value when injected into the pleural cavity. Bleomycin has also been used. Such agents are, however, frequently painful causing an intense pleural reaction.

An alternative method is to put a soft rubber tube in place to drain the effusion and then to keep it in place attached to constant suction for ten days. This is less painful and may be as effective in provoking adhesion of pleural surfaces. Undoubtedly the best method of treating such effusions adequately is to be able to treat the underlying disease effectively. If the underlying tumour is sensitive, appropriate chemotherapy, given systemically, is generally more effective in preventing recurrence of effusion than when given into the pleural cavity. Lymphomatous effusions nearly always occur in association with pressure on lymphatic drainage so that irradiation of the mediastinum may be indicated.

Malignant ascites

The common causes of this most distressing condition are gastro-intestinal cancer and ovarian cancer with widespread peritoneal involvement. Intracavity administration of drugs such as thio-Tepa is even less effective than into the pleural space, and the same principle of adequate specific systemic chemotherapy for the underlying tumour is to be preferred if the tumour is likely to be sensitive. Unfortunately this is a condition which is often not easily relieved so that ever more frequent paracentesis can become necessary to relieve breathlessness and discomfort. This in turn contributes to hypoproteinaemia thus further increasing the need for drainage.

Techniques have been developed recently whereby ascitic fluid can be drained, filtered free of cells and organisms and concentrated before being reinfused into a brachial vein. This ensures that patients do not lose massive quantities of protein and electrolytes when ascitic drainage is necessary. Another method still being assessed is the use of a peritoneovenous shunt using a watertight drain into the peritoneum connected to a one-way valve placed subcutaneously in the abdominal wall, which in turn is connected to a long silastic tube from this valve, laid subcutaneously up to the internal jugular vein into which it drains[25]. This method is particularly successful in alcoholic cirrhosis but has been of great benefit in patients with malignant ascites especially where ascites is the only clinically obvious area of spread.

Neuromuscular disorders
The association of polymyositis and malignant disease is well recognized and indeed over 50% of elderly people who present with polymyositis will be found to have a carcinoma somewhere, usually of lung, breast, large bowel, prostate, uterus or ovary. The clinical features are those of predominantly proximal muscle weakness around the shoulder and pelvic girdles. Combing hair and climbing stairs may become difficult. Painful tender muscles particularly in the arms are a feature but muscle wasting is slight to moderate and appears late; 40% of patients with polymyositis also have a reddish 'butterfly' rash on the face with a similar appearance on forehead, neck, upper chest and arms with or without underlying oedema. These patients have dermatomyositis. Raynaud's phenomenon and an arthritis similar to rheumatoid may be present. Creatine phosphokinase serum levels are raised and light microscopy may show degenerating muscle fibres with infiltration of inflammatory cells, while electromyography may show increases in insertion activity and pseudomyotonic discharges. A similar and possibly identical syndrome of proximal myopathy without histological changes occurs at least as frequently as a fully recognizable polymyositis. Many patients with polymyositis will respond for a time to corticosteroids in doses of 40–60 mg/day prednisolone but the syndrome may equally well be treated by effective treatment of the underlying malignant disease by whatever means, including chemotherapy.

The myasthenic or Eaton – Lambert syndrome is seen sometimes in association with bronchial carcinoma (usually of oat cell histology) although it may occasionally precede the appearance of the bronchial carcinoma by some years. Again there is muscle weakness, particularly in the legs, but it differs from a true myasthenia in that reflexes may be lost and muscles supplied by cranial nerves are rarely affected very much. In an elderly person it is always worth searching hard for an underlying bronchial carcinoma when this complaint appears and once again adequate treatment of the underlying malignancy is most effective. Edrophonium occasionally produces dramatic improvement but anticholinesterases are usually unhelpful. Guanidine in doses of up to 30 mg/kg/day is probably the drug of choice for symptomatic treatment.

Oncological emergencies

Urgent complications of tumours are caused either by the mechanical effects of obstruction, by invasion of contiguous structures or by the metabolic and septic sequelae of dissemination. The following are those which occur with regularity and probably more often in older age groups. They may be mechanical, infective or metabolic.

Cardiac tamponade

Often not recognized, this cause of sudden circulatory collapse from reduced stroke volume and output is most often due to malignant pericardial effusions[26-28]. The incidence of metastases to the heart and pericardium is surprisingly high, up to 10-15% in large cancer autopsy series. The primary is most frequently lung, breast, leukaemia, lymphoma, melanoma or gastrointestinal, and the metastases are usually multiple. The symptoms and signs may be few or be any of those seen in an inflammatory pericarditis. They include dyspnoea, cough, thoracic pain, cardiac enlargement, rales, palpitations and friction rubs. ECG changes are often minimal and chest x-ray may only show cardiomegaly. Therefore diagnosis is difficult and may only be made when acute tamponade with collapse occurs. Other causes of pericarditis are radiation and neoplastic constrictive pericarditis.

Electrocardiography and pericardiocentesis both confirm the diagnosis but often, because of the urgent bedside consultation, the diagnosis is made initially on clinical findings. A combination of dyspnoea, clouded mind, thready pulse or pulsus paradoxus and low systolic pressure suggest the condition. The ECG finding of total or ventricular electrical alternans is an absolute indication for pericardiocentesis.

The immediate treatment is to support the circulation and improve cardiac filling by intravenous fluid, either saline or 5% human serum albumin. A pericardiocentesis must be done immediately, preferably with ECG and blood pressure monitoring. After 100 ml are removed improvement is observed. Either the needle is removed after slow evacuation of fluid, or an indwelling catheter may be inserted. There are favourable reports on the infusion of either thio-Tepa or 5FU and methotrexate via such a catheter. Radioactive phosphorus, yttrium and gold have also been used successfully.

Systemic chemotherapy, if applicable to the primary tumour, is at least as effective in controlling the effusion as intrapericardial drugs and radiotherapy may be considered, as benefit has been described in nearly half the cases reported.

This complication is well worth treating not only for the urgent relief obtained in the tamponade phase but because mean survival time in at least one series has been shown to be 12–16 months.

Superior vena caval syndrome

Whereas this emergency was once most commonly due to syphilitic aneurysms or to tuberculous mediastinitis (40% as recently as 1954), it is now due to bronchial carcinoma in 80–90% of cases and mostly to lymphoma in the remainder[29]. Although a serious development, up to 20% of patients, if actively treated, survive more than 2 years.

The common presenting symptoms are shortness of breath, swelling of the face or of the trunk and arms. Typical signs are thoracic vein distension, neck vein distension, oedema of the face and, in a smaller number, cyanosis and tachypnoea.

It is important to establish the cause, even though emergency treatment is vital, because subsequent treatment depends on accurate diagnosis. Therefore urgent chest x-ray, bronchoscopy and biopsy or washings and node biopsy are necessary. Mediastinoscopy or even thoracotomy are reserved for patients in better condition or until treatment has proved effective.

Urgent supportive therapy includes oxygen administration and tracheal intubation if necessary. Steroids such as dexamethasone have been shown to be of value in reducing inflammatory oedema. Heparin has been used because of the high proportion of patients who have venous thrombosis accompanying this syndrome. The prime treatment is urgent radiotherapy, even without histological proof, if necessary either with conventional or high dose fractions, those with bronchogenic carcinomas receiving doses of five fractions per week up to a full tumour dose of 4000–6000 rads in 5–7 weeks. Chemotherapy has not been found to be an advantage if given at the same time as radiotherapy but is reserved for the post-irradiation period.

Response to treatment can be dramatic with relief of dyspnoea, facial swelling and venous distension, especially in lymphoma (75%) but less with lung tumours (20%). Good responses are obtained in all except about 15% of bronchial carcinomas. Interestingly no lymphomata showed recurrence but 20% of bronchial tumours are liable to have recurrence of this syndrome.

Spinal cord compression

Early recognition and emergency treatment is the key to successful management of patients with this condition[30,31]. Even though there is usually widespread associated metastatic disease, the relief of pain, reversal of neurological deficits and prevention of permanent ones are important as the active and functional portion of the patient's remaining lifespan may be considerably extended.

The prodromal phase is back pain, central with usually radicular radiation to chest or abdomen. This is followed by motor dysfunction and then sensory paraesthesia. Thus there may be unilateral footdrop or weakness or difficulty with balance. If untreated these may cause inability to walk. Cauda equina lesions usually have saddle anaesthesia and partial loss of urethral, vaginal and rectal sensation and disturbance of micturition. The distribution of metastatic pressure is thoracic 70%, lumbosacral 20% and cervical 10%. The common primary tumours are lung, breast, unknown and lymphoma in over 58% of cases. Diagnosis is made by careful neurological examination and myelopathy. Once a diagnosis has been made steroids should be given, starting with large initial doses.

In slowly advancing lesions or those with incomplete block or in cauda equina lesions radiation therapy alone is indicated[32]. In rapidly progressing lesions or those with a complete block laminectomy is preferable with subsequent radiotherapy. In paralysis of short duration emergency laminectomy is necessary but if well-developed, results are so poor that it is not justified.

Radiation therapy alone or combined with surgery should be used in all patients in whom spinal cord tolerance has not been exceeded by previous irradiation and even in patients who are not surgical candidates with well-established paraplegia. Furthermore postoperative radiation relieves pain and helps reduce tumour regrowth.

Chemotherapy is given to patients whose tumours are known to be responsive to particular agents.

Acute infection

The single most important factor which predisposes to acute infection[33,34] is neutropenia. This is defined as a neutrophil count of less than $1000/\mu l$. Neutropenia may be caused by the malignancy itself, or be the result of chemotherapy. At least 75% of acute infections are bacterial, the commonest organisms being Gram-negative aerobes, such as *Escherichia coli*, *Klebsiella spp.* and *Pseudomonas aeruginosa*. Septicaemia due to *P. aeruginosa* is the most severe and is most commonly associated with terminal malignancy. These are commonly endogenous infections, the organisms being derived from the bacterial flora of the patient's large bowel.

Septicaemia due to *Staphylococcus aureus* is also common. The source may be endogenous, the organism being derived from the patient's anterior nares or skin, or the infection may be acquired exogenously from an attendant. The next most common infections are fungal, usually Candida septicaemias which are often preceded by the development of severe oral thrush. Occasionally *Aspergillus* spp. or *Cryptococcus neoformans* cause septicaemia, pneumonia or meningitis.

Desseminated viral infections with one of the Herpes virus group, are frequently seen. These are usually reactivations of latent infections such as Herpes virus hominis (*Herpes Simplex*) or Varicella-zoster virus.

Reactivation of tuberculosis is common and is manifest by caseating nodal disease or widespread pulmonary infection. Differential diagnosis of pulmonary tuberculosis must include infection with the protozoön, *Pneumocystis carinii*, which causes a disseminated interstitial pneumonia.

When neutropenia is present or predicted, prophylactic treatment with a regimen of oral non-absorbable anti-candida and antibacterial agents is of proven value, such as Fracon which is a combination of framycetin, an aminoglycoside active against Gram-negative aerobic organisms (except *P. aeruginosa*), colistin, active against *P. aeruginosa* and nystatin, an anti-candida agent. In addition the use of cotrimoxazole has also been shown to reduce the number of infective incidents in neutropenic patients. Severe oral thrush usually responds to sucking amphotericin B lozenges, 250 mg q.d.s. In established clinical septicaemias after blood cultures have been taken, gentamicin together with another synergistic antibiotic may be given. If there is reason to suspect fungal infection, intravenous micronazole should be added (250–500 mg t.d.s.). In proven fungal infection amphotericin B must be given despite its possible nephrotoxicity. When causative organisms are isolated, antibiotic therapy may have to be modified. For more details see section on septicaemia in Chapter 2.

The investigation of pyrexia of undetermined origin in patients with cancer should include the following infection screen:

(1) Swabs and/or pus from any obvious septic foci (such as, boils, paronychia, anorectal abscess);

(2) Blood cultures – three separate sets taken over the space of an hour irrespective of the height of the fever;

(3) Throat swab;
(4) Sputum;
(5) Midstream specimen of urine;
(6) Stool, if there is diarrhoea;
(7) Serum (10 ml) for fungal agglutinins and precipitins and for viral serology.

These must be repeated frequently for as long as fever persists. If the patient is febrile but not neutropenic, antibiotic therapy may be withheld pending the results of microbiological investigation.

Protective isolation of patients with neutropenia is not of proven value because most infections are endogenously acquired.

A significant recent development is the use of granulocyte transfusion from motivated relatives or friends for patients with neutropenia and proven Gram-negative septicaemia who have not responded to antibiotic therapy within 48 hours. These transfusions are given daily till the neutrophil count has risen above $1000/\mu l$.

Hypercalcaemia

Hypercalcaemia[35-38] is a common and often dangerous complication of malignancy. While the onset of symptoms can be so slow as to be confused with the direct effect of malignant disease it is sometimes sufficiently rapid and unexpected to lead to a patient's early death. It can occur with many types of tumour but is seen very commonly with myeloma, breast cancer, bronchial carcinoma, epidermoid tumours of head, neck and oesophagus and hypernephroma. The mechanism depends principally on direct tumour invasion of bone with release of calcium, the tumour production of inappropriate parathormone-like substances as well as other biologically active substances, and chronic immobilization. Dehydration, which reduces glomerular filtration, worsens hypercalcaemia.

Hypercalcaemia produces symptoms in many systems. Apathy, depression, general malaise and fatigue are often mistakenly attributed directly to the underlying tumour.

Polyuria and nocturia, from a reversible renal tubular defect in fluid conservation, contribute to azotaemia and acidosis. If this persists irreversible renal failure will follow. Hyperuricaemia sometimes occurs in association with hypercalcaemia which does not usually last long enough for the formation of renal stones.

Gastrointestinal symptoms of anorexia, nausea and vomiting, generalized and ill-defined abdominal pain as well as constipation are frequently seen. Unlike nephrolithiasis, acute pancreatitis does occur occasionally with hypercalcaemia due to malignancy as does an increased incidence of peptic ulcer. Other symptoms are bone pain and pruritus.

The heart rate slows, ECG shows a shortening of the QT interval with moderate hypercalcaemia but widening of the T wave at very high levels of serum calcium. Lengthening of the PR interval occurs occasionally with serious arrhythmias. Digitalis effect will be greatly potentiated by hypercalcaemia.

(a) *Treatment* The patient's clinical condition and level of blood calcium dictate what is appropriate treatment. In those patients where hypercalcaemia is life-threatening but who still have reasonable renal function, careful but speedy rehydration with isotonic saline is indicated followed by further infusion with saline and dextrose/saline together with forced diuresis with frusemide 40–100 mg i.v. 2–4 hourly so that a throughput of about 5 l/day is achieved. Great care must be taken to balance fluid input and output after rehydration particularly in the elderly, and detailed fluid and electrolyte balance charts must be kept. Potassium and possibly magnesium supplements should be given with the i/v infusion. A central venous line will give better control of the safe rate of infusion but may not be necessary. Thiazide diuretics should not be used since they tend to worsen hypercalcaemia.

Where renal function is poor intravenous phosphate may be used at a dose of 25–50 mmol over 6–8 hours. There is a risk of resulting hypocalcaemia, hypotension and death if too much is given too rapidly. Calcium may also be precipitated not only in the skeleton but also in the heart, kidney, lens and other soft tissues.

Mithramycin, a toxic derivative from *Streptomyces* sp., lowers blood calcium within 24–48 hours by inhibiting bone resorption or by altering the metabolism of vitamin D. It is given at a dose of 25 μg/kg (body weight) as a rapid infusion. A reasonable maximum dose is 150 μg/kg/per week for a fit young person, but this probably needs to be reduced in the elderly. It is bone marrow-toxic, resulting in thrombocytopenia, and hepatotoxic in too high a dosage, especially when there is renal impairment.

Calcitonin at a dose of 3–6 (MRC) units salmon calcitonin or 2–8 (MRC) units porcine calcitonin/kg (body weight)/day can be given every 6–8 hours intramuscularly but after several days escape from its effect occurs. It is a useful although expensive adjunct to rapid therapy, but, combined with steroids, may well be a safe treatment of choice in elderly patients with impaired renal function.

In those patients with only a moderate hypercalcaemia glucocorticoids such as hydrocortisone 100/mg three to four times daily or prednisolone 40–60 mg/day will lower serum calcium over 3–4 days.

Prolonged use of oral phosphate at a dose of 1·0–3·0 g daily is the treatment of choice but may well give rise to diarrhoea. If this happens more dilute solutions should be used. It is possible that, over the long term, extraskeletal calcium deposition may occur as with i/v phosphate.

Occasionally a false impression may be given of the potential danger of hypercalcaemia since a sample serum calcium estimation does not always accurately reflect the ionized calcium level. For example myeloma protein can bind to calcium giving a very high serum calcium level whereas the ionized calcium level may be much lower in the safer range. Conversely symptomatic hypercalcaemia can exist with apparently normal calcaemic serum levels in the presence of hypoproteinaemia.

Disseminated intravascular coagulation (DIC)

DIC[39,40] is not a disease in itself but a process with many different aetiologies. Malignant disease, which is often responsible for bone marrow infiltration and resulting thrombocytopenia, can be associated less commonly with DIC. The particular types of malignancy are listed in Table 3.

Table 3 Malignant conditions associated with DIC

Carcinomatosis	
Leukaemia	Acute myeloblastic
	Acute promyelocytic
	Chronic myeloid
	Acute lymphoblastic
	Chronic lymphocytic
Neuroblastoma	

In practice there are many instances when abnormal coagulation tests are seen with malignancy but, except with prostatic carcinoma and promyelocytic leukaemia, it is most uncommon for such abnormal tests to be seen in association with a clinical bleeding syndrome which gives rise to an oncological emergency. When this does happen the presentation is that of overt bleeding from such sites as skin or genitourinary tract or from the sites of recent surgery. Infections with fever are commonly present but occasionally clinical shock may arise without any obvious source of bleeding.

It is thought that there are three phases leading to severe bleeding with DIC. In the first phase a 'trigger' leads to tissue damage and a haemostatic response. In stage II accelerated proteolytic activity leads to intravascular coagulation with fibrinolysis. This in turn leads to both consumption of coagulation factors and platelets with consequent bleeding and to disseminated intravascular coagulation with deposition of microthrombi in specific organs.

Since the pattern of coagulation abnormalities changes all the time during an episode of DIC too much reliance should not be placed on tests done at any one time. It is therefore important to establish sequential testing where DIC is suspected. Investigation must be on three levels.

(1) Coagulation studies which determine the pattern of consumption of coagulation factors and measure the phenomenon of circulating fibrin degradation products (FDP)

(2) More general haematological and biochemical tests which give information about haemoglobin and platelet levels together with indicators towards specific organ involvement where severe thrombosis has occurred in the microcirculation.

(3) A search for infection including blood cultures and, if malignancy is suspected, a diagnosis of the nature and extent of the tumour involved.

Treatment This should be directed towards the following.

(1) Supportive therapy to expand blood volume, to correct acidosis and electrolyte imbalance and treatment of the underlying malignancy if this is possible.

(2) Replacement of depleted coagulation factors, if serious bleeding is taking place, with fresh whole blood, fresh frozen plasma, fibrinogen concentrate or cryoprecipitate. The last two should only be used if speed is essential and one of the first two is not available.

(3) The use of heparin is controversial and can only prevent further damage to tissues. Nevertheless it may well stop most distressing haemorrhage where DIC complicates metastatic carcinoma, and it may be temporarily lifesaving in acute leukaemias while chemotherapy has a chance to achieve a more lasting and useful remission. Heparin may be started in a continuous intravenous infusion at a dose of 500–1000 units/hour. This dose may need to be increased to 3000 units/hour depending on laboratory monitoring of the anticoagulant effect and the success in stopping haemorrhage.

Miscellaneous problems

Bowel difficulties
These are notorious and Dorbanex is helpful as a bowel stimulant and softener. Alternately Milpar 10 ml/b.d. or Diotcyl-forte one to two tablets t.d.s. may be alternated with Senokot. Phosphate enemas may be used one to two times weekly.

Local secondary infection
This may be particularly important in the head and neck area, and in ulcerating lesions of breast, chest wall and pelvis. Antibiotic treatment after appropriate sensitivities have been obtained is very helpful in cleaning up such areas, and good nursing care with frequent moist Eusol-soaked dressings will help turn a foul malodorous lesion into a clean tolerably pain-free area. Debrisan powder is very useful for ulcerating lesions but precaution must be taken not to allow it to be in contact with surrounding healthy tissue.

Headache
This may be a troublesome symptom as a result of intracranial deposits. Dexamethasone (Decadron), a glucocorticoid, is very useful for this.

Long continued use of narcotic analgesia is sometimes accompanied by *depression*. It is wise to watch for this even in those having drugs which produce euphoria. In elderly or debilitated patients half the adult dose should be prescribed initially as more may cause confusional states.

SPECIFIC TUMOURS AND THEIR SYMPTOMS

Breast
Breast lumps[41] present in the elderly in exactly the same fashion as in younger patients – a painless lump, a nipple discharge which is usually bloody, or an ulcerated mass tolerated because of fear about its true nature. The differential diagnosis is more narrow in the elderly than in younger patients. Abscesses are few, fat necrosis is seldom seen, and duct ectasia very rare. The long-accepted clinical staging method is unchanged and remains a useful one. Stage I is a mobile tumour of less than 5 cm, non-ulcerated and with no axillary lymph nodes palpable. Stage II is a mobile tumour or one fixed to

skin but less than 5 cm and with palpable axillary lymph nodes. Stage III includes those with wide local spread in the affected breast with deep fixation or in the supraclavicular area. Stage IV is the presence of widespread metastatic disease. Another useful way of assessing breast tumours is to divide them into the 'early' – those with Stage I and II lesions, also described as node negative and node positive, which require a more radical approach, and those that are 'late' – Stage III and IV and which may require lesser degrees of local breast treatment together with radiotherapy, hormone manipulation and chemotherapy. A more precise and uniformly accepted classification is the internationally recognized TNM system which should be used[42] – T is tumour presence and size, N is node involvement clinically and pathologically (Nla or Nlb), and M designates the presence of metastases.

The primary treatment of breast tumours is similar in most respects for elderly patients as it is in younger women[43-46] but there are exceptions when dealing with very old patients who are frail or who have advanced disease. Such patients may benefit more from very limited local treatment and simple measures to relieve distressing symptoms rather than more vigorous treatment which would otherwise be justified.

The operation recommended for those who have early disease (Stage I and II) is removal of the breast together with clearance of the axilla but with preservation of the pectoralis major muscle (Patey mastectomy). This operation causes minimal upset, has almost no mortality and very little morbidity such as small axillary fluid collections or delayed wound healing. Gross arm oedema which can occur after the more radical Halstead mastectomy is rarely seen. Patients are out of bed on the day after operation and may expect to go home at the end of a week or 10 days. It is important that regular arm exercises are begun within 3 or 4 days of operation and that these are continued for several weeks until completely free shoulder movements are achieved and maintained.

One aspect which is sometimes overlooked is the importance of additional support and understanding that is necessary. Not only has the patient to withstand the burden of knowing that she has cancer but also that her breast has been amputated. It is important where possible to have a patient well-adjusted to her mastectomy to talk to the patient before the operation so that the many unspoken fears may be allayed. In our experience most women go through a phase of reactive anxiety and depression but not necessarily immediately after operation. This may occur as long as 6 months later as the gross disfigurement of mastectomy continues to remind the patient of her condition. Medical and family support is therefore of paramount importance from the very beginning. No woman should ever be allowed to leave hospital without some form of breast prosthesis, which will not traumatize the healing wound, and a prearranged interview a few weeks later with a fitter for a more permanent prosthesis. This applies just as much to elderly patients. Eventually patients do come to terms with their condition and to the mastectomy that was necessary.

Even with Stage I or II disease breast cancer must be considered as a systemic disease from the time of presentation. Most women even with 'early' disease eventually die of their disease but this may not happen until 20 years later[47]. Those with initial Stage I disease tend to present with recurrent disease later than those with initial Stage II disease. Recently Fisher and colleagues[48] and Bonadonna and colleagues[49] have shown that chemotherapy, following surgery of the primary disease, may prevent or at least delay recurrence in those women who present with Stage II disease. It is our belief that chemotherapy should also be given following Stage I disease but this needs to be done as part of a properly controlled trial[50]. Since those with initial Stage I disease tend to present with recurrent disease later than those with initial Stage II disease we have fixed an arbitrary upper age limit of 70 years in those with Stage I to be treated with chemotherapy until clearer evidence of benefit is available. Indeed chemotherapy appears to be less effective following surgery of Stage II disease in postmenopausal women generally.

Following trials in Manchester and Scandinavia and in the King's College Hospital/Cambridge trial it appears that there is no place for routine radiotherapy after surgery in early breast cancer[43,51]. Locally advanced Stage III disease may be treated with surgery, radiotherapy and chemotherapy, with radiotherapy and chemotherapy or with radiotherapy alone as circumstances indicate. Again the criterion should be that there will be more disease than can be discovered by chest x-ray, bone scan, liver ultrasound and blood biochemistry which should be done in all cases of breast cancer except in the very frail and very elderly.

In the very old and infirm the finding of a mobile hard non-ulcerated tumour with or without nodes warrants no further treatment, not even a diagnostic biopsy. The pathology is obvious, the biology is of a very slow growing tumour and the prognosis very good or at least only very slowly progressive.

In the other very old but reasonably fit patients the finding of a breast mass deserves excision biopsy and, with histological proof, a local mastectomy only. No radical surgery should be done.

An ulcerated mass represents locally advanced disease. Radiotherapy is the method of choice to dry the exudate area and cause regression of the mass, and is the least upsetting treatment in frail patients.

The more difficult therapeutic problems arise when late manifestations present. These most commonly are bone pain and pathological fractures, fluid collections in the chest and abdomen and liver metastases.

Advanced disease may manifest itself most commonly as:

(1) Local bone disease often in vertebrae. Here radiotherapy provides excellent symptomatic relief. Bone pain may be rapidly relieved by Indomethacin, a prostaglandin synthetase inhibitor, 25–50 mg t.d.s. by mouth.

(2) Chest wall or incisional recurrences: for these, too, local irradiation is a good means of palliation. In a previously irradiated chest wall or where radiotherapy cannot be given for other reasons cryosurgery can be of great benefit in destroying or controlling the lesions before wide ulceration ensues.

(3) The presentation of a discharging ulcerated mass signifies inoperability and therefore radiotherapy is indicated and very helpful in drying these lesions. Chemotherapy is also useful in combination with radiotherapy or where radiotherapy is inappropriate.

(4) More generalized manifestations of advanced disease such as multiple bone and soft tissue secondary spread requires that a judgement should be made between starting cytotoxic chemotherapy immediately or approaching treatment by sequential steps. The first line in the latter approach would be the use of hormonal manipulation; ethinyl oestradiol, 0·1 mg b.d. in the elderly should be given for as long as remission or improvement continues. Nausea may be experienced.

The introduction of the drug Tamoxifen, a so-called antioestrogen, provides another alternative[52]. This is a relatively complication free oral drug used at an initial dosage of 10–20 mg b.d. and may be given before other agents.

Cytotoxic chemotherapy requires specific indications and must be carefully judged in the elderly[53–55]. The indications for its use are widespread late disease (preferably after oestrogen or Tamoxifen has been tried, in otherwise relatively fit patients for a limited period of 2–3 months to judge whether response is occurring without unacceptable morbidity. The other group of patients for whom it is indicated are the elderly who are relatively infirm but in whom there occur specific symptoms and signs such as pain, effusions both peritoneal and pleural, hypercalcaemia or ulcerating lesions already treated by radiotherapy occur. Adriamycin should be used with considerable care because of cardiac toxicity in patients whose cardiac reserve is already compromised. The maximum amount of this drug should not exceed a total of 300 mg/m² in patients over 65 years.

Cancer of the female genital tract

Vulva

Surprisingly, tumours in this region which account for 3–4% of all gynaecological cancers are often diagnosed very late. They occur in the elderly as a rule. Precancerous lesions include Bowen's disease, Paget's disease and papillomatosis, atrophic vulvitis and kraurosis. Most complain of pruritis several years before the malignancy develops. Cytology is helpful. Toluidine blue 1% followed by acetic acid 1% helps identify areas at high risk. Biopsy must be done in any lesion unresponsive to medical treatment after 1 month. The lesions are classified according to the TNM system; nearly 50% of invasive vulval cancer have node involvement mainly of the superficial inguinal nodes.

Where nodes are not involved vulvectomy without node dissection carries a good prognosis – 80% survival at 5 years. With node involvement this figure falls to 30% or less if superficial nodes are involved and 3% if the deep nodes are involved.

Primary vaginal carcinoma is even rarer and is mainly squamous. As the concept of primary multiple malignant condition of the genital tract is more widely accepted, vigilance must be exercised in any woman who has had any other genital cancer. Surgery, at best, carries a 45% 5 year survival rate and consists of radical excision including hysterectomy and pelvic node dissection in the Stage I and II cases. In those where the lesion extends to the pelvic wall and is fixed primary irradiation is indicated usually by intracavity radium with external radiation supplementation.

There are recent reports of the use of adriamycin and methotrexate in advanced squamous cancer of the cervix which shows promise, and this combination may be of value in the vagina as well.

Ovarian cancer

This tumour[57,58] has increased by two to three times in the past 50 years and is the leading cause of death from gynaecological cancer. If found in an early stage treatment is by radical hysterectomy and bilateral salpingo-oophorectomy and omentectomy. In later stages both radiation and chemotherapy have a role. Omental and peritoneal seedings occur early and the mesentery of the bowel may be involved. Thus intestinal obstruction is not uncommon.

The pathology is complex and the International Federation of Gynaecology and Obstetrics has established a histological classification which helps simplify it. This requires in addition the identification of each tumour as benign, potentially malignant or malignant, because of the very wide range of tumour behaviour; 80% of all ovarian tumours are of epithelial origin, the remainder being of mesenchymal origin or from the germ cells.

Poor therapeutic results are due mainly to the absense of characteristic early symptoms. A great number present unfortunately with vague abdominal discomfort and mild digestive disturbance. In later stages there occur the characteristic swelling due to ascites, pain and a palpable mass. The main diagnostic tool is laparotomy based on a high index of suspicion particularly when any adnexal mass is present. Furthermore ovarian tumours can only be staged at the time of laparotomy as only at exploration can the full extent of the lesion be appreciated.

Nearly 10% of ovarian tumours are metastatic arising from the gastrointestinal tract, breast and thyroid.

In Stage I disease complete surgical excision followed by chemotherapy and/or irradiation will produce survival rates of 80–90%. The only means of improving the general survival rates is early diagnosis and treatment and to achieve this a high index of suspicion is necessary in any unusual or unexplained abdominal symptoms. Two other indications for laparotomy should be observed; firstly the ability to palpate an ovary in an older postmenopausal woman; this PMPO (postmenopausal palpable ovary) syndrome is based on the fact that after menopause the normal ovary is about half its previous size and becomes impalpable. Secondly a positive Pap smear without evidence of a vaginal or cervical cancer indicates probable ovarian origin.

Chemotherapy has a definite place and makes a more comfortable terminal period in a moderate number of patients[59]. Alkylating agents have been used in the main, particularly cyclophosphamide 200 mg i.v. for 5 days followed by 50 mg b.d. orally. Some use Melphalan 1 mg/kg weight in divided doses for 5 days post operatively and then monthly to 6 weekly. More recently, combination chemotherapy including the toxic agent *cis*-platinum has begun to show improved results. The management of advanced ovarian carcinoma is often difficult. The commonest complication is ascites. Its pathogenesis is not clear. It is known that ascitic patients have a higher turnover and production of fluid, that there is higher portal pressure and that both normal omentum and small bowel surfaces produce more fluid than usual but the reasons are far from clear.

Simple aspiration is of little value because of rapid reformation. Systemic chemotherapy may be of real benefit. Local instillation is of no greater use in contrast to pleural effusions which can respond well to local infusion of drugs such as nitrogen mustard which probably cause pleural surfaces to adhere.

Intestinal obstruction is common. The surgical treatment must be non-operative initially (suction and i/v fluids) as extensive bowel involvement is common and precise clean surgery usually difficult with external fistula formation not uncommon. When operative intervention is clearly needed the minimum should be done, bypassing where necessary, and only bringing bowel to open on the surface if no other possibility exists.

Cervical cancer

This is no longer the commonest gynaecological cancer and death rates in the United States and United Kingdom from this disease have fallen by nearly half[60,62]. Undoubtedly this is mainly due to early detection by popular education and regular cervical smears. Although the peak incidence occurs in the mid-fifties it is not rare in the elderly. The concept of carcinoma *in situ* is now accepted and its progression, if untreated, to invasive cancer is well documented; 95% are squamous lesions.

Ideally all women should have cytologic studies of cervical smears routinely as malignant cells can be identified in 90% of cases. Certainly in hospital patients the technique should be widely used, and preferably regarded as mandatory as a routine chest x-ray. The technique will then identify *in situ* lesions which are otherwise symptomless. The symptoms of invasive cancer are discharge and bleeding and will require standard examination including biopsy of the cervix.

Staging is arrived at entirely by clinical evaluation, and the most important single feature in prognosis is the extent of the disease when treatment is begun[61]. The classification devised by FIGO is widely adopted. Full examination includes pelvic examination, cystoscopy, proctoscopy, IVP bone X-rays and CT scanning.

Stage O (carcinoma *in situ*) – either cone removal or if it is occult or, in the woman post childbearing, a radical hysterectomy and node dissection.

Stage Ia – early stromal – radical hysterectomy and bilateral node dissection.

Stage Ib – still confined to cervix – radical hysterectomy and bilateral node dissection.

Stage II – beyond cervix but not on side wall – radical hysterectomy and bilateral node dissection.

Stage III – reached sidewall or lower third of vagina – radical hysterectomy and bilateral node dissection and radiation therapy.

Stage IV – involving adjacent organs, bladder, rectum or distant metastases – primary radiation or extenuation in selected cases.

The results of treatment in Stage Ia should not be less than 95% 5 year survival; Stage Ib will have 70–85% 5 year survival.

Chemotherapy has been ineffective. Both nitrogen mustard and methotrexate have had some success in late stage pain relief, but bleomycin has not shown any promise. A preliminary favourable report of the value of adriamycin and methotrexate has been made by Guthrie and Way[62].

Endometrial cancer
This is now the second most common gynaecological cancer. It is a slow-growing adenocarcinoma presenting mainly in the post menopausal groups. Any dysfunctional uterine bleeding must be fully investigated by vaginal smear, endometrial aspiration and curettage. The staging is on the same basis as cervical cancer, Stages O to IV[63].

In the curative Stage O, I and II, total hysterectomy and salpingo-oophorectomy is preferred followed by irradiation. In later phases Stages II and III preoperative irradiation precedes radical hysterectomy. In Stage IV intracavity radium is used.

While mean survival time is good in early stages – 10 years for all ages over 65 – the survival drops markedly with increasing age and, over 80, averages 2·1 years. In Stage 1 tumours 90% of patients are well after 5 years, a figure dropping to 60% in Stage II and to very few in Stage III[65].

(a) *Hormone treatment and chemotherapy*   The discovery of hormone receptors and consequently of the distinction between the hormone-dependent and non-dependent tumours, has opened up a new field of cancer endocrinology[66–68]. These receptors are specific steroid-binding proteins contained by cells which depend on hormones for optimum growth. This phenomenon was first observed in breast cancer cells, but Nordqvist[67] has since shown that when negative patterns for receptors were present only three of the 25 patients achieved remission after hormone treatment, whereas a positive hormone/receptor response was associated with ten of 13 patients having objective remissions.

Further work has shown that oestriol acts as an antagonist to the carcinoma activity of oestradiol and oestrone. It is interesting that Oriental women who have a low incidence of carcinoma in hormone-dependent organs such as the breast, endometrium and ovary, have a high oestriol titre between 15 and 19 years, suggesting that oestriol helps protect the immature cell. There appears to be a relationship between the level of oestrogen precursors and endometrial cancer and the addition of progesterone appears to have a suppressant effect on any carcinogenic activity.

The main hormone used in treatment is intramuscular progesterone in doses of 1250 mg weekly (Delalutin). This is continued indefinitely until the tumour becomes resistant; alternatively Depo-Provera may be given i/m 400 mg over a 50–80 day period followed by a maintenance dose of 800 mg/week. There is also an oral preparation which is equally effective. These drugs produce a 30% response lasting from 12–20 months.

Cytotoxic agents in general have not been as successful in controlling endometrical cancer. If the tumour becomes resistant to progesterone treatment then an alkylating agent may be used. If there is response to this which subsequently fails the patient should be switched back to progesterone treatment which will at least give further symptomatic relief.

Obstruction due to malignant growths

Luminal obstruction due to malignant disease presents either as a life-threatening and dramatic event such as cardiac tamponade, or acute superior vena caval obstruction or, more usually, in the form of a slower onset of obstructive symptoms. The clinical picture varies widely depending on the nature and site of obstruction. In the respiratory, genitourinary and gastrointestinal tracts obstructive symptoms are usually the major presenting syndrome and this particular complication will be dealt with first in each of the discussions in these three systems.

Respiratory tract

Blockage of the airway or of a main bronchus presents with urgency, while tumours in the distal bronchial tree are slow to cause obstructive symptoms.

Upper respiratory tract
Obstruction in this region caused by tumour is very uncommon. The hypopharynx or larynx are seldom significantly obstructed unless the tumour is far advanced. Only 15% of treacheal obstructions are caused by tumour, the majority being caused by prolonged tracheal intubation[69]. Occasionally secondary tumours are responsible for tracheal obstruction by direct invasion from lung or thyroid. Curative treatment is seldom possible and palliation must take the form of an appropriately sited tracheostomy. If the tracheal tumour is discovered early, it is possible to excise up to half of the normal 11 cm length and still achieve primary anastomosis. This procedure is surprisingly effective for long periods. Nine of eleven patients resected survived in one series for 11 years.

Bronchial obstruction[70] is a not infrequent complication of lung cancer and is usually gradual in onset, because it occurs in distal sites. It often presents as an upper respiratory illness and x-ray is usually diagnostic. There is characteristic segmental consolidation or a triangular density based at the pleura. Diagnosis is established by endoscopic bronchoscopy and biopsy, and sputum cytology. Treatment of the primary tumour by surgery is only possible in 20–25% of all lung cancer cases and in fewer than this in obstructed cases[71]. On occasion it is necessary to treat the direct effects of obstruction such as empyema requiring drainage or pneumonia requiring antibiotics. The alternative to surgery is radiotherapy which is at present the most helpful method of treatment. Chemotherapy has a limited role with some tumours being sensitive to agents such as nitrogen mustard, cyclophosphamide, methotrexate and adriamycin. In general bronchial carcinomas of oat cell type can show dramatic responses to chemotherapeutic agents but these are generally shortlived, and, in advanced disease, have not been shown to extend survival. Recent results have been more encouraging where chemotherapy has been combined with surgery and radiotherapy in more limited disease.

Isolated secondary lesions of the lungs are not uncommon; the next most frequent area to harbour a single secondary tumour is the brain, and in both these areas resection of the affected area should be considered as long-term survival has been reported.

Genitourinary tumours
Obstruction of this tract is not an infrequent complication of intra-abdominal malignancy. Since it is caused by the mechanical effects of a discrete tumour mass it is important to know the position of

Table 4   Tumours causing genitourinary obstruction

A *Above the bladder*
 (i) Local growth from without by extension of adjacent tumours, often without
     invasion.
         Cervix
         Ovary
         Colon
         Prostate
         Bladder
         Retroperitoneal glands sarcoma
 (ii) Metastatic nodule in wall of ureter. Not common
         Breast
         Colon
         Stomach
         Lymphoma, etc.
 (iii) Intrinsic tumours
         Renal pelvis much more frequent than ureteral
B *At bladder level*
         Intrinsic bladder tumour in area of trigone
C *Below the bladder*
         Prostatic ⎫
         Urethral ⎬ rare
         Penile   ⎭

---

obstruction and the nature of the tumour mass before deciding on treatment. Table 4 shows how such obstruction may arise.

Above the bladder

The commonest cause of obstruction above the bladder is by local extension of tumour from outside the genitourinary tract. Discrete metastatic nodules within the ureteric wall are not common and are nearly always associated with massive metastatic disease elsewhere. Intrinsic squamous and transitional cell tumours of the genitourinary tract are also a small proportion of the total number of tumours causing obstruction but pelvicalyceal tumours are much more common than ureteral.

Obstruction from malignant disease at this level gives rise to haematuria, which may be gross or microscopic, and pain. This may be a dull ache in one or both loins or an acute severe colic. Frequently the primary disease may be already known but sometimes this may be the mode of presentation of such primary but occult abdominal cancers as ovary, colon and retroperitoneal glands. A mass may be palpable in the abdomen.

An intravenous urogram will give information as to the level of obstruction but frequently will not delineate the cause, and then it is a matter of judgement as to how vigorously an individual patient should be investigated and treated. Ultrasound and CT scan may be helpful. Cystoscopy and retrograde studies may not be justified in an elderly and infirm patient.

If treatment is undertaken this usually lies between radiotherapy and chemotherapy and for this decision the nature of the primary tumour needs to be known. Diversion of the ureters into an ileal conduit is not often justified especially in the presence of massive primary and/or metastatic disease. Indeed in one series only 23% were alive at 6 months after operation and most of these had prostatic carcinoma[73]. Severity of symptoms in the presence of advanced disease as well as the possibility of achieving long remission of the disease as a whole should dictate the lengths to which investigation and treatment should be taken. Obstruction at this level often produces few symptoms by comparison with symptoms from massive disease elsewhere and it may be kinder to allow renal obstruction to be the cause of death than to prolong unnecessary anguish and suffering where the disease as a whole is not amenable to treatment.

At bladder level
Bladder cancer in the area of the trigone can obstruct one or both ureters giving rise to bleeding and pain as with obstruction above the bladder. Once again IVU should help in diagnosis and here cystoscopy is usually justified to visualize the tumour. Obstruction may be relieved with diathermy, or radiotherapy with or without partial cystectomy may be indicated. Occasionally total cystectomy with diversion of ureters into an ileal conduit may be carried out with good results.

Below the bladder
Immediate relief of obstruction can usually be achieved with catheter drainage via the urethra. The cause is nearly always a prostatic tumour, which may be identified *per rectum*. While most prostatic tumours are caused by benign hypertrophy some will be due to carcinoma. Occasionally with prostatic carcinoma it is not possible to pass a catheter via the urethra without risking a false passage and here suprapubic drainage is indicated. In general catheters should be left *in situ* until definitive treatment is undertaken, which may be by transurethral resection together with stilboestrol and/or orchidectomy.

Specific tumours of the kidney, bladder, prostate and testis

Renal carcinoma (hypernephroma)
This disease has an average age incidence between 55 and 60 but can present in all age groups including the elderly[74]. There are no pathognomonic signs or symptoms. The diagnosis is suspected on pyelogram and confirmed by arteriographic findings and surgery. CT scanning and ultrasound are also proving helpful as methods of non-invasive investigation. Treatment of all patients without evidence of local or metastatic spread is by nephrectomy with early control of the renal pedicle prior to handling the tumour.

In those with predominantly bony metastatic disease nephrectomy may also be indicated since this may prolong survival by a significant number of months.

This is one type of tumour where an isolated solitary deposit may be seen commonly in the lung. In this instance serious consideration must be given to surgical removal of the deposit as surprisingly long survival has been frequently reported.

Radiotherapy is sometimes given to those patients where there is no evidence of metastatic disease but where there is a likelihood of residual local disease after nephrectomy. Chemotherapy of metastatic tumour in this disease is most disappointing and, especially in the elderly, it may well be felt that no agents other than progesterone are worth administering.

Bladder
This tumour, about 3% of all malignancies, reaches peak incidence in the seventh decade, the male to female ratio being 3 : 1[75]. Most tumours are transitional cell carcinomas which vary widely in appearance and behaviour. They may be fronded, solid or ulcerated, single or multiple, infiltrating or non-infiltrating. They may remain confined to the mucosa for a long time but some will invade early and metastasize via blood or lymph vessels to bones, liver and lungs.

While the role of industrial chemicals is well recognized in the aetiology of this cancer, both smoking and analgesia abuse have been shown to be factors favouring malignancy at this site.

The staging pathologically is by the TNM system:

T_{1S} carcinoma *in situ.*
T_1 infiltration of the subepithelial tissue
T_2 infiltration of the superficial muscle
T_3 infiltration of the deep muscle
T_4 infiltration of the adjoining organs.

In addition the clinical staging is important as the pathologist is only given a small piece on which to base his observation. Thus the examination of the bladder by cystoscopy and bimanual examination under anaesthesia are essential.

Patients almost always complain of haematuria, but about 20% present with frequency or infection which, in old men, can easily be put down to 'prostatism'. Therefore it is wise to regard every first incident of urinary infection in the elderly as a sign of bladder cancer until proved otherwise.

(a) *Treatment* The early T1 lesions can be adequately dealt with by cystodiathermy and regular follow-up[76]. T2 tumours which involve superficial muscle are now dealt with by megavoltage irradiation. Previously, interstitial radiotherapy was the dominant mode of treatment but this is now only given in a small minority of cases, the ideal situation being a solitary low-grade tumour with a base not exceeding 5 cm and with no premalignant changes in the bladder away from the tumour site. The 5 year survival results of interstitial irradiation range both between 50 and 60%. Once the halfway mark of the bladder muscle has been reached by tumour (that is, a T3 tumour) the prognosis is much more serious. The outlook for these tumours depends upon whether the lesion is confined to deep muscle or whether it involves perivesical fat. The 5 year survival rate is 29% for the former and less than 3% for the latter. The present preferred method is combined treatment consisting of preoperative pelvic irradiation (4000 rads in 4 weeks) followed by radical cystectomy 4 weeks later. This produced 33% 5 year survival in a series of 98 patients. This method is chosen for patients under 65, whereas for those over 65 radical radiotherapy is preferred and cystectomy performed in selected cases only[76].

The role of chemotherapy is of increasing importance. Carter and Wasserman[75] found significant cytotoxic activity against bladder cancer with only 3 agents, adriamycin, 5-fluorouracil and mytomycin-C. Turner *et al.*[77] have reported on the effect of methotrexate which produced an overall objective response of 38% in 61 patients, remissions lasting 2–6 months using intravenous dosages of 50 to 200 mg every 2 weeks with folinic acid rescue at the higher dosages. Therefore methotrexate may have an adjuvant role in deeply infiltrating tumours and the effect of such treatment given prior to irradiation and then as maintenance therapy in 12 months following surgery is being explored.

Inoperable tumours pose a very great problem. Radiotherapy must be considered as it may get rid of local tumour for many months, but it can reduce considerably the volume of the bladder leading to painful and very frequent micturition. Where urinary symptoms become intolerable urinary diversion must be considered. Bleeding and pain may be controlled by Helmstein's distension therapy[78] using a distensible sphere which produces pressure and necrosis or by local hyperthermia.

Prostatic cancer

This is a disease of old men[79], 95% occurring in those over 60. In the Western World the incidence is about 5% of all cancers and 10% of cancers in men over 50, being third in frequency after lung and colorectum. It is much less common in China and Japan. The histological incidence at autopsy is far greater, thus a high proportion are asymptomatic and latent and as the population ages so the incidence of clinical tumours increases. As far as is known there is no relationship to benign prostatic enlargement which usually affects the lateral lobes whereas malignant tumours start in the atrophic glandular epithelium of the posterior lobe.

Its development is dependent on the presence of testosterone since early castration can eliminate the disease. The hormonal imbalance that predisposes to prostatic malignancy is certainly a complex one involving the pituitary–testis–adrenal axis. Androgens and oestrogens are essentially antagonistic in their prostatic effects, the former stimulating secretion while the latter inhibit this and stimulate fibromuscular hypertrophy within the gland.

Almost all prostatic cancers are subcapsular adenocarcinomas; either a fast-growing invasive small cell variety or a more indolent form which is well differentiated. The subcapsular site of origin makes for early invasion of the nerve and copious venous plexuses which in turn communicate with the veins in the pelvis and vertebral column. Lymphatic involvement too is early and widespread. Local involvement occurs in vesicles and bladder base. Bony metastases occur early to the pelvis, lumbar spine and femora and the next most frequent sites are the lungs, liver and aortic nodes.

About half of the prostatic cancers coincide with benign hypertrophy and if a cancer is demonstrated in a resected hypertrophic gland it must be assumed that much residual cancer tissue has been left behind in the subcapsular area.

The natural history is variable as the symptoms only appear when the growth is locally widespread, thus causing pain or bladder neck obstruction or when it has metastasized to bone. In some series 80% show distant spread when first symptomatic and 2 years is an average survival time if untreated. Some survive 10 years or more, but some die in 6 months, mostly of widespread bony disease, anaemia and cachexia, with or without the effects of urinary obstruction.

The diagnosis depends on symptoms, and the finding of a single discrete usually hard prostatic nodule raises suspicion. The nodule may be soft or there may be a more diffuse enlargement which is hard and obliterates the normal contours. As half of all single nodules prove to be cancerous they must be biopsied and the best technique is the transperineal biopsy under local or general anaesthesia using a Silverman needle. Transrectal biopsies should be avoided because of the real risks of urinary tract infection.

Cytology is of no value. Biochemical confirmation of metastatic bone disease from prostatic cancer is obtained in two-thirds of cases by the serum acid phosphatase estimation. Elevation of this measurement is proof of the disease. Blood samples, contrary to widespread belief, may be taken soon after prostatic examination as the reported false rise in levels because of this manipulation has not been substantiated. Alkaline phosphatase levels rise with osteoblastic activity at the periphery of bone metastases and thus is a useful measurement to be followed during treatment.

X-ray studies of bone demonstrate the predominantly osteosclerotic nature of the disease. Only Paget's disease mimics this and although the latter shows increased trabeculation and marked increase in bone density it is often difficult to distinguish the two diagnoses if only the spine and pelvis are involved.

Treatment The only curative treatment[80] is total removal of the entire prostate and vesicles. This approach, practised in the United States, has not generally found favour in Britain. It may be indicated in those cases where cancer is shown to be present in an enucleated or resected gland and where there is no evidence of local spread or metastatic disease. Selected series have yielded a 10 year survival rate of nearly 50% but surgical and urinary complications are high and selection needs to be made with great care. Radical radiotherapy should be considered when local disease causing obstruction is not responsive to oestrogens, and where there is little or no metastatic disease high dose radiotherapy is given. Survival rates are comparable without the serious surgical complications although temporary but substantial proctitis may be encountered. The majority of patients do not fall into a category suitable for the above treatment either because of associated disease, age, or widespread dissemination.

Arrest of tumour growth and relief of pain may be achieved in two-thirds of patients by androgen control. Bilateral orchidectomy alone often produces dramatic remissions of urinary retention, but

2 mg/day of diethylstilboestrol by mouth appears to potentiate this effect. Many prefer oral oestrogens as a first line of treatment reserving orchidectomy for severe pain or poor response to treatment. There is rarely any therapeutic advantage in giving more than 2 mg/day. Indeed the incidence of long-term side-effects of cardio-vascular complications, particularly in the more elderly, rises considerably with higher dosage. It is sometimes held that oestrogen alone is inferior to orchdectomy or a combination of the two, and certainly oestrogen contributes little further to control of the disease after relapse. Since most prostatic cancers are hormone-dependent 70% of patients show improvement in a few days and local cancer as well as metastases and pain frequently 'melt away'. The length of remission is variable, from months to years, with an average of 20 months, but relapses always occur as the tumours eventually lose their endocrine responsiveness.

Persistent urinary obstruction may be managed by transurethral resection and the same technique is useful in dealing with haemorrhage from prostatic cancer. Permanent cystostomy has no place in the treatment of this disease. Careful sedation and judicious use of painkilling drugs and hormone manipulation can make patients very comfortable, particularly in the very elderly.

Other forms of treatment including radioactive gold, adrenalectomy and the systemic use of ^{32}P have very limited application. However cortisone administration can provide useful relief in cases of relapse and recent reports indicate that hydroxyurea may also have a limited role once the tumour has escaped oestrogen control.

Testis
Malignant growths, the majority of which are seminomas, account for less than 1% of all cancers and occur at all ages[81]. Ectopic testes have an incidence of tumour 10 to 20 times as great as those in normal position although the incidence in those testicles brought down into the scrotum surgically is hardly any less. In the very old lymphomata and leukaemic deposits of the testes occur particularly in those patients who have responded well to the chemotherapy of chronic leukaemias.

Testicular tumours present with a hard often painless but heavy swelling of the testicle. But a significant minority (20%) will first present with local oedema, redness and pain suggesting inflammation especially epididymitis. Because early treatment is so important any swelling of the testis that does not subside rapidly must be explored and either a wedge biopsy done to rule out inflammatory disease or orchidectomy performed.

Other diagnostic studies include X-ray of the renal system, lymphangiography to determine the extent if any of lymph node spread, whole lung tomography and CT scanning. Urinary gonadotrophin determinations show increased levels in nearly half the cases because of the frequent histological mixture of various types. Alphafetoprotein assays should be done. Either this marker or gonadotrophins are raised in 90% of patients with metastatic disease[82]. They also help diagnostically as ATP levels are never raised in pure seminomas as are gonadotrophin levels.

Treatment   This is primarily by complete surgical excision with excision or radiotherapy to regional glands. The chemotherapeutic response to testicular tumours is excellent and the prognosis has changed significantly with its use[83]. Seminoma without nodes have 75–90% 5 year survival rate, an average of 60% 5 year survival without nodal involvement and 30% when nodes are involved. The poorly differentiated teratomas with many trophoblasts have also shown improved results.

Gastrointestinal tract

The urgency and severity of symptoms depend on the site and local diameter of the gut lumen. In the capacious caecum the growth will produce no obstructive symptoms whereas at the ileocaecal valve or pylorus symptoms appear early. The situation determines whether relief is possible or easy; a block in the bile duct at the ampulla is most amenable to palliative surgery, whereas widespread secondary tumour masses in the serosa of the small bowel with resultant loss of peristalsis is well-nigh impossible to circumvent. Most patients will be subject to palliative treatment only, but so great is the morbidity and misery produced by duct or luminal obstruction that major surgical procedures may be very worthwhile.

Oesophagus

Malignant growths, which are almost always primary, occur most commonly in elderly men between 70–80 years (5:1 men to women)[84–86]. They are squamous in the upper and middle thirds and often adenocarcinoma at the lower end of the oesophagus. The latter are almost always gastric in origin but give rise to an obstructive picture as they occur at the narrow gastrooesophageal junction.

Dysphagia is the main symptom. It may be slow in onset over 4–6 months, starting with solids like bread and meat and progressing to liquids, or it may arise quite suddenly within a few weeks. Occasionally the early symptoms are subtle and consist of a transitory feeling of food sticking behind the sternum. Eventually there is marked difficulty in swallowing anything, accompanied by obvious weight loss and the effects of aspiration, particularly coughing and pneumonia.

Any swallowing difficulty must be regarded seriously and barium swallow ordered immediately. The differential diagnosis includes peptic stricture which may have a very similar onset, but usually having a history of previous peptic symptoms and heartburn sometimes many years before. Achalasia and motor disorders of a neuromuscular kind should also be considered. X-ray is usually diagnostic and verification is obtained by flexible oesophagoscopy and biopsy with brush cytology. If such verification is unsuccessful, rigid oesophagoscopy under general anaesthesia is necessary, but should be preceded by a lateral X-ray of the cervical vertebrae to indicate the extent of osteophyte formation and therefore the need for care in avoiding unnecessary neck extension with the rigid endoscope. Excessive manipulation may easily cause perforation at the site of the osteophytes.

Operative treatment is technically quite feasible although hazardous, and the long-term results are poor. About 40% prove resectable and 3 year survival overall is about 10–15%. The best results occur with the uncommon squamous cell tumours in the lower third when there are no lymph nodes involved along the left gastric vessels and porta hepatis – a 50% 5-year survival. Adenocarcinomas at this site have a survival rate of half this figure. Middle third lesions have a 5 year survival of about 40% if found early and without nodes, but the majority have nodes involved and at most 15–20% survive 5 years. Above the arch of the aorta the results are even poorer. Only about 20% survive when no nodes are involved.

There is still debate about the role and value of radiotherapy. Some recommend this for all squamous tumours at any level and 5 year survivals of 30% and 16% respectively are reported for cervical and thoracic oesophagus[84]. These, however, are not generally obtainable, and morbidity due to dysphagia, fistula formation and general debility is considerable. Therefore, in our view, the preferable treatment for a squamous lesion in a reasonably fit patient with no major cardiac or pulmonary disease is preoperative radiotherapy over 4–6 weeks which will lessen the dysphagia quite markedly and permit nutritional rehabilitation. High protein and calorie diet of a fluid nature must be carefully supervised by doctor and dietitian. After this has been completed the patient is reassessed. If he is still in good condition with adequate liver and renal function, and no evidence on CT and ultrasound of serious distant spread, resection should be advised for middle and lower third lesions. This is done, despite the generally poor results, because the results of palliation, whether non-resectional palliative intubation or oesophagojejunal bypass, are much worse in terms of survival and are far from ideal in relieving symptoms. Thus one is weighing on the one hand an average 20–25% operative mortality, a further 25% postoperative morbidity (atelectasis, empyema, cardiac failure, etc.) with a limited number of months (9–30) for survivors, against on the other hand the results of palliative intubation which will provide no survivors at all by 1 year. Immediate mortality of intubation is high, at least 10%, and more often closer to 25–33%. The survivors are able to take pureed and liquid food but this is only for a period of 3–4 months on average.

If resection is not possible the preferred method of intubation is by a traction technique using a Celestin tube. Dilatation of the carcinomatous stricture is carried out via a rigid oesophagoscope and passage of a narrow plastic introducer into the stomach. It is followed by a gastrostomy and gentle traction on the introducer to which has been sutured at the upper end the gradually bevelled Celestin tube. This is then gently drawn into the stomach across the tumour and, with 5 cm left protruding, the remainder is cut off. The protruding end is then sutured to the stomach wall to prevent upward dislocation and the stomach and abdomen closed. Immediately after operation a chest x-ray is taken to note any perforation shown by air in the mediastinum or pleural fluid. Such a complication is usually fatal. If all has gone well a liquid diet is started and finally soft foods. The patient is taught to take carbonated drinks at the end of each meal to help clear the tube of debris.

With full knowledge of the generally poor results of radiation and surgery treatment it is nevertheless advised in those elderly patients who are reasonable fit physically and mentally.

Unfortunately there is little benefit from any form of chemotherapy at present.

A not infrequent clinical problem is the very old emaciated patient with almost complete oesophageal obstruction. Saliva dribbling is the most distressing immediate problem. The treatment alternatives are palliative radiotherapy if this is feasible, to provide some shrinkage and therefore partially re-establish a lumen which will allow at least a liquid diet. If a palliative intubation operation is not feasible then a cervical oesophagostomy is a last resort, the fistula so created being drained into a colostomy-type bag. Whether or not this should be supplemented by a feeding gastrostomy is for individual judgement – it is not often indicated but should be considered in an otherwise starving and dehydrated patient.

Stomach

Obstruction within the stomach[87,88] may occur from a lesion arising at the cardia or oesophagogastric junction. At the pylorus, the obstruction may be caused by a primary gastric neoplasm or from pressure on the duodenum caused by an extrinsic tumour.

A quarter of all stomach tumours present as obstructions, and many more will eventually develop these symptoms if untreated. Men predominate 2 : 1 and the sixth decade is the peak period in which they occur. Extensive tumours affecting the duodenum most commonly arise from the pancreas but may arise from colon, gallbladder, kidney or retroperitoneum. The early symptoms are anorexia together with epigastric fullness and discomfort arising from a partial block at the pylorus and eventually retention and pain due to vigorous peristaltic attempts to overcome the obstruction. Vomiting, often non-bilious, then occurs, usually of much undigested food of the previous day or night. A mass is easily palpable in about half the cases, while in others a succussion splash may be elicited. Intubation demonstrates large residual volumes of over 500 ml which contain undigested food. After lavage the diagnosis can be confirmed by endoscopy and biopsy if a gastric lesion is present. A barium meal is more helpful where an extrinsic tumour is present.

Unfortunately outlet obstruction is often a symptom of late disease. Nevertheless wherever possible it should be relieved surgically[89]. The first choice is resection even when there is a large tumour and where lymph node disease may have to be left behind. This is advisable not only because obstruction is relieved, but the removal of a large mass of tumour tissue will usually make surviving patients feel much better; they are able to eat, surrounding gastritis is removed and they are freed from continuing slow bleeding from the tumour surface. Resection is technically feasible in 50% of patients. The mortality is not unduly high at 10–15% and the postoperative morbidity is of the same order of frequency. Survival in comfort for the remainder should average 12–18 months.

Where the tumour is unresectable a bypass gastroenterostomy may be carried out. In such cases a loop is brought in front of the colon and anastamosed well above and away from the tumour either in the form of a loop or in a Roux-en-Y fashion. This method will give relief from vomiting but the presence of bleeding tumour tissue will continue to weaken the patient and survival is only a matter of months[90]. Gastrostomy has no role in management.

Radiotherapy with fast neutrons may well have a place and this is presently being investigated. Conventional radiotherapy only has a role where there is an ulcerating tumour on the surface of the abdominal wall.

Chemotherapeutic agents including 5-fluorouracil, mitomycin C, adriamycin, the nitrosoureas and vincristine used singly have all shown some activity in advanced disease, but their potential role in combination for minimal residual disease after resection of the primary tumour still needs to be evaluated, and this is the subject of a number of clinical trials[91].

Every effort must be made to relieve these patients surgically unless the whole stomach is involved such as occurs in a contracted linitis plastica with maximal pyloric involvement. Here the alternatives lie between a major operation, an oesophagojejunostomy by the Roux-en-Y technique which is a considerable procedure suitable only perhaps for thin patients, or a fine indwelling nasogastric tube brought out via a pharyngostomy to avoid nasal ulceration and discomfort. We would advise the latter as survivals are few following major gastric resection in this condition. At the same time pain and anxiety must be relieved by appropriate analgesia and largactil to avoid the absolute misery of this condition. Dryness of the mouth must be attended to by glycerin sticks or small amounts of ice water but no attempt at adequate fluid replacement or antibiotics is indicated.

Small intestine
Small bowel obstruction is a common surgical emergency[92-95]. The majority are due to adhesions or hernial obstruction, but nearly a quarter are caused by malignant disease. Most of the latter are due to metastatic disease from colorectum (45%), ovary (17%), cervix (15%), and other sites 24%. These result from direct extension or generalized intra-abdominal carcinomatosis[91]. Secondary tumour from lymphoma and melanoma may also occur.

Primary tumours of the small bowel are much less common being 1-5% of all gastrointestinal tumours and include adenocarcinoma, carcinoid, sarcoma, lymphoma and melanoma. Carcinoid tumours are especially liable to cause obstruction even with small tumours as they spread submucosally.

The symptoms of small bowel obstruction are usually slow in progression and without great discomfort at the onset; cramp-like abdominal pains occur at irregular intervals and there is gradual abdominal distension[95]. These symptoms become more severe, and eventually nausea, vomiting, loss of appetite and constipation become marked. At this stage all the typical signs of obstruction are present including distension, visible peristalsis and sometimes one or more masses. Confirmation is made by erect and supine x-rays of which the erect films show multiple fluid levels. Barium enema should be done and finally upper gastrointestinal contrast studies, preferably in the form of a small bowel enema, are arranged to delineate as accurately as possible the site and nature of the obstruction.

The aim of treatment is to attempt non-surgical means of relief and to avoid operation, but surgical intervention will be necessary if 2–3 days of conservative treatment fails. Non-surgical management means intravenous fluids and the use of a long decompression tube, the best being the Cantor tube. This tube with a mercury-filled bag is introduced via the nose, carefully placed by the radiologist at the pylorus and the patient turned on to the right side and given sips of water every 5–10 min. While still in the X-ray department the progression of the tube along the bowel is noted fluoroscopically half-hourly for 1–1½ hours unless return of clear duodenal bile indicates passage past the pylorus; 80% of tubes will pass the pylorus within 4–6 hours and then slowly progress until the tube reaches the site of obstruction. It is important to leave a free loop of tube at the nasal orifice to allow steady downward passage of the tube; if strapped to the nose it cannot of course go down any further. The use of this type of decompression tube has proved invaluable and has saved many patients an operation. It requires practice and attention to detail and, above all, patience. It is no use leaving it to the most junior staff who may have little experience in its use, as most of the tube will still be in the stomach after 24 hours unless properly handled. As much information as possible should be gathered about the extent of tumour growth and spread, either during the intubation period or after successful relief of the obstruction. This should include ultrasound scans of the liver, and CT scanning if available. Such information helps make the decision about further radical or palliative surgery.

By this conservative means about a third of patients will have the obstruction relieved, as evidenced by passage of flatus and general abdominal decompression, and after 4–6 days the tube may be gradually withdrawn. The relief may last for many months. Many reobstruct and unless rapid decompression by a long tube can be achieved surgical intervention is necessary. Mortality is of necessity high, probably around 20%. The following general principles should be applied during the operation; single or multiple adjacent lesions should be resected and the ends anastomosed and if this is not possible an internal bypass should be done whenever possible so as to avoid ileostomy or colostomy. If necessary multiple side to side, small bowel anastomoses, may be made. As much small bowel as possible should be preserved and the ileocaecal valve should not be sacrificed if possible. It is important for the clinician to appreciate that obstruction, which occurs in a patient with a known previous tumour, is by no means incurable and may be helped considerably for long periods. Such patients may in fact, have simple band obstruction or indeed may have a second new primary growth amenable to resection. This occurred in 25% of one series in which over a third sustained a long survival. Furthermore internal bypass is frequently effective as palliation and may give long relief.

The average survival after such surgery for metastatic tumours is about a year. The prognosis is better for primary tumours of the small bowel which are resected, about 15% 5 year survival. The best prognosis is for carcinoid tumours where nearly half survive for 5 years.

Colorectum
(a) Colon   Colonic obstruction is almost always due to malignant growths[96]. About 20% of colon tumours present as obstructions and fully half of these are near complete or complete. Of considerable diagnostic significance is the fact that two-thirds of obstructing lesions lie distal to the splenic flexure and one of three will be in reach of the sigmoidoscope. It has become clear how important it is that every older patient who has any complaints relating to bowel dysfunction should have a sigmoidoscopy and barium enema, the former preceded by a lower bowel washout or a good bowel movement. Extracolonic causes of large bowel obstruction are few and consist mainly of tumours of ovarian or cervical origin.

If obstruction is incomplete, symptoms start slowly and progress inexorably. There is colicky pain, gradual distension, and a tendency to constipation and eventually weight loss and vomiting. Rectal bleeding may occur but is more usual in distal lesions.

Complete obstruction may present quite suddenly with its accompanying four cardinal signs and symptoms of colicky pain, absence of wind or faeces, distension and vomiting. If allowed to progress the patient becomes quite rapidly dehydrated and exhausted, or if the ileocaecal valve is competent, a closed loop obstruction results and the caecum bears the brunt of the increased pressure. There is a very real danger of caecal perforation in such cases and an x-ray diameter of 10 cm or greater must be regarded as a sign of imminent catastrophe. Decompression by caecostomy should be done forthwith.

On examination a mass is palpable in nearly two-thirds of patients by careful abdominal and rectal examination. Even in the presence of considerable abdominal distension, ballotting the abdominal wall with one hand will often demonstrate a hard mass that may not be felt on ordinary pressure. Erect and supine X-rays will demonstrate both fluid levels, and the lower limit of air in the distal colon. It is necessary in almost all cases to do an immediate barium enema. Treatment is dictated by the urgency of the obstruction. If chronic and incomplete, the patient should be intubated with a long Cantor tube, and intravenous fluid, mineral and calorie replacement started. Other assessments, including those of cardiovascular, pulmonary and renal function should be undertaken in the next 2–3 days and laparotomy then follows in a suitably prepared patient. Bowel preparation must be carried out in the form of two thorough soap and water enemas on successive days if possible. This at least ensures a clean distal bowel, and usually the proximal colon will not be packed with faecal material. If the lesion is not obstructing to any great degree the mechanical washing is surprisingly effective in cleaning the bowel.

Controversy surrounds the preferred method of treatment for an obstructed left colon. The safest method particularly for the more occasional colon operator is the classic three-stage method of preliminary colostomy to provide decompression, followed in 10–14 days by planned resection, after which the colostomy is closed in 4–6 weeks when a barium enema has demonstrated an intact healed suture line. Despite the multiplicity of operations and anaesthesia the overall mortality in most hands is lower than in one-stage resections, although carefully selected series have been published favouring the latter. An alternative is a two-stage method comprising resection of the tumour with appropriate amount of proximal and distal bowel being brought out from the site of the tumour in the form of a colostomy (Paul – Mickulicz procedure). This is then closed in 14–21 days so that there is no suture line at risk during this time. The mortality following operation for obstructive lesions is in the order of 25% and the 5 year survival rate is correspondingly small (15–30%).

Right-sided lesions require a one-stage ileo-colic anastomosis after removal of 15 cm of terminal ileum and up to one-third of the transverse colon. Transverse colon lesions require resection of the whole transverse colon, if necessary mobilizing both flexures to avoid tension in the suture lines.

(b) *Rectum*   Carcinoma of the large bowel is the second commonest cause of death from cancer in the United Kingdom and of these about half occur in the rectum, equally distributed in upper, middle and lower third[97]. It is more common in men than women, a ratio of approximately 3 : 2 compared to the colon where the ratio is almost the exact opposite. Half occur over 60 years and the commonest decade is 60–69, but nearly a third occur between 70 and 80. The recognized aetiological factors include (1) polyps, particularly villous, of which at least a third are malignant, and adenomas, of which fewer become or are malignant but which represent a sign of possible epithelial instability; and (2) ulcerative colitis of more than 10 years duration and especially where the entire large bowel is involved.

Rectal tumours may be polypoid or ulcerated and progress to an annular growth. Spread may be direct in the bowel wall and anteriorly to involve prostrate and bladder or cervix, or by lymphatics in an upward direction, usually sequentially up the lymph node chain. Spread by blood stream along the venous channels also occurs.

Tumours of the rectum have been classified by Dukes[97], as follows:

(1) degree of differentiation – low, average and high grade
(2) degree of spread   – 'A' confined to the bowel wall
                            'B' spread to extra rectal tissues
                            'C' lymphatic node metastases.

Both clasifications are extremely useful and probably reflect the predictable, sequential and slow growth rate of the majority of rectal tumours.

The symptoms are straightforward and clear; the tragedy is that this most curable of tumours is frequently missed. Bleeding, mucous discharge, bowel irritability are the early hallmarks – all typical of piles and it is for this latter condition that some patients are mistakenly treated for many months. Therefore these common symptoms require rectal examination, proctoscopy, sigmoidoscopy, biopsy if necessary and barium enema in that order, which must be followed without any exception whatsoever. Other symptoms including those of severe tenesmus, pain and loss of weight, are indicative of advanced disease.

The best chance for cure of cancers in the mid and lower rectum in all but widespread metastatic disease, is by radical abdominoperineal resection of the rectum and a permanent colostomy. This operation is well tolerated even in older patients, and has better end results than almost any major cancer operation in the body. Age is not a major consideration but the condition of the cardiovascular renal and pulmonary systems is. The resection even as a palliative treatment for large tumours or patients with early liver metastases, rids the patient of a fungating painful tumour and makes life much more tolerable. The present mortality is less than 5%. For tumours of the upper rectum, that is more than 10 cm from the anal verge, the tumour may be excised and the sphincters preserved intact by an anterior resection as there is so rarely downward spread for more than 2–3 cm.

The results of treatment are impressive – 90% of all tumours are resectable; 'A' cases have over 90% chance of 10 year survival, and 'B' cases have a 70% 10 year survival; in 'C' cases the 5 and 10 year survival is 30 and 25% respectively. Some of those who undergo resection but who already have liver metastases can survive up to 2 years and maintain good health for most of this time.

There are two additional methods of treatment that must be considered. Radiotherapy is of value as a supplement in anaplastic growths or where removal has been incomplete, and particularly when patients refuse surgical treatment or are frail and otherwise unfit. It can provide significant palliation and has a definite place in treatment.

Of considerable significance, especially for the very old and infirm patient, is the method of diathermy fulguration of rectal tumours. Originally introduced by Strauss in 1935[98] the method has received support from Turnbull[99], Jackman[100], and Madden[101]. Turrell[102] has most recently reviewed the indications for this method: (a) Duke's 'A' category, an early localized tumour confined to bowel wall; (b) poor surgical risks in all Duke stages, that is advanced senility or systemic disorders; (c) blind or institutionalized patients unable to care for themselves; (d) bleeding inoperable lesions where life-expectancy is short, and recurrence at suture lines following resection[102].

The technique consists of diathermy fulguration via a wide proctoscope or by retractors, using a needle electrode to fulgurate the whole surface of the tumour[101]. The resultant coagulum is scraped off and bleeding ceases once all the tumour tissue is removed. A second session follows 14 days later and then re-examination is needed monthly for 6 months and any doubtful area biopsied and fulgurated. Madden cites nine of every ten patients alive 5 years later and one in three alive by 5 years after fulguration of inoperable tumours.

These impressive end results in selected cases, operable and inoperable, rival those following surgery. Whether this is due to an induced immunological response (which has been demonstrated experimentally) is not proven. It is a method which must be constantly considered in every rectal cancer and particularly in the older age groups.

If obstructive symptoms override the possibility of radiotherapy or fulguration, urgent surgery is sometimes necessary. In the old and infirm, the minimum should be done and either the tumour should be exteriorized and a proximal and distal loop separately developed, or a terminal colostomy established.

The single most useful agent in chemotherapeutic treatment for colorectal tumours is 5-fluorouracil[103], but activity has been demonstrated for mitomycin C and the nitrosoureas. It is doubtful whether any of these agents used singly will induce a response in more than one in five tumours. Imidazole carboxamide (DTIC) may also have some activity and has been used in combination with 5 FU, BCNU and vincristine[104] where 43% were reported as responding. A similar response rate has been found with 5 FU, vincristine and methyl-CCNU.[105,106]. Unfortunately these improved response rates have not been translated into significantly improved survival times. Where there is significant hepatic disease intravenous chemotherapy does not often exert beneficial effect although arterial perfusion with 5 FU has improved both survival and response. Even so it is questionable whether chemotherapy should often be used in the elderly until more significant improvement has been seen in the younger age groups.

Pancreaticobiliary tumours
Obstruction of the biliary outflow causing jaundice is due to a wide variety of intrinsic and extrinsic tumours[107,108]. The prognosis is usually poor because of the nature of the tumours, their relative anatomical inaccessibility, the closeness of vital structures which cannot be resected, and their tendency to infiltrate widely and metastasize. A small proportion of obstructing biliary tumours are intrahepatic (3–5%). The most common of these are the bile duct carcinomas, and these may produce jaundice early if situated at, or slightly proximal to, the bifurcation of the hepatic ducts.

Extrahepatic obstruction occurs much more commonly (75% of cases) and is due in most cases to tumours around the ampulla. The large majority (85%) of these are due to a cancer in the head of the pancreas. Unfortunately most of these have already spread regionally by the time jaundice appears. About 10% arise in the ampulla itself, and it is this group in which surgical resection achieves its best results (20–40% 5 year cures). This is probably due to the fact that jaundice is an early symptom and regional spread has not yet occurred in many. The remaining 5–10% of periampullary tumours occur in the duodenum itself or in the distal bile duct. Of the bile duct tumours about half lie proximally and are unresectable. Carcinoma of the gall bladder, although occurring almost five times as frequently as bile duct tumours, only causes jaundice in about a third of cases and they represent only 8% of all cases of biliary obstruction.

The symptoms which accompany jaundice of malignant origin are weight loss, anorexia and, very commonly, pain. The jaundice is progressive and unremitting and pruritis complicates the picture. Pain occurs commonly under the right costal margin or in the epigastrium. It is constant and frequently radiates through to the back. It is seldom colicky but tends to be dull and is constantly present and of boring character. The degree of anorexia and lessened food intake largely explains the invariable weight loss. On examination there is almost always a mass in the right subcostal area or epigastrium, which represents either tumour or a dilated gall bladder or an enlarged liver. The biochemical evidence is usually clear: a total bilirubin of 15–30 mg/100 ml and an increase in alkaline phosphatase to high levels. Serum transaminase may be normal or slightly elevated but gamma-glutamyl transpeptidase levels are increased.

X-ray studies of the biliary tract in the form of oral cholecystography or i/v cholangiograms are unhelpful because of the level of jaundice and poor liver excretory function. Apart from barium meal examination which will demonstrate an ampullary lesion in 50–60% of cases, the helpful diagnostic studies, if available, are: (1) CT scanning which demonstrates pancreatic lesions particularly well; (2) percutaneous transhepatic cholangiography, a procedure which is much safer now a fine needle (Chinba) technique is used, and which has an added advantage in that a temporary soft drainage catheter may be introduced by this means over a wire guide; (3) ERCP with pancreatic juice collection and cytology is a reliable and accurate method even less hazardous than the percutaneous needle technique and provides definitive diagnosis in 60–70% of cases; (4) ultrasound will usually demonstrate a dilated biliary tree behind the obstruction and will delineate masses within the porta hepatis and also in the pancreas in 50%.

Once the diagnosis has been made and confirmed patients must be explored. Most will be beyond cure. A few (10–25%) may be suitable for major surgical resection, a subtotal pancreatectomy. This treatment is particularly applicable to ampullary carcinomas which are more localized.

Subtotal or total pancreatectomy, the Whipple operation, is a *tour de force* which is nevertheless limited in its scope because of the close proximity of tumours to vital structures, particularly the portal vein. It consists in removal of the pancreas and duodenum and lower quarter of stomach with reconstitution of anatomy by joining the gall bladder to a loop of jejunum and stomach to an adjoining jejunal loop. If the distal third of the pancreas is left, which has the advantage of preserving endocrine function, then the dilated pancreatic duct needs to be anastomosed to the jejunal loop close to the gastrojejunal junction. This suture line represents one of the great hazards of the procedure. Not only is the technique demanding but the gains in terms of survival are too small to justify the operation except in the most ideal localized situations. Therefore the vast majority require (a) relief of their jaundice, (b) prophylaxis against later duodenal obstruction. If the tumour is a pancreatic head cancer then a double system bypass procedure is necessary[109]. The distended gall bladder is anastomosed to a loop of jejunum either by a Roux-loop or a simple jejunal loop with an entero-anastomosis done 30 cm below the gall bladder junction. The second part of the double bypass procedure consists in a gastrojejunostomy done in antecolic fashion. This is an essential component of the operation. The inevitable enlargement of the tumour will produce duodenal obstruction and in a third of cases this will require a second operation within a matter of months unless the prophylactic bypass is performed while the patient is still reasonably fit and well. Prognosis following this palliation is 4–12 months and death ensues due to inexorable liver failure and ascites. Fortunately this occurs fairly quickly in the terminal stages after many months of comfortable palliation.

The role of chemotherapy in this tumour is beginning to look less hopeless. Isolated cases have been reported of 24 months survival following chemotherapy and then resection. We have recently used Melphalan. In one patient there was impressive palliation for 24 months with almost total disappearance of the tumour on CT scan at one time. In another two there was marked improvement of symptoms and wellbeing for some 5 months but no objective evidence of tumour regression. Intra-arterial perfusion of the tumour with a sufficiently high dose of 5-fluorouracil and other drugs may have a place, and with satisfactory techniques of infusion (pump and catheter) its role must be further explored. Here again we have experienced impressive regression as measured on CT scan with the patient surviving 19 months.

If the tumour is intraluminal and unresectable, diversion in the form of a permanent indwelling stent or an internal fistula as described by Smith is necessary[110]. The survival of patients with gall bladder carcinoma is 3–5 months and most are unresectable.

Head and neck tumours (intraoral, parotid, thyroid and laryngeal)

Intraoral tumours
These include those of the floor of mouth, alveolar and mandibular lesions and tongue and are almost always squamous cell cancers. They all occur in the older age groups, and any ulcer, thickening or painful area within the mouth must be regarded as malignant and therefore biopsied, usually under local anaesthesia.

The important considerations in this area are the extent of the tumours, the degree of differentiation, and the type of reconstruction that may be required. As a general rule if the tumour is exophytic then local and regional resection may be less extensive whereas if they are infiltrative and cross the midline, bilateral regional node dissection must be considered. If the tumour is well differentiated small local resection may be all that is required whereas the poorly differentiated ones require regional node dissection. As an example, a small 2 cm lesion of the tongue, near the tip or laterally, but only superficially infiltrative and well differentiated, requires no more than local resection with adequate tumour-free margins. If the lesion is larger and more infiltrative, then suprahyoid dissection is required in addition with extension to radical neck dissection if nodes are found to be positive.

Radiotherapy has a definite role especially for lesions not involving bone or nodes, and treatment in the elderly should be planned from the beginning with radiotherapeutic consultation.

Parotid tumours
In recent years the pathology of these tumours has become more clearly defined[111]. In essence there is a clearcut group of primarily malignant tumours, about 20%, which include adenocarcinomas, epidermoid carcinomas and undifferentiated carcinomas. The bulk (over 80%) are benign because only inadequate removal may be followed by recurrence. The commonest type is the pleomorphic adenoma (75%), for many years called 'mixed tumour', and the next commonest are Warthin's tumour (papillary cystadenoma lymphanetosum) 15–20%, and lymphoepithelial tumours.

The age incidence in large series shows the frequency of these tumours in older age groups. Nearly 50% of cancers occur between 60 and 80 years and over a quarter of the benign lesions are in this group. The typical presentation of the benign tumours is a slow-growing painless lump or mass, almost always without facial nerve involvement. Most are obviously situated in or over the parotid gland. A significant number however present as smaller masses around the parotid region below or behind the ear, in the upper anterior triangle of the neck or far forwards towards the submental region. Any lump in these sites, especially in the elderly, must be regarded as likely to be of parotid origin, and not as lymph nodes to be biopsied under local anaesthesia.

Malignant tumours most frequently have features of rapid growth, facial paralysis and pain as primary symptoms.

Treatment of parotid tumours is now based on well-established principles[112]. Pleomorphic adenomas require either superficial or complete parotidectomy, and not merely local excision. The pleomorphic adenomas occur in the superficial lobe in 80% of cases, 15% in the deep lobe. Recurrence rate after local and inadequate excision is nearly 10%, but less than 2% when the whole lobe or gland is removed. Radiation adds nothing to the success after adequate excision but has a place when recurrent tumours occur.

Treatment of malignant tumours is by more radical excision often with deliberate sacrifice of the facial nerve. Facial paralysis, complete or incomplete, occurs in about one-third of patients who have required this form of treatment. Recurrence rates are in the region of 33%, being highest with the squamous cell type, and the 5 year per cent survival is between 70–90% except in the undifferentiated and squamous cell varieties where the figure is between 25–40%.

Because of the recurrence rate the role of irradiation is being reassessed and must be considered as a postoperative therapy. Chemotherapy so far has no clear role in treatment.

Thyroid tumours

Malignancy of this organ is occasionally seen in older patients[113,114]. The pathology of these tumours is best classified by the system proposed by Woolner *et al.* namely papillary (60%) follicular (20%) anaplastic (15%) and medullary (5%). Papillary carcinoma is in most cases a disease of younger people under 40, but about one in five occur in older patients. Papillary and follicular tumours are treated by total lobectomy on the side of the lesion and subtotal lobectomy on the opposite side – in papillary lesions because of multifocal disease, and in follicular lesions because of the need to remove as much iodine-absorbing tissue as possible, so that the metastases will be able to absorb radioactive iodine. In addition papillary lesions require that nodes on the side of the tumour be carefully examined at operation, because of the propensity to spread there, and if involved they need to be removed by a modified neck dissection with preservation of the sternomastoid muscle.

Total thyroidectomy is seldom necessary as long-term results show no improvement over the more conservative methods. Furthermore the risk of permanent hypoparathyroidism is greatly increased: at least 5% and in many other series up to 12% or even 30% have been reported. This compares with less than 1% after conservative procedures.

Medullary tumours are treated by total thyroidectomy with block dissection of regional nodes if necessary. There is no effective treatment for anaplastic carcinomia. Biopsy is necessary and in a few cases total thyroidectomy may be done if the tumour appears to be locally resectable. In most cases radiotherapy is indicated and may give temporary relief and palliation. Chemotherapy has been attempted and there are reports of the use of adriamycin with temporary benefit.

An important observation has been made concerning the large goitres seen in elderly women which are mainly of recent development. These are usually small cell tumours and were regarded as anaplastic but are now increasingly recognized to be malignant lymphomata. Generally the prognosis is poor but subtotal and total thyroidectomy combined with external irradiation may be of much benefit with survival of several years.

All post-thyroidectomy patients should be given suppressive doses of thyroid hormone to prevent myxoedema and to help limit cancer recurrence.

Thus in older patients the likely diagnosis of a newly developed mass in the region of the thyroid is an anaplastic carcinoma or a malignant lymphoma with a small number being medullary or even more rarely follicular tumours. A longstanding goitre is most likely to be a non-toxic multinodular goitre.

Laryngeal tumours

Glottic tumours occur in the vocal cords and the anterior commissure joining them[115]. The area is a small one with a vertical diameter of at most 2 cm from the upper cricoid border below to the ventricle above. They are the commonest laryngeal tumours, two out of three occurring in this site. The early symptom is hoarseness which persists, and the experienced ear is able to distinguish the quality of voice disturbance from other problems such as polyps or paralysis. Indirect laryngoscopy and biopsy are essential and observations should be made concerning cord mobility, limitation or not to one cord, the anteroposterior extent of the growth and the presence and size of cervical lymph nodes. *In situ* cancers are treated by intraoral surgical removal and less than 5% require further treatment. Irradiation, although equally successful, results in almost 40% who require further treatment. Some of these even require laryngectomy. Early invasive cancer (Stage I) may be treated by endoscopic transoral means or by conservative surgery (laryngo-fissure and cordectomy, or hemilaryngectomy) or irradiation with equal success in 90% or more over 5 years. The advantage of radiation in preservation of the voice as opposed to the distortion of glottic tone after surgery, is offset by the increased number of patients, 30% or more, who require subsequent treatment after completion of irradiation. In older patients irradiation is usually to be preferred and certainly this is true in poor-risk patients.

In Stage II cancers (invasive) the same options are available. Either treatment may be used and the retreatment necessary after irradiation is even higher. In Stage III and IV laryngectomy appears to be the method of choice. Cervical node dissection is advisable in all patients with palpable nodes. These occur in less than 15% in Stage III, in a third of cases in Stage IV disease.

Supraglottic cancer occurs in the epiglottis, false cords and medial aryepiglottic folds. These are less easy to diagnose, and therefore likely to be more advanced, and more likely to invade both sides of the neck. Patients may have vague discomfort in the throat or marked pain, or they may have no symptoms at all until a lump occurs in the neck.

The therapeutic decisions revolve around supraglottic resection with or without laryngectomy, the latter depending on the degree of vocal cord fixation. In early growths either of the two methods bring about equal results both being superior to radiation therapy. Certainly for those growths involving the larynx as indicated by glottic fixation, laryngectomy is much superior to irradiation. Unless there is great infirmity the surgical alternative is to be preferred. Neck dissection is still surrounded by controversy. In general the procedure should be done when nodes are palpable and this may be necessary bilaterally.

Lymphomas
This group of diseases, along with leukaemias, tend to have a disproportionate importance in relation to their incidence, in any

discussion of malignant diseases. Although lymphomas account for only 5% of all cancers, intensive study over 20 years has brought more advance in the understanding and management of this group of malignant diseases than in any other. They are broadly divided into Hodgkin's disease and non-Hodgkin's lymphomas.

Hodgkin's disease

A decade ago this disease[166,177] was accepted to be nearly always a fatal condition. Early Stage I and IIA disease is now curable in most cases with radiotherapy. Even Stage IV disseminated disease responds in most cases to chemotherapy and survival of 80% for at least 5 years is reported. There is a biphasic peak incidence of the disease at age 25 and again at 70. It is classified according to histological type[118] in Table 5 and can be staged according to the Ann Arbor method in Table 6.

Table 5   Pathological classification of Hodgkin's disease[118]

Lymphocyte predominance
Nodular sclerosing
Mixed cellularity
Lymphocyte depletion

Table 6   The Ann Arbor staging of Hodgkin's disease[117]

Stage I	Disease limited to lymph nodes of one anatomical region
I_E	Involvement of a single extranodal site other than lung (L) liver (H) or bone marrow (M)
II	Disease limited to two non-contiguous lymph node regions but all on the same side of the diaphragm.
II_E	Involvement of one lymph node region plus a single extranodal extension other than L, H or M
III	Lymph node involvement on both sides of the diaphragm
III_E	Lymph node involvement on both sides of the diaphragm plus a single extranodal extension other than L, H or M
IV	Secondary involvement of any non-single extranodal site or the lung, liver or spleen

Each stage may be A = absence or B = presence of constitutional symptoms such as fever, night sweats and generalized pruritus. Recently there has been a suggestion that pruritus should be removed from the B category since it may not carry the worse prognosis that generally goes with this category.

It is the supreme example in malignant disease of how prognosis has been improved by a rational combined approach of treatment modalities based on accurate staging of the disease with the appropriate therapy that follows from that staging.

Patients with Stage I and II disease do better than those with Stage III disease who in turn have a better prognosis than those with Stage IV disease. Those with category 'B' disease with generalized symptoms fare worse than those with category 'A' without symptoms. Lymphocyte-predominant and nodular sclerosing disease carries a better prognosis than mixed cellularity and lymphocyte-depleted disease, so that it is also true to say that there is a higher proportion of the latter two histological categories in those with Stage IIIB and IV disease.

Such staging requires extensive investigation including blood counts, liver and renal biochemistry together with chest and lateral postnasal space x-ray. Laparotomy and splenectomy are indicated in all cases of suspected Stage I, II and IIIa disease. Abdominal lymph nodes may be biopsied and at the same time bone marrow trephine and liver wedge biopsies are taken. We believe that CT scanning will eventually replace more invasive and uncomfortable lymphagiography for demonstration of abdominal lymph nodes. Staging laparotomy with the need for histological evidence of lymph node and spleen involvement remains necessary for demonstration of abdominal lymph nodes. CT scanning also has the added advantage of demonstrating lymph nodes just above and below the diaphragm, an area where lymphangiography is of little use.

Treatment of Hodgkin's disease is with splenectomy and radiotherapy for Stages I, II and IIIA disease. Chemotherapy may well have a place following radiotherapy in those with IIIB disease but when used following radiotherapy in Stage IIIA disease no improved survival has been obtained even though there has been an improved disease-free interval after such combined treatment.

Stage IIIB and IV disease should be treated with chemotherapy, initially with the MOPP regime[119].

Non-Hodgkin's lymphomas

This is a difficult group of diseases to treat but therapeutic advances are being made now so that it too has become a focal point of research effort[120,121]. Unlike Hodgkin's disease there is no universally accepted pathological classification and all those put forward have drawbacks. One classification which has found favour is that of Rappaport[122] since there is a degree of relation to prognosis. It may be said that those patients whose lymph node histology shows a fair degree of nodularity and whose cell type is well differentiated have a better prognosis. Those with diffuse well-differentiated node histology nearly all develop a frank chronic lymphocytic leukaemia. It is particularly a disease of older patients but carries a relatively good prognosis if managed well. Nearly all other diffuse pattern non-Hodgkin's lymphomas are poorly differentiated and carry a worse prognosis. The poorly differentiated diffuse lymphocytic type sometimes becomes indistinguishable from acute lymphoblastic leukaemia with the same problems of insidious CNS involvement. Thus non-Hodgkin's lymphomas represent a spectrum from nodular well-differentiated lymphocytic lymphoma (formerly known as giant follicular lymphoma) with the need for minimal treatment and an excellent prognosis, to the adult type of lymphoblastic leukaemia with a poor prognosis.

In the absence of any better staging system it is appropriate to use the 'Ann Arbor' staging as for Hodgkin's disease. Patients with non-Hodgkin's lymphomas tend to present initially with more advanced disease and at least 25% have involvement of extranodal sites. Advanced disease may be missed unless a resolute search is made with chest and postnasal space X-rays, full blood count, bone marrow trephine and examination of the marrow clot, together with biochemical estimations of renal and liver function, uric acid and calcium estimations. Since abnormal immunoglobulins may be produced with consequent renal failure and hyperviscosity syndrome as in myeloma, serum protein electrophoresis and immunoglobulin measurements should be made. Reticulocyte count and a Coombs test should be carried out.

As with Hodgkin's disease, these lymphomas require extensive assessment of their lymph node status if it appears that they have disease limited to lymph nodes. This may be achieved with bipedal lymphangiography but again, if available, CT scanning, especially with the new generation of 'faster' scanners, may well be a preferred alternative especially in the older, more ill patient. CT scanning is becoming more important anyway in order to show sequentially the effects of treatment.

Because the majority of non-Hodgkin's lymphomas present with late stage disease in an older age group, who are often not very well, laparotomy is not indicated for staging purposes but may be necessary occasionally to obtain histological evidence and to deal with obstruction due to extranodal gut lymphoma.

The treatment of non-Hodgkin's lymphomas is less well defined than in Hodgkin's disease. The exact role of radiotherapy is not clear and there are a large number of chemotherapeutic regimes from which to choose. Apart from nodular well-differentiated lymphocytic lymphoma which requires minimal radiotherapy or single agent chemotherapy alone, the better prognosis, apparently localized nodular disease (Stages I, I_E, II, and II_E), should receive radiotherapy to the involved regions and should perhaps receive chemotherapy after a short interval with nothing more vigorous than single agent chlorambucil or CVP chemotherapy[123] (with cyclophosphamide, vincristine and prednisolone). These patients should not be overtreated. Apparently localized disease of diffuse histology should also be treated with local radiotherapy but such lymphomas relapse much earlier – diffuse histiocytic lymphomas very often within a year. More vigorous chemotherapy with CMOPP[125] or CHOP[124] may be given following radiotherapy to the poor prognosis group so that the disease-free interval may be prolonged, but great care should always be exercised in the more elderly patient especially with adriamycin as part of CHOP.

Stage III and IV may be treated with chemotherapy with possibly prior radiotherapy to particularly large or symptomatic masses: CVP is appropriate for the better prognosis group while CMOPP and CHOP will temporarily benefit from 30–60% of those with poor-prognosis diffuse disease. About half the patients with favourable histology will die within 5–10 years. A smaller proportion survive 5 years with diffuse unfavourable histology although there is a small subgroup of patients with diffuse histiocytic lymphoma confined to lymph nodes who may be cured. Evaluation of whole body irradiation is being carried out but it is still too early to say what place in treatment this technique has, if any, in elderly patients.

Myeloma is a slowly progressive disease of plasma cells which may be found in elderly people. Diagnosis is made on the findings of Bence–Jones proteinuria, a monoclonal band on serum electrophoresis and an increased proportion of presumably abnormal plasma cells in bone marrow aspirate. Occasionally the abnormal cells may be identified by developing an antibody to the abnormal protein that is produced and using it to cause fluorescence of the plasma cells in the marrow that produce the protein. Prognosis has improved a little in the last 10 years, and there is now more than 3 years median survival in treated patients. While a search goes on for improved chemotherapeutic regimes, 5 day intermittent courses of prednisolone and melphalan at 6 weekly intervals are probably best in elderly patients together with radiotherapy to locally painful and fragile bone areas. Hyperviscosity syndrome and impending renal failure may be treated with regular plasmapheresis for a while but unless the disease is likely to come under control with chemotherapy this is not indicated.

Leukaemias

Along with lymphomas, acute leukaemias which account for less than 5% of all malignancies are best managed in specialist centres. Patients can become acutely ill during the phase of remission induction and often require an established and expensive commitment to support systems such as intensive chemotherapy, platelet and granulocyte transfusions, necessitating access to a cell separator. They usually require a high degree of nursing and medical time if a high proportion are to survive this induction period.

Leukaemias may be divided into acute and chronic with further subdivisions according to cell type. Patients usually present with non-specific symptoms of fever, malaise, tiredness or weight loss or with haemorrhage from mucous membranes, intracranial vessels or uterus. Sternal and periarticular pain are also features which are found. Anaemia is a common finding. Enlarged lymph nodes, spleen and liver are more commonly found in lymphoblastic and lymphocytic leukaemia than in leukaemias of the myeloid series.

Acute leukaemias

(a) *Acute myeloblastic leukaemia (AML)* This is nearly always found in adults, a third of whom are over 60 years of age[126]. The prognosis is generally very poor in the very elderly, most patients dying within a few weeks of diagnosis. Over the age of 60 probably less than 25% will achieve a complete remission on treatment. Low platelet counts, low haemoglobin, high peripheral blood blast counts and a coagulation disorder are all factors for poor prognosis. Diagnosis is made from peripheral blood and bone marrow aspirate from the sternum or iliac crest. Morphological interpretation of bone marrow can be difficult and usually requires the use of special stains. The findings of more cytoplasm than in acute lymphoblastic leukaemia (ALL) with fine lace-like chromatin, Auer rods (in 20–30%) and Sudan black or peroxidase-positive staining of primitive cells confirm the diagnosis. Leukocyte alkaline phosphatase will be low and electron microscopy can be useful in those remaining cases which are difficult to differentiate. Myelomonocytic forms with folded, indented nuclei may be found while megaloblastosis and red cell dysplasia points to di Guglielmo's disease (erythroleukaemia.)

(b) *Acute lymphoblastic leukaemia (ALL)* This is usually a disease of children but 20% present as adults with an increasing incidence with age. Unlike children only 40% will achieve remission and indeed the disease in adults and particularly old age carries a worse prognosis with a much shorter survival. Diagnosis is made in the same way as in AML but here there is a high nuclear-cytoplasmic ratio in blast cells with only one to two nucleoli in round nuclei. The cell population is more homogeneous. There is clumped chromatin with coarse granules and block positivity on PAS stains. Again low platelet counts, low haemoglobin and a high circulating blast count are poor prognostic factors but coagulopathies do not occur as often. As with AML bone marrow examinations need to be repeated at appropriate intervals to assess progress.

Treatment Patients and their families need to be told of their disease and of the implications of treatment which are unpleasant. Nearly all patients develop an aplastic marrow picture with pancytopenia before normal marrow elements can regenerate. This means that most patients become very ill for from 1–4 weeks with infective episodes and haemorrhagic disorders. A minority of patients will elect not to be treated and this is probably a wise decision in the elderly. A comprehensive discussion of the relevant chemotherapeutic regimes is not appropriate here but the addition of cytosine arabinoside, daunorubicin and adriamycin (hydroxydaunorubicin) has improved treatment both in terms of remission induction and survival. Following induction it is clear that patients need to have maintenance chemotherapy. Except for one maintenance study in AML, immunotherapy has not been found useful in treatment.

There is a group of elderly patients who have what might be termed a preleukaemia. Their marrow is dysplastic and they usually fail to produce one of the normal elements of blood in adequate quantity. Such patients eventually develop a frank leukaemia but this may not happen for some years and they should not be treated in the interim period. There are other patients with AML who never achieve a complete remission, which is usually essential for long survival, and yet who also survive for long periods on minimal treatment.

(c) *Meningeal leukaemia* As with children it is clear that remissions longer than 6 months in ALL are associated with leukaemic meningeal infiltration. This is also true in a smaller proportion of those with AML. Prophylactic craniospinal irradiation and intrathecal methotrexate are of proven value in children but this is not necessarily so in adults. Nevertheless it is current practice to employ craniospinal irradiation in adults after remission induction in ALL and poorly differentiated diffuse lymphocytic lymphoma.

Chronic myeloid leukaemia
This disease presents only occasionally in the elderly being more of a disease in younger people between 30–50. It is characterized by malaise, a large spleen and high peripheral granulocyte count. The

Philadelphia chromosome is found in 85% of patients while the leukocyte alkaline phosphatase is 0 or very low. This is important since it helps distinguish the disease from a leukaemoid reaction where there is a high leukocyte alkaline phosphatase. The treatment of choice is busulphan at dosages of 4–6 mg/day until the peripheral granulocyte count is reduced, at which point the drug should be stopped remembering that it has a half-life of more than 3 weeks. Courses may be repeated as appropriate. This drug should be used with great care since a small proportion of patients develop persistent marrow aplasia. Median survival is about $2\frac{1}{2}$–3 years after which transformation to acute myeloblastic leukaemia occurs (acute blast cell crisis). This is usually refractory to treatment. Under 10% die with a picture like that of myelofibrosis.

Chronic lymphocytic leukaemia
This is predominantly a disease of old people with a picture of large spleen, large liver and large lymph nodes[127]. Peripheral blood shows a high leukocyte count of which 80–90% are small lymphocytes, nearly always 'B' lymphocytes. Humoral immunity is impaired, immunoglobulin levels may be low and haemolysis may be present together with thrombocytopenia. Again it is important not to overtreat these patients. The majority have chronic indolent disease which requires continuous single alkylating agent such as chlorambucil 4–6 mg/day or intermittent courses at a higher dosage. Treatment should be stopped when relief of symptoms and signs is achieved while no great emphasis should be placed on reducing high lymphocyte counts too far. As with the other leukaemias, where there is a moderate to high tumour burden, allopurinol should be given as part of treatment to prevent urate nephropathy.

Haemolytic and autoimmune episodes may require high dose prednisolone at 40 mg/day for a while. It used to be thought that this disease generally carries a good prognosis but while 20% may survive 10–15 years the majority die much sooner. An ethical problem is arising therefore as to how vigorously this disease should be treated in the elderly in whom it occurs. As yet no effective vigorous treatment has been devised but more interest in investigating this has been generated in recent years.

Sarcomas
Apart from osteosarcomas which may arise in a proportion of those with Paget's disease this group of malignancies is rarely seen in old age. Treatment of sarcomas is by radical surgery, if this is possible, and radiotherapy may play a part in combined treatment. Since

sarcomas metastasize early, chemotherapy after removal of the primary tumour may also play a role. Methotrexate is of proven use with minimal residual disease in osteosarcoma in younger patients and may also be of value in older patients. Soft tissue sarcomas tend to spread along muscle bundles and sheaths and are nearly always more locally extensive than is realized requiring very wide excision indeed to avoid local recurrence. CYVÁDIC, a regime utilizing cyclophosphamide, vincristine, adriamycin and DTIC and developed at the M. D. Anderson hospital in Texas by Gottlieb *et al.*[128] is of proven benefit in more advanced disease of soft tissue sarcomas and may confer long-term remission and survival in over half the patients. It is, however, a debilitating regime even in younger patients and therefore the accompanying morbidity may be unacceptable in the elderly.

Primary skin cancer
These are amongst the commonest tumours and are probably the most frequent cancers seen by general practitioners. They occur primarily on exposed areas and are those readily accessible for treatment. Nevertheless there are many that are left until late because they often present as apparently benign lesions.

Amongst the predisposing factors are pale, fair and dry skins and those who are exposed to sunlight because of environment and occupation for long periods.

Squamous cell cancer
These are frequently seen in older patients. They often mimic keratoses and frequently occur in areas of previous skin change such as old burn scars, etc. Some start in an area of leukoplakia or as a 'fever blister'. The transformation to a squamous cancer is detected by thickening ulceration or crusted overgrowth. These tumours are quite malignant from the beginning and may metastasize early to lymph nodes. This is especially so for tumours in oral cavities. Any recent lesion must be removed for biopsy usually under local anaesthesia. If the diagnosis is clear from the outset wide excision is necessary. In older people these often occur as an ulcer over the bridge of the nose, near the inner canthus, or adjacent to the nostril. Because of proximity of adjacent cartilage, eyelid or lobe of ear plastic surgical advice is usually necessary.

Basal cell cancers
These are local malignant growths, often highly so and very often treacherous in their presentation. They may behave like benign les-

ions in their early stages and unless removed widely will recur, and gradually erode all tissues in their path. They occur most frequently in the midportion of the face and usually without a previous skin alteration such as keratoses. Not only are they indolent in their early stages but they frequently crust over, which allays the patient's concern and medical advice may be deferred.

There are a number of varieties of this condition, the commonest presentation being a firm slightly elevated edge which may be grey blue or pearly surrounding a shallow central ulcer. The lesion is indurated and looks and feels like a button. Other varieties include a large flat lesion with an active edge, being serpiginus and irregular. This spreads actively and rapidly. Another type is the invasive rodent ulcer which although innocuous on the surface shows extensive invasion beneath the skin. These lesions must all be biopsied promptly.

Small lesions are treated by excisional biopsy. While irradiation is very effective, in most instances wide surgical excision is usually the treatment of choice.

Other skin cancers include intraepithelial cancers or carcinoma *in situ*. One example of this is Bowen's disease which resembles a basal cell lesion. Other lesions which are locally malignant and should be treated by excision are adenocanthoma which is a verrucous lesion seen on the face and the ears; calcifying epithelioma of Malherbe is a circumscribed indurated solitary tumour attached to the skin but mobile over underlying tissues. This too occurs on the face and upper extremities and should be removed.

Malignant melanoma

Pigmented skin lesions are very common indeed in elderly people. In the past decade much light has been thrown on the pathology and prognosis of this unpredictable cancer, and a clearer understanding of the nature of these lesions has been gained[132,133].

The older the patient the more likely a pigmented lesion is to be a melanoma and the larger the lesion the greater its potential for malignancy. It occurs about six times as frequently in men as in women. In about two-thirds of patients the melanoma arises in a pre-existing skin blemish but in 30% of patients the tumour occurs *de novo*. The commonest feature, which draws the patient's attention to the lesion, is an increase in size. Sometimes the increase consists in a spreading pigmentation or it may become slightly raised. Colour changes and bleeding are the next commonest manifestations of malignancy and sometimes the lesion may become itchy. The type of naevus likely to become cancer is the flat dark brown, black or bluish junctional naevus which is usually smooth, well demarcated and often hairless. In particular naevi of the feet and genitalia have a higher potential for malignancy, although their occurrence is uncommon in these sites.

Hutchinson originally described the *senile freckle* now called Hutchinson's melanotic freckle in 1867. Clark[134] introduced his classification of melanoma and this has now been adopted as the basis for the international classification. (Table 7).

Table 7 Classification of melanoma

1. *Lentigo maligna melanoma* (Hutchinson's melanotic freckle)
   This is often large with an irregular outline, flat with many shades of brown. Spread occurs in the epidermis up to 1 cm beyond the gross limits.
2. *Superficial spreading melanoma*
   This is a raised lesion, 1–4 mm above the skin and at least a part of the outline is regular. There may be a number of nodules. The colour is shades of brown, grey or pink.
3. *Nodular*
   There is no flat component: it is uniformly invasive.

The melanotic freckle often enlarges and regresses over the years and may disappear completely only to return again. It occurs most commonly in the sun-damaged skin of the malar region and also on the hands and wrists.

The superficial spreading melanoma is more circumscribed than the freckle. It starts as a macule growing fairly rapidly until a nodule appears after about 12–18 months. These occur in both covered and exposed parts and also on the mucosal surfaces. About two-thirds of patients with this type of lesion have a pre-existing pigmented lesion. The commonest presenting symptom is enlargement often 'spreading like a stain' and the spreading margin is almost always palpable in contradistinction to that of the melanotic freckle.

The nodular variety is frequently polypoid or dome-shaped and is more frequently ulcerated than the other two types. There is usually no preliminary spreading pigmentation.

The prognostic features of melanoma have been clarified by Clark's description of the microscopic levels of invasion.[134]. He has described five such levels:

(1) *In situ*, confined to the epidermis;
(2) Invading the papillary zone of the dermis;
(3) Filling the papillary layer and abutting upon the interface between the papillary and reticular layers without actual invasion of the reticular dermis;

(4) Invading the reticular zone of the dermis;
(5) Invading the subcutaneous fat.

This taken in conjunction with mitotic activity, provides a reasonably accurate assessment of the likely mortality rate.

Grade I:
      fewer than 1 mitosis/high power field – 80% 5 years survival
Grade II:
      1–3 mitosis/high power field – 55% 5 years survival
Grade III:
      5 or more mitosis/high power field – 41% 5 years survival

The mortality for the various levels of invasion have been assessed by a number of authors: 8% with level 2, 35% with level 3, 46% with level 4 and 52% with level 5.

Thus the prognosis varies according to its clinical and histologic type; the melanotic freckle has the best prognosis, the superficial spreading type occupies an intermediate position and the nodular melanoma has the worst prognosis.

Every suspected melanoma should have the diagnosis confirmed by frozen section, thus permitting either limited removal or wide resection with grafting if necessary. The commonest non-melanomatous conditions which may be mistaken clinically are:

(1) Lentigines: these are usually flat pigmented macules which in section show increased pigment but not of melanocytes.
(2) Seborrhoeic warts or keratoses: these raised nodules occur on the face, temple or back.
(3) Basal cell carcinoma.
(4) Histiocytoma. This occurs frequently on the leg with increased pigmentation.
(5) Melanoacanthoma.
(6) Pigmented squamous cell carcinoma.
(7) Bowen's disease: the lesions are occasionally pigmented.

None of the above are difficult to separate from true melanomas.

The superficial spreading variety should have a wider margin of excision because of the adjacent intraepidermal component. The question of lymph node resection is a controversial one but there is a body of opinion which considers this to be appropriate treatment where possible in all Grade II and III mitotic activity that have invaded to level 3 or beyond, or in lesions which measure, in paraffin section, 1·5 mm in depth.

Chemotherapy in disseminated malignant melanoma has been generally disappointing. In addition, since this disease is so very variable, objective results have been difficult to assess. Combinations of BCNU, hydroxyurea and DTIC or vincristine and DTIC have from time to time apparently caused substantial regression of disease although there has evidently been some variation in response of different metastatic disease areas in the same patient. Because of the cumulative toxicity of BCNU this drug should be used with great caution in elderly patients.

A number of other rare primary skin lesions occur. The guiding principle, especially in the old, is that any new or persistent skin lump or ulcer or 'scab' or pigmented area must be treated as a cancer and immediate biopsy done. This is almost always possible under local anaesthesia.

SKIN MANIFESTATIONS OF MALIGNANCY

There are well-recognized harbingers of cancer which appear on the skin as a first pointer to the generalized underlying disease[129,130]. Invasion of the skin is the commonest skin manifestation of cancer, usually a late development and occurs commonly in the scalp, chest wall and abdominal wall. Primary sites are usually breast and lung.

Definite skin markers include:

(1) Acanthosis nigricans – a dry brown-black hyperplasia with a velvety texture that occurs in the axilla and may spread to neck, groins and abdominal wall. If occurring in an adult who is not obese it is a certain sign of cancer, nearly always adenocarcinoma, usually of the stomach or an other abdominal viscus including genitourinary sites. The prognosis is very poor indeed.

(2) Dermatomyositis – an inflammatory condition of skin and muscles often with necrosis and fever . The rash in the form of a reddish-blue discolouration starts around the eyes and spreads to light exposed areas of face, neck and arms. Myopathy is largely proximal and may involve pharynx and tongue. The common primary sites are breast, ovary, cervix, bone or tumours of retroperitoneal origin and in men may be stomach, kidney or lung, or nasopharyngeal. Leukaemias may also be related to this manifestation.

Clinical suspicion of malignancy should be raised by a number of unusual skin presentations.

(1) Skin inflammation, particularly if severe, or if it is an atypical infection. These include severe cases of herpes zoster, fungal infections or extensive staphylococcal boils.

(2) Petechiae and purpuric eruptions occur as a result of the platelet deficiencies in lymphomas, leukaemias and bone marrow secondaries. Diffuse erythemas occur in the carcinoid syndrome and may lead to permanent cyanotic flush of the face and neck. Localized erythemas in the form of migratory thrombophlebitis in unusual situations such as the neck, chest, pelvis and limbs are well recognized. Multiple attacks of deep venous thrombosis also occur.

(3) Clubbing (pachydermoperiostosis) of recent origin may signal a lung tumour either primary or secondary. An interesting clinical observation is the relief of pain after resection of the lung tumour or after denervation of the lung root.

There are a number of specific associations of skin changes with malignant endocrine disorders. Examples are ectopic ACTH secretion, usually due to tumours in the lung, thymus and pancreas and which cause diffuse hyperpigmentation and cushingoid states.

Genetic syndromes include the epidermoid cysts in Gardner's syndrome (autosomal dominant), and Peutz–Jegher's syndrome. This condition is characterized by pigmented macules around the mouth, benign small intestinal polyps, and, in some, colonic polyps which are potentially malignant.

One common skin lesion in the elderly is Campbell de Morgan spots – reddish, raised or flat lesions 1–3 mm irregularly scattered over the chest and abdomen. Widely regarded as harbingers of malignant disease by generations of medical students, there is in fact no such proven association.

CANCER AS A CHRONIC GENERALIZED DISEASE

For many years it was believed that, where it seemed that a solid tumour was confined to the primary site, later recurrence was due to the dissemination of tumour cells at the time of operation for removal of the tumour. Little progress has been made in improving the disease-free interval and survival in many solid tumour malignancies. Current belief recognizes that tumour cells may indeed be disseminated at the time of surgery but holds that other factors are more important.

(1) By the time a primary tumour is removed micrometastatic disease almost certainly exists in those patients who appear to have no further disease at this time but who subsequently develop a recurrence.

(2) The earlier the stage of disease at the time of surgical removal of the primary the less likely it is for recurrence to occur later.

(3) The earlier the stage of disease when the localized primary is removed the longer the disease-free interval appearance of overt recurrence in those patients who do eventually develop more widespread disease[135].

The tumour–host relationship again is poorly understood but it is undoubtedly true that with some tumours such as melanoma and breast cancer a very long interval indeed can elapse before metastatic disease, identical to the primary tumour, appears. After removal of a breast cancer patients can suddenly develop rapidly progressive metastic disease after 25 years of health. It is inconceivable that steady growth of micrometastatic disease has taken place since the primary was first treated. Presumably a dormant period intervened for a variable length of time before the disease began to progress once more.

A number of conclusions may be drawn that have relevance with regard to treatment of these primary tumours which usually metastasize early.

(1) Before undertaking treatment accurate staging is usually essential in order to ascertain whether there is any detectable metastatic disease.

(2) If the disease is apparently confined to the primary tumour, with or without involvement of regional lymph glands, it is certain that local treatment confined solely to these areas, no matter how radical, will fail to cure the disease in a proportion of cases depending on the type of primary tumour.

(3) If it is decided, after accurate staging, that no evidence exists of overt metastatic disease some form of additional treatment such as cytotoxic chemotherapy may be appropriate at this stage if a higher proportion of 'cures', or at least a lengthening of the disease-free interval, is to be achieved. This is dependent on the availability of drugs of proven benefit in the specific malignant disease being treated. Most treatment of this nature is at present carried out in a research environment so that definitive information can be obtained.

It is also true that such multimodal treatment may not be appropriate in the elderly person with very early malignant disease if the time-interval before development of metastatic disease is likely to be relatively long. In this instance simple local treatment may be all that is indicated, remembering, however, that in those with a much higher risk of early recurrence systemic treatment should be given as early as possible after local treatment.

(4) In general, cytotoxic chemotherapy is more effective in low-volume disease than with disease that is of a size that can be seen, felt and identified radiologically[136]. Waiting until the disease has overtly recurred probably diminishes the chances of the disease's useful regression.

COMBINED MODALITY TREATMENT IN SOLID TUMOURS

It is now better understood that, with most malignant diseases, surgical removal of the primary tumour is unlikely to effect a cure in the majority of patients and that this is almost certainly due to the presence of established metastatic disease. It follows, therefore, that it is of great importance even in elderly people to search carefully for evidence of such metastatic disease throughout the body in order to arrive at an accurate staging of disease.

Early disease
It is true to say that great effort is often expended on local treatment with surgery and radiotherapy in apparently early disease, while ignoring the statistical probability with many solid tumours that micrometastatic disease already exists elsewhere even when it cannot be discovered immediately.

Since it is likely that growth fractions in such metastatic tumours may be at their highest at this stage it may represent the only time when systemic measures such as cytotoxic chemotherapy may be really effective. Modern belief is strengthening that chemotherapy and/or hormonal manipulation should be used earlier than when massive recurrence of disease has occurred. Definite benefit, however, has only been proven in younger patients where careful treatment trials have been carried out in particular diseases such as breast cancer or osteogenic sarcoma.

With most of the more common solid tumours such as those of bronchus or gastrointestinal origin it is true to say that drug regimes have not yet been devised that are even reasonably effective in most patients with advanced disease, and experience shows that until this occurs it is unlikely that such drugs will produce great benefit at an earlier stage of the disease. Because of these factors great caution should be exercised in the elderly. The time has not yet come when the majority of patients with cancer should automatically be submitted to 'adjuvant' chemotherapy following surgery and/or radiotherapy for their early primary disease. Even in the presence of limited morbidity from chemotherapy the likelihood of death from causes other than the underlying disease must be carefully balanced against the probability of recurrence of tumour within a defined period of time.

Advanced disease

Providing drug combinations exist which are statistically likely to produce regression of tumour of worthwhile duration there is no reason why such chemotherapy should not be given in old age, always accepting that regimes may have to be modified to take account of the increased likelihood of toxicity from such drugs as adriamycin (cardiomyopathy) and vincristine (neuropathy). Here again, if it is feasible, tumour should be 'debulked' with surgery and/or radiotherapy before commencing chemotherapy. If radiotherapy has been necessary, particularly to areas where subsequent chemotherapy may have an adverse effect, further care should be taken in modifying dosages and schedules of chemotherapeutic treatment. Bone marrow reserve can be seriously impaired by radiotherapy before marrow-toxic drugs are given and there is some evidence that adriamycin is more toxic to heart muscle following radiotherapy. Chemotherapy and/or radiotherapy are not always given to obtain measurable regression of tumour and useful extension of worthwhile life. There are instances where distressing specific conditions such as severe pain, pleural effusion, ascites, the syndrome which accompanies superior vena caval obstruction and others may be relieved thereby improving the quality of life remaining. In this context radiotherapy may be particularly useful in keeping a patient on his feet where a metastatic deposit appears in a long bone or vertebra even though no pain may be present.

References

1 Copeland, E. M. and McBride, C. M. (1973). Axillary metastases from unknown primary sites. *Ann. Surg.*, **178**, 25
2 Kubler-Ross, E. (1972). On death and dying. *J. Am. Med. Assoc.*, **221**, 174
3 Dunphy, E. (1976). On caring for the patient with cancer. *N. Engl. J. Med.*, **295**, 313

4 Saunders, C. (1976). Care of the dying. *Nurs. Times,* **72,** 1003
5 Saunders, C. (1977). On dying and dying well. *Proc. R. Soc. Med.,* **70,** 290
6 Few, E. (1975). Nursing the dying at home. In: R. Raven (ed.). *The Dying Patient.* (Tunbridge Wells: Pitman Medical) pp. 63–75
7 Editorial. (1976). Cell life and death in human tumours. *Br. Med. J.,* **1,** 177
8 Tubiana, M. and Malaise, E. P. (1976). In: T. S. Symington (ed.). *Scientific Foundations of Oncology.* (London: Heineman)
9 Steel, G. G. and Lamerton, L. F. (1966). The growth rate of human tumours. *Br. J. Cancer.,* **20,** 74
10 Cline, M. J. (1971). Cancer chemotherapy in major problems. In: W. H. Smith (ed.). *Internal Medicine.* (Philadelphia: W. B. Saunders and Co.), pp. 1–41
11 Brulé, G., Eckhardt, S. J., Hau, T. C. and Winkler, A. (1973). *Drug Therapy in Cancer.* (Geneva: World Health Organization)
12 Bagshawe, K. D. (1979), Cancer chemotherapy: successes, failures and hopes. *J. R. Soc. Med.,* **72,** 152
13 Frei, E. III. (1974). Combination chemotherapy. *Proc. R. Soc. Med.,* **67,** 425
14 Bruce, W. R., Meeher, B. E. and Valeriotte, F. A. (1967). Comparison of the sensitivity of normal haematopoietic and transplanted lymphoma colony-forming cells to chemotherapeutic agents administered *in vivo. J. Natl. Cancer Inst.,* **37,** 233
15 Valeriote, F. A. and Bruce, W. R. (1967). Comparison of the sensitivity of haemopoietic colony-forming cells in different proliferative states to vinblastine. *J. Natl. Cancer Inst.,* **38,** 393
16 Cassady, J. R., Richter, M. P., Piro *et al.* (1975). Radiation – adriamycin interactions: Preliminary clinical observations. *Cancer,* **36** (3), 946
17 Rigby, D. J., Wallace, H. J., and Holland, J. F. (1973). *Cis-*diaminedichloroplatinum (NSC 119875): A phase I study. *Cancer Chemother. Rep.,* **57,** 465
18 Johns, D. A. and Bertino, J. R. (1973). Folate antagonists. In: J. F. Holland and E. Frei III (eds.). *Cancer Medicine.* (Philadelphia: Lea and Febiger, pp. 739–754
19 Vogler, W. R., Cooper, L. E. and Groth, D. P. (1974). Correlation of cytosine arabinoside-induced increment in growth fraction of leukaemic blast cells with clinical response. *Cancer,* **33,** 603
20 Kremer, W. B., Vogler, W. R. and Chan, Y. K. (1976). An attempt at synchronisation of marrow cells in acute leukaemia. *Cancer,* **37,** 390
21 Price, L. A., Hill, B. T., Calvert, A. H., Shaw, H. J. and Hughes, K. B. (1975). Kinetically-based multiple drug treatment for advanced head and neck cancer. *Br. Med. J.,* **3,** 10
22 Barranco, S. C., Ho, D. H. W. and Drewinko, B. *et al.* (1972). Differential sensitivities of human melanoma cells grown *in vitro* to arabinosylcytosine. *Cancer Res.,* **32,** 2733
23 Moertel, C. G. and Reitemeier, R. J. (1969). Treatment of nausea and vomiting. In: *Clinical Management of Advanced Gastro-intestinal Cancer.* (New York: Hoeber), pp. 30–40
24 Moertel, C. G. and Reitemeier, R. J. (1969). Treatment of oedema and ascites. In: *Clinical Management of Advanced Gastro-intestinal Cancer.* (New York: Hoeber), pp. 22–29
25 LeVeen, H. H., Wapnick, S., Grosberg, S., and Kinivey, M. (1976). Further experiences with peritoneovenous shunt for ascites. *Ann. Surg.,* **184,** 574
26 Kilpatrick, Z. M., Chapman, C. B. (1965). On pericardiocentesis. *Am. J. Cardiol.,* **16,** 722

27 Smith, F. E., Lane, M. and Hudguns, P. T. (1974). Conservative management of malignant pericardial effusion. *Cancer*, **33**, 47

28 Goudie, R. B. (1955). Secondary tumours of heart and pericardium. *Br. Heart J.*, **17**, 183

29 Perez, C. A., Presant, C. A. and Van Amburg III A. L. (1978). Management of superior vena cava syndrome. *Sem. Oncol.*, **5**, 123

30 Harries, B. (1970). Spinal cord compression. *Br. Med. J.*, **1**, 611

31 Brice, J. and McKissock, W. (1965). Surgical treatment of malignant extradural spinal tumours. *Br. Med. J.*, **2**, 1341

32 Khan, F. R., Glicksman, A. S. and Chu, F. C. H. *et al.* (1967). Treatment by radiotherapy of spinal cord compression due to extradural metastases. *Radiology*, **89**, 495

33 Budey, G. P. (1975). Infections in cancer. *Cancer Treat. Rev.*, **2**, 89

34 Cartwright, R. Y. (1975). Antifungal drugs. *J. Antimicrob. Chemother.*, **1**, 141

35 Muggia, F. M. and Heinemann, H. O. (1970). Hypercalcaemia associated with neoplastic disease. *Ann. Intern. Med.*, **73**, 281

36 Elias, E. G. and Evans, J. T. (1972). Hypercalcaemic crisis in neoplastic diseases. Management with mithramycin. *Surgery*, **71**, 631

37 Vaughan, C. B., Vaitkevicius, K. (1974). The effects of calcitonin in hypercalcaemia in patients with malignancy. *Cancer*, **34**, 1268

38 Easty, G. C., Dewsett, M., Powles, T. J., Easty, D. M., Gazet, J. C. and Neville, A. M. (1976). Hypercalcaemia in malignant disease. *Proc. R. Soc. Med.*, **70**, 191

39 Kwaan, H. C. (1972). Disseminated intravascular coagulation. *Med. Clin. N. Am.*, **56**, 177

40 Sharp, A. A. (1977). Diagnosis and management of disseminated intravascular coagulation. *Br. Med. Bull.*, **33**, 3, 265

41 Handley, R. S. (1972). Observations and thoughts on cancer of the breast. *Proc. R. Soc. Med.*, **65**, 437

42 Sicker, K. and Waterhouse, J. A. H. (1973). Evaluation of TNM classification of carcinoma of the breast. *Br. J. Cancer*, **28**, 580

43 Leader (1976). Management of early cancer of the breast. *Br. Med. J.*, **1**, 1035

44 Hughes, L. E. and Forbes, J. F. (1978). Early breast cancer. Parts I and II. *Br. J. Surg.*, **65**, 753

45 Frazier, T. G., Copeland, E. M., Gallager, H. S., Paulus, D. D. and White E. C. (1977). Prognosis and treatment in minimal breast cancer. *Am. J. Surg.*, **133**, 697

46 Baum, M. (1978). Role of local treatment for primary carcinoma of breast. *Ann. R. Coll. Surg. Engl.*, **60**, 479

47 Duncan, W. and Kerr, G. P. (1976). The curability of breast cancer. *Br. Med. J.*, **2**, 781

48 Fisher, B., Glass, A., Redmond, C., Fisher, E. R., Barton, B., Such, E., Carbone, P., Economon, S., Foster, R., Frelick, R., Lerner, H., Levitt, M., Margolese, P., Macfarlane, J., Plotkin, D., Shibata, H. and Volk, H. L. (1977). Phenylatamine mustard (L-PAM) in the management of primary breast cancer. *Cancer*, **39**, 2883

49 Bonadonna, G., Rossi, A., Valagussa, P., Banfi, A. and Varonesi, U. (1977). The CMF program for operable breast cancer with positive axillary nodes. *Cancer*, **39**, 2904

50 Systematic chemotherapy in early breast cancer – Statement by British Breast Group (1976). *Br. Med. J.*, **3**, 861

51 Clinical trials of the treatment of breast cancer in Britain and Ireland – Report by co-ordinating committee (1977). *Br. Med. J.*, **1**, 361

52 Legha, S. S. and Carter, S. K. (1976). Anti-estrogens in the treatment of breast cancer. *Cancer Treat. Rev.*, 3, 205

53 Hancock, Kathleen, Peet, B. G., Price, J. J., Watson, G. W., Stone, Joan, Turman, R. C. (1977). Ten year survival rate in breast cancer using combination chemotherapy. *Br. J. Surg.*, 64, 134

54 Rubens, R. D., Knight, R. K. and Hayward, J. L. (1975). Chemotherapy of advanced breast cancer: A controlled randomized trial of cyclophosphamide versus a four-drug combination. *Br. J. Cancer*, 12 (6), 730

55 Jones, S. E., Duric, B. G. M. and Salmon, S. E. (1975). Combination chemotherapy with adriamycin and cyclophosphamide for advanced breast cancer. *Cancer*, 36, 90

56 Way, S. (1976). The vulva and vagina. In: T. F. Nealon, Jr. (ed.). *Management of the Patient with Cancer*. (Philadelphia: Saunders and Co.), pp. 674–681

57 Clark, D. G. C., Hilaris, B. S. and Ochoa, M., Jnr. *et al.* (1974). Interdisciplinary approach to advanced ovarian cancer. *Surg. Clin. N. Am.*, 54, 897

58 Greenwald, E. F. (1975). Ovarian tumours. *Clin. Obstet. Gynaecol.*, 18, 61

59 Young, R. C., Hubbard, S. P. and DiVita, V. T. (1974). The chemotherapy of ovarian carcinoma. *Cancer Treat. Rev.*, 1, 99

60 Nealon, J. H., Jnr. and Nikrui, N. (1976). The cervix. In: *Management of the Patient with Cancer*. (Philadelphia: W. B. Saunders), pp. 658–681

61 Peterson, O. (1956). Spontaneous course of cervical precancerous conditions. *Am. J. Obstet. Gynecol.*, 72, 1063

62 Guthrie, D. and Way, S. (1974). Treatment of advanced carcinoma of the cervix with adriamycin and methotrexate combined. *Obstet. Gynecol.*, 44, 586

63 Kistner, R., Krants, K. E. and Leisher, T. B. (1973). Endometrial cancer: Rising incidence, detection and treatment. *J. Reprod. Med.*, 10, 53

64 Reagan, J. W. (1974). The changing nature of endometrial cancer. *Gynec. Oncol.*, 2, 144

65 Morrow, C. P., Disaia, P. J. and Townsend, D. T. (1973). Current management of endometrial carcinoma. *Obstet. Gynecol.*, 42, 399

66 Barber, H. R. K. and Kwon, T. H. (1976). The endometrium. In: T. F. Nealon (ed.). *Management of the Patient with Cancer*. (Philadelphia: W. B. Saunders and Co.) pp. 641–657

67 Nordquist, S. (1969). Hormonal responsiveness of human endometrial carcinoma studied *in vitro* and *in vivo*. (Lund: Sweden Student Literature)

68 Gusberg, S. B. (1973). The dysfunctional and the neoplastic clinical investigation in the cervix of patient care in endometrial cancer. *Ann. J. Obstet. Gynecol.*, 116, 175

69 Grille, H. C. (1973). Obstructing lesions of the trachea. *Ann. Otol. Rhinol. Laryngol.*, 84, 770

70 Evans, E. W. T. (1973). Resection for bronchial carcinoma in the elderly. *Thorax*, 28, 86

71 Laing, A. H., Berry, R. J., Newman, C. R., Peto, J. (1975). Treatment of inoperable carcinoma of bronchus. *Lancet*, II, 1161

72 Turney, S. Z. and Haight, C. (1971). Pulmonary resection for metastatic neoplasm. *J. Thorac. Cardiovasc. Surg.*, 61, 784

73 Brin, E. N., Schiff, M. and Weiss, R. M. (1975). Palliative urinary diversion for pelvic malignancy. *J. Urol.*, 113, 619

74 Moore, C. (1970). *Cancer of the Kidney. Synopsis of Clinical Cancer*. (St Louis: C. V. Mosby Co.), pp. 161–166

75 Carter, S. K. and Wasserman, T. H. (1975). The chemotherapy of urologic cancer. *Cancer*, 36, 729

76 Bloom, H. J. G. (1979). Treatment of infiltrating bladder cancer. *J. R. Soc. Med.*, **72,** 203

77 Turner, A. G., Hendry, W. F., *et al.* (1977). The treatment of advanced bladder cancer with methotrexate. *Br. J. Urol.*, **49,** 673

78 England, H. R., Rigby, C., *et al.* (1973). Evaluation of Helmstein's distension method for carcinoma of the bladder. *Br. J. Urol.*, **45,** 593

79 Murphy, J. J. and Schoenberg, H. W. (1976). The genito-urinary tract. In: T. F. Nealon (ed.). *Management of the Patient with Cancer.* (Philadelphia: W. B. Saunders Co.), pp. 593–597

80 Moore, C. (1970). Cancer of the prostate. In: *Synopsis of Clinical Cancer.* (St Louis: C. V. Mosby Co.), pp. 167–174

81 Dixon, F. J. and Moore, R. A. (1952). Tumours of the male sex organs. In: *Atlas of Tumour Pathology*, Section VIII, Fasc. 31B & 32. (Washington, DC: Armed Forces Institute of Pathology), pp. 48–120

82 Lange, P. H. and Fraley, E. E. (1977). Serum alphafetoprotein and human chorionic gonadotrophin in the treatment of patients with testicular tumours. *Urol. Clin. N. Am.*, **4,** 393

83 Einhorn, L. H. and Donohue, J. P. (1977). Chemotherapy for disseminated testicular cancer. *Urol. Clin. N. Am.*, **4,** 407

84 Gunnlaugsson, G. H., Wychulis, A. R., Roland, C. and Ellis, H., Jnr. (1970). Analysis of 1657 patients with carcinoma of oesophagus and cardia of the stomach. *Surg. Gynecol. Obstet.*, **130,** 997

85 Pearson, J. G. (1969). Value of radiotherapy in management of esophageal cancer. *Am. J. Roentgenol.*, **105,** 500

86 Duvoison, G. E., Ellis, F. H. and Payne, W. S. (1967). Value of palliative prosthesis in malignant lesions of esophagus. *Surg. Clin. N. Am.*, **47,** 827

87 Hawley, P. R., Westerholm, P. and Morson, B. C. (1970). Pathology and prognosis of carcinoma of the stomach. *Br. J. Surg.*, **57,** 61

88 Lawrence, W., Jnr. and Terz, J. J. (1977). Management of gastro-intestinal cancer. In: *Cancer Management.* (New York: Grune and Stratton), pp. 202–219

89 Gilbertsen, V. A. (1969). Results of treatment of stomach cancer. *Cancer*, **23,** 1305

90 Moertel, C. G. (1975). Clinical management of advanced gastrointestinal cancer. *Cancer*, **36,** 675

91 Comis, R. L. and Carter, S. K. (1974). A review of chemotherapy in gastric cancer. *Cancer*, **34,** 1576

92 McPeak, C. J. (1967). Malignant tumours of the small intestine. *Am. J. Surg.*, **114,** 402

93 Lawrence, W., Jnr. and Terz, J. J. (1977). Management of gastrointestinal cancer. In: *Cancer Management.* (New York: Grune and Stratton), pp. 236–241

94 Glass, R. L. and Ledue, R. J. (1974). Small intestinal obstruction from peritoneal carcinomatosis. *Am. J. Surg.*, **125,** 316

95 Ketcham, A. S., Hoye, R. C. and Pilch, Y. (1970). Delayed intestinal obstruction following treatment for cancer. *Cancer,* **25,** 406

96 Welch, J. P. and Donaldson, G. A. (1974). Recent experience in the management of colon and rectum. *Am. J. Surg.*, **127,** 258

97 Lockhart-Mummery, H. E. (1969). In: B. C. Morson (ed.), *Disease of Colon, Rectum, Anus.* (New York: Appleton-Century-Crofts), pp. 114–128

98 Strauss, A. A., Strauss, S. F., Crawford, R. A. and Strauss, H. A. (1935). Surgical diathermy of carcinoma of the rectum: its clinical end results. *J. Am. Med. Assoc.*, **104,** 1480

99 Turnbull, R. B., Jnr. (1969). The coagulation radon, seed implantation for certain cancers of the rectum. In: R. Turell (ed.). *Disease of Colon and Anorectum*. (Philadelphia: Saunders), pp. 528

100 Jackman, R. J. (1961). Conservative management of selected patients with carcinoma of rectum. *Dis. Colon. Rectum.*, **4**, 429

101 Madden, J. L. and Kandaleft, S. (1967). Electrocoagulation. A primary and preferred method of treatment for cancer of the rectum. *Ann. Surg.*, **166**, 413

102 Electrocoagulation of rectal cancer updated. *Mt. Sinai J. Med.*, **43**, 263

103 Carter, S. K. (1976). Large bowel cancer – the current status of treatment. *J. Natl. Cancer Inst.*, **53**, 3

104 Falkson, G, Van Edin, E. G. and Falkson, H. C. (1974). Fluorouracil midazole carboxamide dimethyltriazeno, vincristine and *bis*-chloroethylintrourea in colon cancer. *Cancer*, **33**, 1207

105 Moertel, C. G., Schutt, A. J. and Hahn, R. G. *et al.* (1975). Therapy of advanced colorectal cancer with a combination of 5-fluorouracil, methyl 1-, 3-*cis*(2-chloroethyl) 1-nitrosourea and vincristine. *J. Natl. Cancer Inst.*, **54**, 69

106 Falkson, G. (1976). Fluorouracil, methyl-CCNU, and vincristine in treatment of large bowel cancer. *Cancer*, **38**, 1468

107 Warren, K. W. and Jefferson, M. F., Carcinoma of the exocrine pancreas. In: L. C. Cary (ed.). *The Pancreas*. (St Louis: C. V. Mosby Co.), pp. 243

108 Warren, K. W., Mountain, J. C. and Lloyd-Jones, W. (1972). Malignant tumours of the bile ducts. *Br. J. Surg.*, **59**, 501

109 Crile, G., Jnr. (1970). Advantage of bypass operations over radical pancreaticoduodenectomy in treatment of pancreatic carcinoma. *Surg. Gynecol. Obstet.*, **130**, 1049

110 Smith, R. (1973). Progress in the surgical treatment of pancreatic disease. *Am. J. Surg.*, **125**, 143

111 Foote, F. W., Jnr. and Frazell, E. L. (1954). Tumours of major salivary glands. In: *Atlas of Tumour Pathology*, Section IV, Fasc. II. (Washington, DC: Armed Forces Institute of Pathology)

112 Edis, A. J. (1977). Surgical treatment of thyroid cancer. In: J. E. Woods and O. Deehos. *Symposium of Head and Neck Surgery. Surg. Clin. N. Am.* (Philadelphia: Saunders), **57**, No. 3, 533

113 Buckwalter, J. A. and Thomas, C. G., Jnr. (1972). Selection of surgical treatment for well differentiated thyroid carcinomas. *Ann. Surg.*, **176**, 565

114 Woods, J. E., Weiland, L. H., Chong, G. C. and Irons, G. B. (1977). Pathology and surgery of primary tumours of the parotid. In: J. E. Woods and O. Deehos. *Symposium of Head and Neck Surgery. Surg. Clin. N. Am.* (Philadelphia: Saunders), **57**, No. 3, 565

115 De Santo, L. W., Devine, K. D. and Lillie, J. C. (1977). Cancer of the larynx: glottic cancer. In: J. E. Woods and O. Deehos. *Symposium of Head and Neck Surgery. Surg. Clin. N. Am.* (Philadelphia: Saunders), **57**, No. 3, 611

116 Hamilton Fairley, G. and Freeman, J. E. (1974). Treatment of the lymphomas. *Br. Med. J.*, **4**, 761

117 Carbone, P. P., Kaplan, H. S., Musshof, K., Smithers, D. W. and Tubiana, M. (1971). Report of the committee on Hodgkin's disease staging classification. *Cancer Res.*, **31**, 1860

118 Lukes, R. J. and Butler, J. J. (1966). The pathology and nomenclature of Hodgkin's disease. *Cancer Res.*, **26**, 1063

119 DeVita, V. T., Serpick, A. A. and Carbone, P. P. (1970). Combination chemotherapy in treatment of advanced Hodgkin's disease. *Ann. Intern. Med.*, **73**, 881

120 Crowther, D. and Blackledge, G. (1977). Lymphomas other than Hodgkin's disease. In: E. Besser (ed.). *Advanced Medicine*. (Tunbridge Wells: Pitman Medical), p. 68 ˙

121 Bonadonna, G., Lattuada, A. and Banfi, A. (1976). Recent trends in the treatment of non-Hodgkin's lymphomas. *Eur. J. Cancer*, **12**, 661

122 Rappaport, M., Winter, W. J. and Hicks, S. B. (1956). Follicular lymphoma: A re-evaluation of its position in the scheme of malignant lymphomas based on a survey of 253 cases. *Cancer*, **9**, 792

123 Bagley, C., DeVita, V. T., Berard, C. W. and Canellos, C. P. (1972). Intensive cyclical chemotherapy with cyclophosphamide, vincristine and prednisone. *Ann. Intern. Med.*, **76**, 227

124 McKelvey, E. M., Gottlieb, J. A., Wilson, H. E., Hant, A., Talley, R. W., Stephens, R., Lane, M., Gamble, J. F., Jones, S. E., Grozea, P. N., Gutterman, J., Coltman, C., Jnr. and Moon, T. E. (1976). Hydroxyldaunorubicin (adriamycin) combination chemotherapy in malignant lymphoma. *Cancer*, **38**, 1484

125 DeVita, V. T., Canellos, C. P., Chabner, B., Schein, P., Hubbard, S. and Young, R. C. (1975). Advanced diffuse histiocytic lymphoma, a potentially curable disease. Results with combination chemotherapy. *Lancet*, **i**, 248

126 Keating, M. J., Freireich, E. J., McCredie, K. B., Bodey, G. P., Hersh, E., Hester, J. P., Rodrignex, V. and Hart, J. (1977). Acute leukaemia in adults. *Cancer*, **27**, 1, 2

127 Silverstein, M. N. (1977). Managing chronic leukaemias. *Postgrad. Med.*, **61**, 1, 212

128 Gottlieb, J. A., Baker, L. H., O'Bryan, R. M., Sinkovic, J. G., Hoogstraten, B., Quagliana, J. M., Rivkin, S. E., Bodey, G. P., Rodrignez, V. T., Blumenschein, G. R., Saiki, J. H., Coltman, C., Burgess, M. A., Sullivan, P., Thigpen, T., Bottomley, R., Balcerzak, S. and Moon, T. E. (1975). Adriamycin (NSC-123127) used alone and in combination for soft tissue and bony sarcomas. *Cancer Chemother. Rep.*, **3**, 6, 271

129 Dobes, W. J., Jnr. and Kierland, R. K. (1973). Dermatologic effects of cancer. In: J. Holland, and E. Frei III (eds.). *Cancer Medicine*. (Philadelphia: Lea and Febiger), pp. 1067

130 Staughton, R. C. D. (1978). Cutaneous manifestation of malignancy. *Br. J. Hosp. Med.*, **July**, 38

131 de Graciausky, P. (1967). Weber–Christian syndrome of pancreatic origin. *Br. J. Dermatol.*, **79**, 278

132 McGovern, V. J. (1976). *Malignant Melanoma: Clinical and Histological Diagnosis*. (New York: Wiley Medical Publication)

133 Milton, G. W. (1972). The diagnosis of malignant melanoma. In: McCarthy, W. H. (ed.). *Melanoma and Skin Cancer. Proc. of Int. Cancer Conf. Sydney 1972*. (Int. Union Against Cancer and Australian Cancer Soc.)

134 Clark, W. H., Jnr. (1967). A classification of malignant melanoma in man correlated with histogenesis and biologic behavior. In: W. Montagna and Funan Hu (eds.). *Advances in Biology of the Skin, The Pigmentary System*, 1st ed. vol. 8. (London: Pergamon Press Ltd.)

135 Duncan, W. and Kerr, G. P. (1976). The curability of breast cancer. *Br. Med. J.*, **2**, (6039) 781

136 Eagle, H. and Foley, G. E. (1956). The cytotoxic action of carcinolytic agent in tissue culture. *Am. J. Med.*, **21**, 739

Index

abscess 61–5
absorption of drugs 7–9
acanthosis nigricans 407
acetanilide 14
acetohexamide 179
  formula 180
acetylcholine
  drug-improved brain levels 309
  and memory 298, 299
acetylcholinesterase 299, 309
actinomycin D 343
α-adrenergic blocking drugs 299–301
β-adrenergic blocking drugs 23, 24, 107
  adverse drug reaction 150, 151
  in hypertension 150
β-adrenergic stimulants 301, 302
adriamycin 343, 375
  adverse drug reaction 345, 411
adverse drug reactions
  β-adrenergic blockers 150, 151
  amantadine 231
  antiarrhythmic drugs 107
  anticholinergics 229
  antiepileptics 282
  biguanides 188–90
  chloramphenicol 62
  co-trimoxazole 46
  cytotoxic drugs 344, 345
  digoxin 22, 83
  diuretics 85–7, 147
  dopa decarboxylase inhibitors 236, 237
  in hospital 3, 4
  incidence 1, 2, 4
  intestinal 3
  methyl dopa 149

monoamine oxidase inhibitors 273
  narcotics 289
  papaverine 303
  penicillins 43
  phenothiazines 269–71
  potassium chloride 90
  rauwolfia 148
  resulting in hospitalization 2, 3
  tetracyclines 41, 46
  tricyclics 276
ageing
  brain changes 260, 261
  and depression 272
  and drug elimination 13–15
  and gastric absorption 7
  glucose tolerance 161
  heart 78, 79
Alcaligenes spp. 71
alcohol 267–70, 273
  and biguanides 189
alcoholism 50
allergy 43, 193
allopurinol 344
aluminium 261
Alzheimer's dementia 222, 243, 260, 261, 297, 299, 311
amantadine 73, 231, 250
  adverse drug reaction 231
American Universities Group Diabetics Program Trial 178, 179
Ames reflectance meter 171
amikacin 45, 58, 71
amiloride 91
aminoglycosides 36, 45
  resistance to 70

aminophylline 306
aminopyrine 80
amitriptyline 20, 241
  metabolism 275
amoxycillin 37, 39, 48–50, 62
  in cystitis 52
amphetamines 314, 315
amphotericin B 58, 69, 96, 357
ampicillin 41, 42, 50, 58, 60, 62
  macular skin rash 43
amylobarbitone sodium 17, 263
anaphylaxis 43
androgens 343
angina 84
  pectoris 109
  treatment 109, 110
antibiotics in elderly 35–73, 357
  and abscesses 61, 62
  absorption 37, 71
  aminoglycoside 45
  bone and joint infection 67, 68
  cephalosporins 43, 44
  cholecystitis 63
  cholera 63
  colitis 63
  comparability 37, 38
  co-trimoxazole 46
  diverticular disease 64
  dosage 38, 39
  drug interactions 39, 40
  endocarditis 57–9
  food poisoning 62
  fungal infection 68–70
  furtive therapy 70–2
  liver abscess 64
  liver excretion 40
  penicillin type 42, 43
  peritonitis 64
  properties 42–7
  in renal failure 40, 41
  resistance 59, 60
  respiratory tract infection 47, 48
  routes of administration 37, 38, 66
  see-saw profile 38
  septicaemia 54, 55
  skin infection 65–7
  tetracyclines 46
  urinary tract infections 52–4
anticoagulants 20, 21, 97–102, 297
  antibiotic interaction 40
  coumarin 185
antihypertensives 24, 26

antipyrine half-life and age 12–14
aortic valve disease 77, 79
arecoline 311
arterial thrombosis and embolism 12
arteriosclerosis and Parkinsonism 217,
    221, 243
Aspergillus spp. 69, 357
aspirin 13, 14, 348
atherosclerosis 110, 111, 174
ATP, cerebral 298
atrial fibrillation 93

Bacillus cereus 61
bacteria
  anaerobic 61
  investigations of infections 35–7
  survival of cell wall-deficient 52
Bacteroides spp. 42, 44
  septicaemia 55
  B. fragilis 61
  B. melaninogenicus 61
ballistocardiography 22
barbitone 263
barbiturates 17, 263, 264
  contraindications 263
  drug interactions 263
Bayliss effect 133
BCNU 343
benaprizine 230
bendrofluazide 146
benserazide 235–7, 249–51
benzodiazepines 264, 265
  anticonvulsant 283
  metabolites 265, 266
  pharmacodynamics 17, 18, 81
benzothiadiazines 146
benztropine 230
benzylpenicillin 15, 36, 41, 57–9, 64
  half-life 42
  spectrum 42
betahistine 304
bethanidine 26, 275
biguanides 177, 186–90
  formula 186
  and lactic acidosis 188–90
  mode of action 187
bladder obstruction 372, 373
blastomycosis 69
bleomycin 343
blood–brain barrier 9, 12
blood glucose, home monitoring
    197

blood pressure *see also* hypertension
  and age 118–21
  circadian rhythm 138
  diastolic 119–21, 143
  levels needing treatment 143, 144
  and obesity 140, 141
  systolic 119–21, 143
    arterial pressure wave 122
  variability 138
blood viscosity in disease 296
bone and joint infections 67, 68
Boston Collaborative Drug Surveillance
    Program 18, 20
  diazepam study 18
  potassium supplement efficacy 89, 90
Bowen's disease 404
bradykinesia 219
brain infarction 133
bromocriptine 238–40, 251
  contraindications 239
  dose 238
Brompton Cocktail 288, 291, 349
bronchiectasis 51
bronchitis 48, 49
bronchopneumonia 49
brucellosis 57
buformin 188
Build and Blood Pressure Study of
    Society of Actuaries 123
bumetanide 85, 91
burns 65
butyrophenones 272, 289

caffeine 305, 306
calcitonin 359
Campbell de Morgan spots 408
cancer *see also* carcinoma, malignant
    disease
  bowel difficulties 362
  and disseminated vascular coagulation
    360
  generalized 408–10
  hypercalcaemia and 358–60
  malignant ascites 352, 353, 368
  malignant plural effusion 351, 352
  nausea and vomiting 350, 351
  and neuromuscular disorders 353,
    354
  and neutropenia 356, 357
  oedema 351
  pyrexia investigation 357, 358
  treatment of advanced 346–62

Candida spp. 46, 57, 58, 357
  deep infections 69
Cantor tube 384
carbamazepine 207, 282
  adverse drug reaction 282
carbenicillin 38, 41, 42, 53
  adverse reactions 43
carbenoxolone 10
carbidopa 235–7, 249–51
carbon dioxide, partial pressure and
    cerebral blood flow 133
carbromide 267
carcinoma *see also* . cancer, malignant
    disease, tumour
  basal cell 403
  bladder 373–6
    clinical staging 374
    treatment 375
  breast 351, 358, 362–6
    clinical staging 362–4
    cytotoxic drugs 365, 366
    radiotherapy 364, 365
    surgery 363
  cervical 366, 368, 369
  colon 385, 386
  endometrial 369, 370
  gastrointestinal 379–89
  genitourinary 371–3
  intraoral 392
  larynx 394, 395
  leukaemia 400–2
  lymphoma 395–9
    Hodgkin's 396, 397
    non-Hodgkin's 397–9
  myeloma 399
  oesophageal 379–81
  ovary 366–8
  pancreaticobiliary 389–92
  parotid 392, 393
  prostatic 373, 376–8
    and castration 376
    diagnosis 377
    surgery 377, 378
  rectum 386–9
    classification 387
    therapy 387–9
  renal 374
  respiratory tract 370, 371
  small bowel 383, 385
    treatment 384, 385
  squamous cell 403
  stomach 382, 383

carcinoma (*continued*)
  testis 378, 379
  thyroid 393, 394
  vulva 366
cardiac amyoidosis 78
cardiac arrhythmias 79, 103–9
  causes 104
  conduction disorders 107, 108
  DC current conversion 105
  and digoxin 83
  and drugs 104
  ECG monitoring 104
  supraventricular 105
  treatment 105, 106
  ventricular 106, 107
cardiac atherosclerosis 103
cardiac failure 81–94
  acute 91
  complications 94
  diagnosis 90
  and digoxin 81–4
  and diuretics 84–8
  potassium supplementation 88–90
  treatment 90–4
cardiac glycosides
  dose and age 22, 23
cardiac surgery 102, 103
cardiac tamponade treatment 354, 355
cardiomyopathy 78
cardiovascular disease *see also* cardiac
    failure, endocarditis
  congenital 77
  and diabetes 179
  drug therapy and age 79–81
  heart ageing 78
  heart failure 80
  and ischaemic heart disease 109–11
  risk of death and hypertension 126–7
  surgery 102, 103
  treatment in elderly 77–111
carfecillin 72
cataracts 206
catheterization 53, 54
  therapy 54
cefotaxime 44, 70
cefoxitin 44, 63, 70, 71
cefuroxime 70
cellulitis 66
cephaleridine 40, 41
  nephrotoxicity 44
cephalexin 41, 44, 53
cephalosporins 36, 58

development of 70
  properties 43, 44
cephalothin 40, 41
  nephrotoxicity 44
cephamycins 44
cephazolin 41, 44, 49
cephradine 44
cerebral autoregulation 133–7, 295
  and blood flow 133, 295, 296
  in hypertension 134–7
cerebral blood flow 295–314
  and dementia 297, 298
  in old age 296–8
  vascular resistance 296
  vasoactive drugs 299–314
cerebral haemorrhage 131, 132
cerebral metabolism
  in dementia 298, 299
  improving drugs 309–14
Charcot–Bouchard aneurysms 131, 143
Chicago Heart Association Detection
    Project in Industry 122
Chicago Stroke Study 123, 144
chiropodist 167
Chlamydia spp. 45, 51, 95
chlormethiazole 265, 266, 285
chloral hydrate 266, 267
chloramphenicol 36, 37, 40, 41, 46, 61, 62
  adverse reactions 62
  in meningitis 60
  topical 48, 65
chlordiazepoxide 8, 11, 264
  clearance and age 13, 14, 17
chlormethiazole 10, 11, 19
  clearance 13, 14
chlorothiazide 148
chlorpromazine 217, 268, 269, 350
chlorpropamide 179, 183, 184
  alcohol sensitivity 183
  avoidance in elderly 182
  formula 180
cholangiitis 63
cholecystitis 63
cholera 63
choline 310
choline acetyltransferase 225, 261, 299
cinnarizine 308, 309
  adverse reactions 309
clavulanic acid 70, 71
clindamycin 36, 37, 40, 41, 60
  and colitis 45
clinical pharmacology and elderly 1–26

clofibrate 185
clonazepam 264
clostridia 42
Clostridium difficile 64
 C. welchii 55, 56, 62
cloxacillin 37, 41, 42, 56, 58, 60
CNS-active drugs 259–293
 incidence of use 259
coccidiomycosis 69
codeine 288, 348
co-dergocrine mesylate 299
 clinical review 300
 and EEG studies 300
colistin 41, 46
coma
 diabetic 199–203
 hyperosmolar non-ketonic 201–3
compliance 4, 5
 digoxin therapy 93
 and diuretics 88
 epileptics 284
computerized axial tomography (CAT)
 243
conduction disorders
 Mobitz type heart blocks 108, 109
conjunctivitis 48
Corynebacterium diphtheriae 48
cotrimazine 46
co-trimoxazole 36, 40, 41, 49, 52, 53, 62
 in endocarditis 58
 folate deficiency 46
 properties 46
Coxiella burnetti 45, 46, 50, 51, 57
Coxiella spp. 95
creatinine clearance 16, 23, 39
 in severe renal failure 41
Cryptococcus neoformans 69, 70, 357
cyclandelate 303, 304
cyclizine 241
cyclobarbitone 263
cyclopenthiazide 146
cyclophosphamide 367
cystitis 52, 53
cystodiathemy 375
cytosine arabinoside 343, 344
cytotoxic drugs 341–5, 365, 366
 classification 343
 and cancer 383, 391, 401, 403, 407
 effectiveness 410
 and excretion 344
 multiple treatment 343–5
 and neutropenia 356

daunorubicin 343
deanol 310, 311
debrisoquin 26, 275
deep vein thrombosis 97–102
 diagnosis 97
 and heparin 98–100
 incidence 98
 and warfarin 100–2
dementia 243, 244, 260, 297, 298
 and cerebral metabolism 298, 299
 multi-infarct 297
 senile 261, 297
dental extraction and endocarditis 57,
 97
deprenyl 240
depression 272–9
 causes 278
 management in elderly 278, 279
 and neurotransmitters 273
dermatitis, infected 65
dermatomyositis 407
desipramine 20, 275
desmethyldiazepam 10, 11
desmethylimipramine 13, 14, 18
dexamethasone 362
dextran 309
diabetes 150, 159–208
 amyotrophy 208
 biguanides and 186–90
 care, organization of 165–73
  community care 170, 171
  diabetic clinic 166–9, 195
  follow-up 168
  GP role 171
  hospital 166
  miniclinics 170, 171
  patient education 168–70
 coma 199–203
 complications 198–208
 diagnosis 161
 diet 169, 173–5
 drug interactions 169, 185, 186
 emotional impact 172, 173
 exercise 175
 eye disorders 205
 florid 165
 foot care 203–5
 glucose tolerance 161–5
 glycosylated haemoglobin 196,
  197
 incidence and age 162
 ketoacidosis 198–202

diabetes *(continued)*
  longterm supervision 194–8
  maculopathy 205, 206
  maturity onset 177
  monitoring 195
    at home 197
  neuropathy 207, 208
  oral hypoglycaemic agents 176–90
  and pancreatic neoplasm 165
  retinopathy 205
  stability 175
  sulphonylureas 180–6
  types I and II 161
  and urinary tract disease 207
  urine tests 194, 195
diamorphine 347, 349
diathermy fulguration 388, 389
diazepam 10, 11, 13, 14, 264, 283, 284,
    347
  clearance, dose and age 17, 18
  and smoking 17, 18
dichloralphenazone 266
diet and diabetes 169, 173–5
digoxin 8, 11, 15
  absorption 9, 82
  action 82
  adverse reaction 22
  clearance 16
  and heart rate 82
  intoxication 83
  pharmacokinetics 22
  prescribing 23
  radioimmunoassay 82
  regime 83, 84
  and renal function 22
  toxicity 83
dihydrocodeine 289
dihydroergocristine 299–301
diphenylhydantoin 281
disopyramide 107
disseminated intravascular coagulation
    360, 361
  malignant associations 360
diuretics 84–8
  complications 86, 87
  and hypertension 146, 147
  loop 85, 146
  potassium supplements 88–90
  salt loss 87
  side-effects in elderly 87, 88
  spironolactone 86
  thiazide 85, 93, 146, 147, 358

triamterine 86
  and urinary symptoms 88
diverticular disease 64
dopa decarboxylase inhibitors 235–7
  adverse reactions 236, 237
dopamine
  regulation 224
  release and Parkinsonism 217
  synthesis 223, 224
doxycycline 40, 41
drug therapy 1–26
drugs *see also* antibiotics, diuretics *etc.*
  absorption 7–9, 81
  antiarrhythmic 106, 107
  antidepressant 272–9, 317
  antiemetic 292
  antiepileptic 279–85
  antiparkinsonism 3
  antipsychotic 20
  blood concentrations 5
  in cardiovascular disease 79–81
  cerebral activating 299–318
  cerebral metabolic improvers 309–14
  cerebral stimulants 314–6
  cholinomimetics 311
  clearance 7, 14–16
  CNS active 259–93
  cytotoxic 341–5
  distribution 9–11
  -induced Parkinsonism 217, 218
  interactions 39, 40, 44, 169, 184, 185,
      187, 263, 276
  metabolism 12–14
  microcirculation 309
  muscle relaxant 292
  narcotic analgesic 285–92
    antagonists 290
    indications 290, 291
  organ distribution 12
  in pain 348, 349
  Parkinson's disease 226–40
  plasma half-life 6, 7
    and age 12, 13, 17, 39
  polarity 10, 12
  products 72
  protein binding 10, 81
  psychotropic 262–79
  renal elimination 14, 15
  responses 15–27
  vasoactive 299–314

Eaton–Lambert syndrome 353

electrocardiogram (ECG) 129
  age changes 79
  monitoring of arrhythmias 104
electroconvulsive therapy 279
empyema 51
endocarditis 57–9, 94–7
  anaerobes 58
  antibiotic assay 58
  brucellosis 57, 58
  fungal 96
  infective 94–7
    prevention 97
    treatment 95–7
  organisms 57, 94, 95
  therapy 58, 59
enteric fever 62
Enterobacter spp. 42, 49
enterocolitis 63
epilepsy
  barbiturates in 263
  compliance 284
  grand mal 280, 281
  Jacksonian 280
  management 283
  precipitating factors 279, 280, 283
  status epilepticus 284, 285
  therapy 280–3
erysipelas 66
erythromelalgia 239
erythromycin 36, 40, 41, 48, 52, 60
  lactbionate 38
  spectrum 45
Escherichia coli 49, 53, 95, 356
ethacrynic acid 85
ethopropazine 230
European Working Party on Hypertension in the Elderly 24, 26, 148

fenatyl 289
fencamfamin 315, 316
fibrinogen leg scanning 98
flucloxacillin 37, 42, 48, 66
  fractures 68
5-fluorocytosine 58, 69
fluorazepam 19, 264
5-fluorouracil 343, 350, 375, 389, 391
flupenthixol 277
fluphenazine 269, 271
fluphenazine decanoate 217
focal neurological disease 297
folate deficiency 46, 281, 282

food poisoning 62, 63
fractures 68
Framingham Heart Study 124–9, 140
  risk of death 126–8
frusemide 40, 85, 89, 91
fucidin 36, 37, 60
fungal infections 68–70
fusidic acid 41

gamma-amino butyric acid 224
  metabolism 281
Gardner's syndrome 408
gas gangrene 43, 55, 67
gentamicin 41, 43–5, 49, 53, 57, 58, 65
  dose 56
  in septicaemia 56
  topical 65
glibenclamide 177, 179
  duration 182
  formula 180
glibornuride 179, 182
  formula 180
glimidine 179
glipizide 179, 182
glomerular filtration rate 15, 39
glucose tolerance and age 161–5
glutethimide 267
glyceryl trinitrate 109
glycosuria 161–3
gout 147
guanethidine 26, 275
guanidine 354

haemoglobin, glycosylated 196, 197
Haemophilus influenzae 42, 44, 48, 49, 59, 61, 67
  meningitis 60
haloperidol 217, 272
  in schizophrenia 272
heart *see also* coronary
  ageing 78, 79
  disease 125
  rate 104
Helmstein's distension therapy 376
heparin 20, 21, 98–100, 361
heroin 289
Herpes simplex 66, 357
  and Parkinsonism 216
hexamethonium 137
hexobendine 306
histoplasmosis 69
HLA 161

Hodge seat   247
Hodgkin's disease   396, 397
homovanillic acid   224
hormone neuropeptides   312
Huntington's chorea   261, 272
hydrallazine   151, 152
hydrochlorothiazide   146, 147
hydrocortisone   359
3-hydroxyamylobarbitone   17
hydroxyurea   343
hyperaldosteronism   86, 93
hypercalcaemia in malignancy   357–60
hyperglycaemia   147, 198–200
hypertension *see also* Framingham heart
      study
  and age   118–21, 123–30
  assessment in elderly   137–45
  associated abnormalities   141, 142
  in aviators   118, 119
  cerebral autoregulation   134–7, 145
    in elderly   135–7
  clinical assessment   141–5
  crisis   274
  death rate ratio   124
  definition   117
  diastolic   119, 120, 124, 125, 130
  effects of treatment   130–3
  essential symptomless   131
  management in elderly   117–53
  mortality   129, 131
  and obesity   140, 141
  organ damage   139
  and risk of death from coronary
      disease   126–31
  and sex   119, 120, 125–8
  systolic   119, 120, 141
    definition   122
    and mortality   123, 124, 129, 130
    risks   122–30
  treatment   145–52
    β-blockers   150, 151
    contraindications   144, 145
    diuretic experience   147, 148
    'gentle seduction'   145
    steps   1–3, 146–52
    thiazides   146, 147
  and urban life   118
Hypertension–Stroke Cooperative Study
      Group   132
hyperuricaemia   147
hypoglycaemia   40, 150
  in elderly   183

hypokalaemia   23, 43, 90, 147
hyponatraemia   87
hypotension, postural   135
hypothermia   198
hypothyroidism   198

imipramine   14, 20, 241
  dose   20
  metabolism   275
immunodeficiency   68, 69, 73
indomethacin   8, 14
infusion sites, infected   66
inositol nicotinate   304
insomnia management   267, 268
insulin   177, 190–4
  administration problems   192
  allergy   193
  antagonists   200
  antigenicity   192, 193
  in coma   200
  drug interactions   185
  drug stimulated release   181
  duration of action   191
  lente   190
  isophane   171, 190
  molecular weights   193
  purified   191–4
  resistance   193
  use in elderly   190, 191
interferon   73
intestinal and biliary infections   62–5
iproniazid   273
ischaemic heart disease   81
  and digoxin   81
isocarboxazid   273
isoniazid   14
isoprenaline   24
isoxsuprine   301, 302

Jacob–Creutzfeld syndrome   222
jaundice   389, 390

kanamycin   15, 45
ketoacidosis   198–202
Klebsiella spp.   42, 49, 53, 356

β-lactamase   42, 44, 70
β-lactam nucleus   42
lactic acidosis
  and biguanides   188–90
  and renal failure   189
lecithin   310
Legionnaire's disease   45, 52

leukaemia 400–2
  acute lymphoblastic 400, 401
  acute myeloblastic 400
  chronic lymphocytic 402
  chronic myeloid 401, 402
  meningeal 401
levodopa 226–9, 232–5
  and dementia 213, 214
  drug combinations 235–7
  longterm effects 237, 238
  on–off phenomena 237
levorphanol 289
lignocaine 11, 13, 14, 107
  adverse reactions 107
  dose 107
lipoatrophy 193
Listeria spp. 60
lithium 278
lorazepam 10, 11, 14, 264
lung abscess 51
lymphoma 395–9

malignant disease *see also* cancer,
    carcinoma, leukaemia, lym-
    phoma, melanoma
  advanced 346–62
  chemotherapy 341–5, 365, 366
  diagnosis 334
  home nursing 338
  informing patient 335–7
  management in old age 333–411
  obstructions 370–85
  pain treatment 348, 349
  skin 403–7
  skin manifestations 407, 408
  terminal management 337–9
manganese poisoning 218
maprotiline 277
mecillinam 39, 44
meclofenoxate 313, 314
medazepam 264
mefanamic acid 207
megaloblastic haemopoiesis 46
melanoma 404–7
  chemotherapy 407
  differential diagnosis 406
  invasion rate 406
  lentigo maligna 405
  nodular 405
  prognosis 405
  superficial spreading 405
melphalan 367

Ménière's disease 292, 304
meningitis 59–61
meprobamate 267
6-mercaptopurine 343
metaclopramide 350
metformin 177, 179
  duration of action 187
  formula 186
  lactic acidosis 188–90
methadone 207, 287, 290
methaqualone 267
methenamine mandelate 41
  and catheters 54
methoin 282
methotrexate 343, 345, 403
methyldopa 26, 136
  adverse reactions 149
  and hypertension 148
methylphenidate 315
  adverse reaction 315
methylxanthines 305–8
metronidazole 37, 40, 47, 51, 61, 63, 64
mexiletine 107
mianserin 277
miconazole 69, 357
miosis 288, 289
mithramycin 343, 359
mitomycin 343, 375, 389
monoamine oxidase inhibitors 185,
    234, 273, 274
  drug interactions 274
morphinans 287
morphine 12, 287, 288, 349
  distribution in elderly 16, 17
Mucor sp. 70
myasthenia gravis 353
Mycoplasma pneumoniae 45, 50, 51
myeloma 399
myocardial infarction 107, 110

naftidrofuryl 307, 308
naladixic acid 40
Neisseria gonorrhoea 57, 58
  N. meningitidis 42, 59
    sulphonamide resistance 59
neomycin 48
nepenthe 348
neuropathy 207
  autonomic 208
neutropenia 356–8
nicotinic acid 304, 305
  derivatives 304, 305

nicotinyl alcohol tartrate   304, 305
nigrostriatal degeneration   221
nitrazepam   12, 14, 81, 264
  dose and age   18, 19
  performance test   19
nitrofurantoin   40, 41
nortriptyline   13, 14, 275
nylidrin   302
nystatin   68, 69

obesity   140, 141, 160, 173
oesophagectomy   51
oestrogens   343, 370
olivopontocerebellar degeneration   221
ophthalmologist   167
opium   288
oral hypoglycaemic agents   176–90
  continuing management   178
  contraindications   177
  drug interactions   185
  and hypoglycaemia   183–5
  lactic acidosis   188–90
  and maturity-onset diabetes   177, 178
  and weight   177
orphenadrine   229–231, 248
osteomyelitis   67, 68
otitis externa   48
oxazepam   11, 264
oxiperomide   240
oxpentifylline   306, 307
oxprenolol   150
oxygen
  and cerebral metabolism   298
  and cognitive function   316

pacemaker   108, 109
pain   286
  in cancer   346–50
  chronic   291
  physiology   285–7
  terminal illness   291, 292
  treatment   286, 287, 291, 348, 349
pancreatic β-cell stimulation by sulphon-
    ureas   181
pancreatectomy   176
papaveretum   288, 348
papaverine   302, 303
paracetamol   8, 9, 11, 13, 14, 348
paraldehyde   266, 285
Parkinsonism   20
Parkinson's disease
  causes   216

clinical tests   219, 252, 253
  and dementia   243, 244
  differential diagnosis   221, 222
  dopamine deficiency   223, 224
  drug-induced   217, 218, 270, 271,
    277
  epidemiology   215, 216
  familial   216
  idiopathic   216, 217
  incidence   215, 216
  management in elderly   215–53
  mental score test   220
  mortality   226
  neurochemistry   222–5
  nigral cell loss   226
  pathology   222
  postencephalitic   217
  prognosis   225, 226
  signs and symptoms   218, 219
  and social services   247
  symptomatic   217, 218
  therapy programmes   245–7
  treatment
    alkaloids   228
    amantadine   231
    anticholinergics   229–31
    bromocriptine   238, 239
    drugs   226–40
    levodopa   226–9, 232–8, 244
    mild   248, 249
    moderate   249–51
    new drugs   240
    severe   251, 252
    supporting drugs   241, 242
    surgery   240, 241
Parkinson's Disease Society   246–8
paronychia   66, 69
pemoline   312, 313
penicillin   10
  phenoxymethyl-   37, 42, 47
penicillin-type antibiotics   42, 43, 96
  allergy   43
pentazocine   289
pentifylline   306
pentobarbitone   263
Pentz–Jegher's syndrome   408
peritonitis   64
pethidine   10, 11, 274, 288, 289, 348
  adverse reactions   16
  group   287
pharmacodynamics, altered in elderly
  1, 15–27

pharmacokinetics, altered in elderly 1, 6–15, 79, 80
phenazocine 289, 349
phenazone 8, 11
phenformin 179
  duration of action 187
  formula 186
  lactic acidosis 188–90
phenobarbitone 10, 15, 17, 80, 263, 280
phenoperidine 289
phenothiazines 20, 224, 268–71
  adverse reactions 269
  classification 269
phenylbutazone 10, 11, 185
  clearance and age 13, 14
phenytoin 10, 14, 80, 107, 280–2, 285
Phycomyces spp. 70
physostigmine 309, 310
piracetam 311, 312
pivmecillinam spectrum 44, 45
plasma protein, drug binding 10, 81
cis-platinum 343, 367
pneumococci 42
Pneumocystis carinii 357
pneumonectomy 51
pneumonia 49–52
  bacteraemia in pneumococcal 36
  Gram-negative 49
  hospital 50
  lobar 50
  mycoplasma 51
  postoperative 50
polymyositis and cancer 355
potassium
  chloride 89, 90
  loss and diuretics 87
  supplements 88–90
povidone iodine 55, 65
practolol 8, 15, 151
  elimination and age 24
prazosin 151
prednisolone 359
prednisone 343
pressure sores 66, 67
primidone 281
procainamide 107
procarbazine 343
prochlorperazine 220
procyclidine 230
progesterone 343
  and endometrial cancer 370
promazine 269, 271

promethazine 267
propicillin 8, 10, 11, 15
propoxyphene 8
propranolol 110, 150, 151
  adverse reactions 24
  clearance and age 13, 14
  in diabetes 185
  dose and age 23–5
  in Parkinsonism 242, 249
protamine sulphate 98
Proteus spp. 49, 53
pseudomembraneous colitis 45, 63, 64
  treatment 47, 64
Pseudomonas spp. 42, 43, 45, 53, 71
  pneumonia 50
  P. aerusinosa 356
Psittacosis spp. 46, 50
psychic pillow test 220
pulmonary embolism 97–102
  diagnosis 98
  and heparin 98–100
  and warfarin 100–2
pyelonephritis 53, 68, 139

Q fever 95
quinalbarbitone 263
quinidine 10, 11, 107
quinine 8, 13, 14

radiotherapy 343, 355, 356, 392
  bladder cancer 375
  breast cancer 364, 365
  hypernephroma 374
  oesophageal cancer 380, 381
  stomach cancer 382
Raynaud's phenomenon 151, 353
renal failure and antibiotic dose 40, 41
renal function
  and antibiotics 38
  and digoxin therapy 23
reserpine 217, 224
  adverse effects 26
respiratory tract infections 47–52
  bronchitis 48, 49
  lung abscess 51
  pneumonias 49–51
  sinusitis 48
  upper 47, 48
retinopathy 205
rheumatic heart disease 77, 102
ribovarin 73

rifampicin 47, 52
RNA, brain levels and drugs 312, 313

salicylate 10
Salmonella paratyphi 62
  S. typhi 62
    chloramphenicol resistance 63
sarcomas 402, 403
schizophrenia 272
septicaemia 54, 55
  fungal 68, 69
  source 56
  treatment 56
serotonin 224, 281
Serratia spp. 71
Shy–Drager syndrome 222
silver sulphadiazine 65
sinusitis 48
sinus rhythm 92
sisomicin 71
skin infections 65–7
smoking
  and blood pressure 140
  and drug half-life 13, 17, 18
social workers and diabetics 167
sodium loss and diuretics 87
sodium valproate 282, 283
spinal cord compression 356
spironolactone 86, 147
sporotrichosis 69
Staphylococcus aureus 45, 48, 49, 55, 57,
    61, 62, 65–7, 357
  persisters 36, 37
  resistance 70
  septicaemia 56
  S. epidermidis 57, 58, 65
  S. pyogenes 95
Steele–Richardson syndrome 221
Stokes–Adams attacks 108
Streptococcus spp.
  β-haemolytic 42
  Lancefield's Groups 47, 55, 58, 66
  S. bovis 57
  S. faecalis 42, 47, 57, 58, 64
    endocarditis 58, 59, 95
  S. milleri 61
  S. mitior 57
  S. pneumoniae 44, 48, 49, 61
    antibiotic resistance 60
  S. pyogenes 47, 48, 55, 58, 66
  S. sanguis 57
streptozotocin 343

stroke 125, 131, 138, 297
  and antihypertensive treatment 132,
    133
  and hypertension 133–7
suloctidil 306
sulphadiazine 46
sulphadimine 41
sulphamethizole 8, 15
sulphamethoxazole 46
  adverse reactions 41
sulphonamides 36, 40
sulphonylureas 177, 180–6
  and body weight 177
  formula 180
  and hypoglycaemia 183–5
  interactions 184–6
  mode of action 181
  and pancreatic β-cell stimulation 181
  toxicity 182
sulthiame 283
superior vena caval syndrome 355
systemic lupus erythematosus 152

talampicillin 37, 42, 50, 72
tamoxiphan 365
temazepam 264
tetrabenazine 270, 272
tetracycline 8, 9, 36, 40, 41, 46, 65
  nephrotoxicity 40, 41, 46
tetranicotinyl fructose 304
theophylline 9, 11, 80, 305
thiazides 85, 93, 146, 147
  adverse reactions 147
6-thioguanine 343
thiopropazate 271
thioridazine 241, 269, 271
thio-Tepa 354
thyrotoxicosis 104
tobramycin 45
tofenacin 277
tolazamide 179
tolbutamide 10, 11, 40, 80, 182
  and diabetes 179
  formula 180
transient ischaemic attacks 297, 301
tranylcypromine 273
tremor 221, 242
triamterene 86, 91, 147
tricyclic antidepressants 274–6
  cardiotoxicity 20
  classification 276

dose and adverse drug reaction 20, 276
trifluperidol 272
trimethoprim 46
L-tryptophan 241, 251, 277
tumour *see also* cancer, carcinoma, malignant disease
  cell kinetics 339–41
  chemotherapy 341–5
    additive effects 344
  doubling time 340, 341
  drug resistance 345
  emergencies 354–62
  gastrointestinal 379–89
  genitourinary 371–3
  –host relationships 409
  solid, combined modality treatment 410, 411

urinary tract infections 52–4
  Candida spp. 68
  and diabetes 207

vaginitis 69
vancomycin 41, 47, 64
  toxicity 47

varicella-zoster 357
vasopressin 312
ventricular hypertrophy 129
Veterans Administration Cooperative Study Group 130
vinblastine 343
vincristine 343, 345
  adverse reactions 411
vitamin B_6 234
  B_{12} malabsorption 188
  D deficiency 281
  K-dependent clotting 21
  drug supplement 315
vitreous haemorrhage 206

warfarin 10, 14, 40, 80, 100–2
  dose and age 21, 101
  mode of action 100–2
  protein binding 101
Webster timed test 219, 253
  rating scale 253
Wechsler Adult Intelligence Scale 243
wound infections 67

xanthinol nicotinate 305
X-ray 50, 92